MW00380417

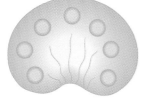

ATLAS OF LYMPHOID HYPERPLASIA AND LYMPHOMA

ATLASES IN
DIAGNOSTIC SURGICAL PATHOLOGY

Consulting Editor

Gerald M. Bordin, M.D.
Department of Pathology
Scripps Clinic and Research Foundation

Published:

WOLD, McCLEOD, SIM, AND UNNI:
ATLAS OF ORTHOPEDIC PATHOLOGY

COLBY, LOMBARD, YOUSEM, AND KITAICHI:
ATLAS OF PULMONARY SURGICAL PATHOLOGY

KANEL AND KORULA:
ATLAS OF LIVER PATHOLOGY

OWEN AND KELLY:
ATLAS OF GASTROINTESTINAL PATHOLOGY

VIRMANI:
ATLAS OF CARDIOVASCULAR PATHOLOGY

RO, AMIN, GRIGNON, AYALA:
**ATLAS OF SURGICAL PATHOLOGY OF THE MALE
REPRODUCTIVE TRACT**

WENIG:
ATLAS OF HEAD AND NECK PATHOLOGY

WENIG, HEFFESS, AND ADAIR:
ATLAS OF ENDOCRINE PATHOLOGY

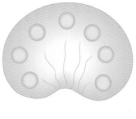

ATLAS OF LYMPHOID HYPERPLASIA AND LYMPHOMA

Judith A. Ferry, MD
Associate Professor of Pathology
Harvard Medical School
Department of Pathology
Massachusetts General Hospital
Boston, Massachusetts

Nancy L. Harris, MD
Professor of Pathology
Harvard Medical School
Director of Anatomic Pathology
Massachusetts General Hospital
Boston, Massachusetts

W.B. SAUNDERS COMPANY
A Division of Harcourt Brace & Company
Philadelphia ■ London ■ Toronto ■ Montreal ■ Sydney ■ Tokyo

W.B. SAUNDERS COMPANY
A Division of Harcourt Brace & Company

The Curtis Center
Independence Square West
Philadelphia, Pennsylvania 19106

Library of Congress Cataloging-in-Publication Data

Ferry, Judith A.

Atlas of lymphoid hyperplasia and lymphoma / Judith A. Ferry,
Nancy L. Harris—1st ed.

p. cm.

ISBN: 0–7216–5907–1

1. Lymphomas—Atlases. I. Harris, Nancy L. II. Title.
   [DNLM: 1. Lymphoma—pathology—atlases. 2. Lymph Nodes—pathology—atlases.
   3. Hyperplasia—pathology—atlases.   WH 17 F399a 1997]

RC280.L9F47 1997   616.4—dc20

DNLM/DLC   96–29401

Atlas of Lymphoid Hyperplasia and Lymphoma   ISBN: 0–7216–5907–1

Printed in the United States of America.

Last digit is the print number: 9   8   7   6   5   4   3   2   1

To

David, Cynthia Clio, Deborah Alexis, Jay, Matthew, and Daniel

PREFACE

This Atlas is intended as a quick reference guide to the diagnosis and classification of neoplastic and reactive conditions in lymph nodes and selected extranodal sites. The majority of lymphomas are diagnosed using the biopsy findings from enlarged lymph nodes or extranodal masses. Diagnostic problems can involve distinction of benign from malignant lymphoid processes, subclassification of neoplasms to determine prognosis and therapy, and determination of etiology of non-neoplastic processes to permit appropriate management. We have attempted to cover briefly the majority of such conditions that may be seen in daily practice. The Atlas is organized by disease entities, rather than by morphologic features, such as patterns, that may be useful in the differential diagnosis. Although the latter method is helpful to beginners in learning how to analyze lymph node biopsy material, we find that in the long term, it is better to understand the spectrum of morphologic manifestations of a specific disease entity, rather than to artificially group disparate entities because of superficial morphologic similarities.

The classification of lymphomas has undergone a relatively recent evolution, with the proposal of the Revised European American Lymphoma (R.E.A.L.) classification of lymphoid neoplasms. The R.E.A.L. classification is an attempt to select from the Working Formulation and the Kiel classification, as well as from the published literature, all the specific disease entities that can and are being recognized by expert hematopathologists in daily practice that appear to have distinctive clinical features. This classification, i.e., R.E.A.L., utilizes a combination of morphologic features, immunophenotypic and genetic features, and clinical features to define and classify disease entities. Although the immunophenotypic and genetic features are an important part of the definition of an entity and provide objective data that make a consensus on classification possible, most typical cases of lymphoma can be diagnosed by experienced pathologists using only routine sections. In difficult cases, or if the pathologist lacks experience, immunophenotyping studies can be very helpful. The major uses of immunophenotyping are (1) distinguishing benign from malignant lymphoid infiltrates (most commonly follicular lymphoma from hyperplasia and extranodal lymphocytic infiltrates); (2) distinguishing lymphoid from nonlymphoid neoplasms (lymphoma from myeloid leukemia, carcinoma, melanoma, sarcoma, and germ cell tumor); and (3) subclassification of lymphoma. In the last category, several major areas exist in which immunophenotyping can be helpful: (1) lymphoblastic versus mature B- or T-cell neoplasms; (2) T- versus B-cell lymphomas; (3) subclassification of small B-cell neoplasms (follicle center versus small lymphocytic versus mantle cell versus marginal zone/MALT lymphomas); and (4) distinction between Hodgkin's disease and non-Hodgkin's lymphomas.

Although flow cytometry and frozen-section immunohistochemistry have been the standard for immunophenotyping, the availability of new monoclonal antibodies and antigen retrieval techniques has expanded the utility of paraffin section immunohistochemistry, so that most clinically relevant diagnoses can be made without the need for fresh tissue. The majority of diagnoses can be established with a combination of morphology and immunophenotypic studies. Molecular genetic studies are needed in 5% of cases or fewer—but when needed, they can be extremely helpful. The constellation of clinical features is an important part of the definition of a disease entity and may be useful in establishing the diagnosis in individual cases.

Although the R.E.A.L. classification recognizes over 20 distinct lymphoid neoplasms, only a few of them, in fact, are common enough to be seen by most general pathologists and oncologists who practice outside referral centers. Three entities—diffuse large B-cell lymphoma, follicular lymphoma, and classic Hodgkin's disease—account for over 60% of all lymphoid neoplasms diagnosed using lymph node biopsy in the United States and Europe. Recognition of these entities is usually straightforward, once reactive processes and nonlymphoid tumors are excluded. General pathologists can become familiar with the diagnostic criteria for these entities, and most general oncologists are familiar with their treatment. Other, less common entities are nonetheless clinically distinctive, and their existence and distinctive features should be recognized so that they are not "lumped in" with the more common entities for treatment purposes. Thus, practicing general pathologists should be sufficiently familiar with the morphologic features of the nonfollicular small B-cell lymphomas (particularly mantle cell lymphoma and marginal zone/MALT lymphoma) and the peripheral T-cell lymphomas (particularly anaplastic large cell lymphoma and angioimmunoblastic T-cell lymphoma) to realize that they are dealing with something different. If they are not satisfied with a specific diagnosis, expert consultation can be sought. In this Atlas, we have tried to present diagnostic criteria for each of these diseases, with an indication of which special studies may be useful in differential diagnosis and when.

In addition to the neoplasms, there are a variety of non-neoplastic disorders that manifest themselves in lymph nodes. Although probably the most common diagnosis on a lymph node biopsy sample that does not show a neoplasm will be nonspecific reactive hyperplasia, there are several conditions in which a specific diagnosis can be made that will either dictate treatment or at least spare the patient further evaluation. We have attempted to describe and illustrate many of these specific conditions and provide criteria for differential diagnosis. We have also included a section on the pathology of lymphoid tissues in immunosuppressed patients. Although these conditions are unusual, they often cause problems in differential diagnosis, and we hope this section is a good reference source.

The pathology of lymphoid tissues is a difficult area because of the wide variety of processes that can be seen, the subtlety of some of the morphologic analysis required, the relative rarity of some of the diseases, and the high clinical "stakes" associated with the diagnosis of lymphoma. We hope that this Atlas helps to demystify this field for the beginner and provides some quick reassurance to the general pathologist confronted with these cases in daily practice.

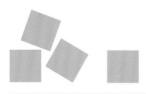

ACKNOWLEDGEMENTS

This Atlas could not have been prepared without the assistance of many others. We would like to take this opportunity to thank Bruce Kaynor, Sharon Campbell, and Marcia Levy for their technical expertise in immunohistochemistry; Steve Conley and Michelle Forrestall for their many hours of assistance with photography; Bernadette Vijayakanthan for her care in preparation of the manuscript; and our residents, fellows, and other colleagues for their help in identifying interesting cases and for their moral support.

CONTENTS

CHAPTER 1

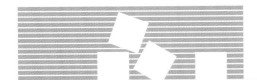

Normal Lymph Nodes: Histology and Immunohistology

B and T lymphocytes are believed to originate from bone marrow–derived precursors. In lymph nodes (or in organized lymphoid tissue in extranodal sites), lymphocytes are exposed to antigen and develop into cells capable of immunologic response (Figs. 1–1 and 1–2). The normal lymph node has a cortex (which includes follicles and a paracortex), medullary cords, and sinuses all enclosed within a fibrous capsule (Fig. 1–3).

FOLLICLES

Follicles are typically present in the cortex—the peripheral portion of the lymph node. Their primary function is to generate the T-cell-dependent late primary and secondary immune responses to a specific antigenic challenge, with subsequent production of memory B cells and plasma cells.

Primary Follicle

A relatively small, round aggregate of small lymphoid cells with round to slightly irregular nuclei, the primary follicle has not been stimulated to respond to antigen. It is composed of B cells (CD19+, CD20+ and CD22+) that express polytypic immunoglobulin (Ig) (mixture of κ and λ+ cells) of IgM and IgD type, and follicular dendritic cells (FDC), which are the antigen-presenting cells of the lymphoid follicle. The FDCs are CD21+, CD23+, and CD35+, and they stain for Ig in a coarse dendritic pattern.

Secondary Follicle

The secondary follicle has been stimulated to respond to antigen; it consists of a germinal center and a mantle zone. The mantle zone is composed of cells identical to those of the primary follicle.

   The appearance of the germinal center changes with time. Although the earliest stage of germinal center formation is rarely observed in humans, it is believed to begin with the entry into the primary follicle of only three to ten B cells that have been transformed into IgM+ blasts in the paracortex.

   The IgM+ blasts differentiate into sIg− centroblasts (large, noncleaved follicle center cells) with vesicular nuclei, one to three peripherally located nucleoli, and scant cytoplasm that is basophilic with Giemsa stain. Centroblasts differentiate into centrocytes (cleaved follicle center cells), which are small to intermediate-sized lymphoid cells with dispersed chromatin, inconspicuous nucleoli, and scant cytoplasm that express sIg, usually IgG or IgA type. Centrocytes may differentiate into memory B cells or plasma cells. Reactive follicles characteristically show a zonation phenomenon ("polarization") (Fig. 1–4). In the pole of the germinal center toward the capsule, centrocytes and FDCs accumulate to produce the "light zone" (Figs. 1–5 and 1–6). In the opposite pole, centroblasts predominate, and form the "dark zone" (Fig. 1–7). The mitotic rate is high, and tingible body macrophages are abundant in the dark zone. The mitotic rate is low in the light zone. Occasionally, B immunoblasts (which have vesicular nuclei, prominent central nucleoli, and basophilic cytoplasm that is more abundant than that of centroblasts) and plasma cells may also be found in germinal centers. Small lymphocytes are present in various numbers, and these are predominantly T-helper cells (CD4+). End-stage follicles become hyalinized (also called "burnt out" or "regressively transformed").

   B cells may leave the germinal center to form a marginal zone around the periphery of the mantle zone. Marginal zone cells are small cells with slightly irregular nuclei and moderate amounts of pale cytoplasm. A marginal zone is not always recognizable. It tends to be prominent in mesenteric lymph nodes, Peyer's patches, and spleen (Fig. 1–8). Bands of monocytoid B cells (previously called immature sinus histiocytes) that have slightly larger, oval, indented, or bean-shaped nuclei and abundant pale cytoplasm may be found within or adjacent to subcapsular and cortical sinuses and are sometimes continuous with marginal zone cells. Monocytoid B cells are believed to be related to marginal zone cells (Fig. 1–9).

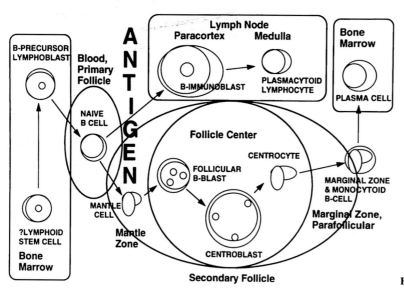

Figure 1–1. Postulated pathway of B cell differentiation.

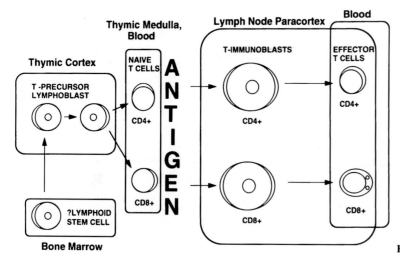

Figure 1–2. Postulated pathway of T cell differentiation.

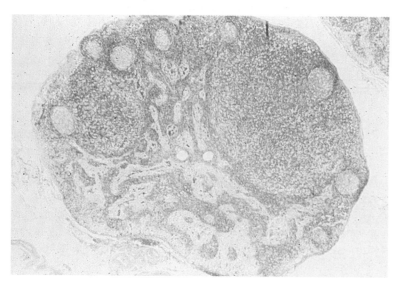

Figure 1–3. Lymph node with nonspecific reactive hyperplasia. Around the periphery of the node are secondary lymphoid follicles with pale germinal centers surrounded by dark blue, narrow mantle zones. The paracortex, located between and deep to the lymphoid follicles, has a mottled appearance because of its mixture of small lymphocytes and pale antigen-presenting cells. Sinuses are patent. Narrow medullary cords extend from the paracortex to the hilus, at the bottom of this figure (H&E stain).

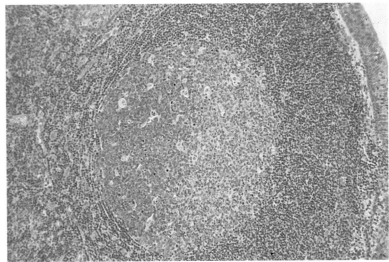

Figure 1–4. Secondary follicle with polarization into light and dark zones (H&E stain).

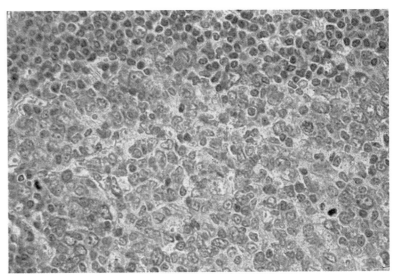

Figure 1–5. Light zone of germinal center. Centrocytes (small cleaved cells) predominate, and the mitotic rate is relatively low (Giemsa stain).

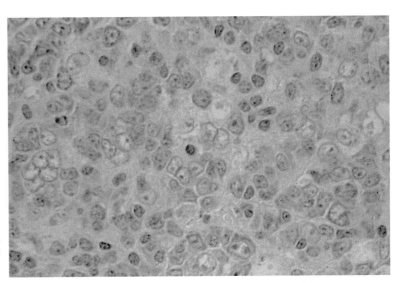

Figure 1–6. Follicular dendritic cells (FDCs). Several bi-, tri-, and multinucleated FDCs, with pale nuclei showing nuclear molding, small nucleoli, and inconspicuous cytoplasm, are present (Giemsa stain).

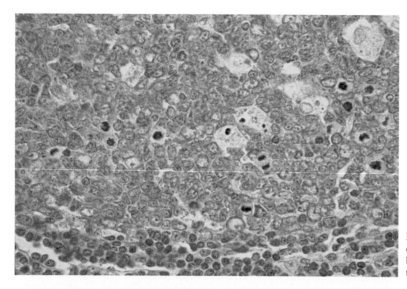

Figure 1–7. Dark zone of germinal center. Blast cells predominate. The mitotic rate is high, and scattered tingible body macrophages are present, producing a starry-sky pattern (Giemsa stain).

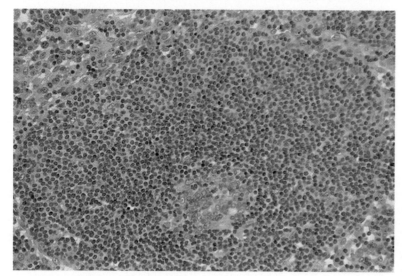

Figure 1–8. Follicle with prominent marginal zone in a mesenteric lymph node. The periphery of the upper portion of this follicle shows a broad arc of small lymphocytes, which have minimally irregular nuclei and slightly more cytoplasm than the mantle-zone lymphocytes immediately around the small germinal center (H&E stain).

Progressively Transformed Germinal Center (PTGC): A PTGC is an enlarged secondary follicle in which mantle zone–type lymphocytes are sprinkled evenly throughout the germinal center. PTGCs are usually found in small numbers in a background of typical follicular hyperplasia. Occasionally, lymphadenopathy in boys and young men is caused by reactive hyperplasia with prominent PTGC. PTGCs may also be found in association with Hodgkin's disease, usually the lymphocyte-predominant type. In rare cases (mainly in children), PTGCs are encircled by small clusters of epithelioid histiocytes (Figs. 1–10 to 1–12).

Follicle Lysis: In follicle lysis, the follicular dendritic cell (FDC) meshwork is broken up, resulting in small clusters of germinal center cells surrounded by FDCs, which appear to "float" in a background of small lymphocytes. Follicle lysis is a nonspecific change most often seen in florid follicular hyperplasia. It may be especially prominent

in the lymphoid hyperplasia of early HIV infection (Fig. 1–13).

PARACORTEX

The paracortex occupies the area between follicles and extends deeper into the lymph node toward the medulla. The paracortex is the site of activation of T cells and of B cells in T-cell-independent reactions and in early primary immune responses. In the B-cell reactions, naive B cells are transformed into IgM+ blast cells, which may differentiate into the IgM-secreting plasma cells of the primary immune response or may enter follicles to initiate the formation of a germinal center. When T cells are activated, their appearance changes from that of a small lymphocyte to an immunoblast. The paracortex contains small lymphocytes, a variable number of immunoblasts, interdigitating dendritic cells (IDC; the antigen-presenting cell of the paracortex),

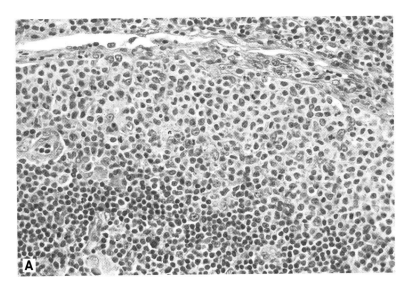

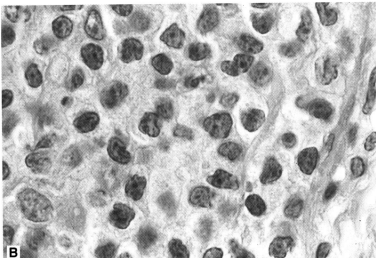

Figure 1–9. Monocytoid B cells in a case of toxoplasma lymphadenitis. *A,* A subcapsular band of monocytoid B cells appears with abundant pale cytoplasm (H&E stain). *B,* Monocytoid B cells have oval or indented nuclei with relatively fine chromatin and abundant pale to clear cytoplasm (H&E stain).

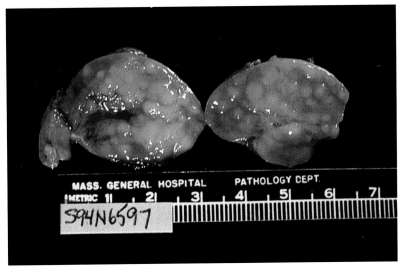

Figure 1–10. Lymph node with extensive progressive transformation of germinal centers (PTGCs). The cut section of this inguinal lymph node from a 16-year-old boy shows multiple tan nodules, each of which is a lymphoid follicle with PTGC.

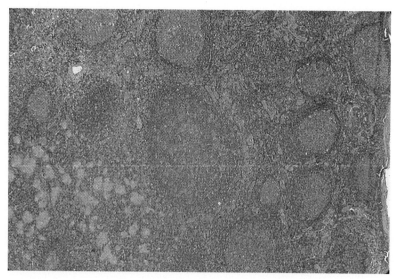

Figure 1–11. A single large, dark follicle with progressive transformation of its germinal center is seen in a background of follicular hyperplasia. Small clusters of epithelioid histiocytes are present *(lower left)* (H&E stain).

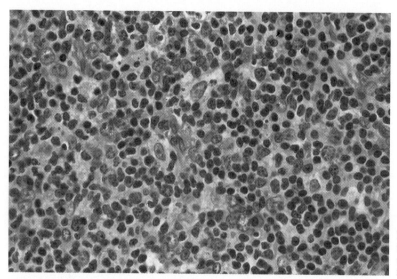

Figure 1–12. Progressive transformation of a germinal center. On high power examination, there is a predominance of small lymphocytes of mantle zone type, with only scattered residual germinal center cells (H&E stain).

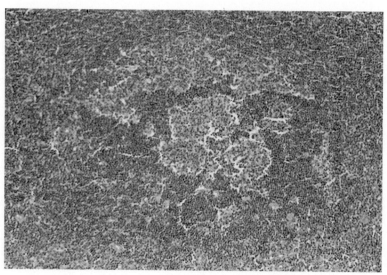

Figure 1–13. Follicle lysis in a patient with rheumatoid arthritis. Irregular bands of small lymphocytes disrupt a germinal center (H&E stain).

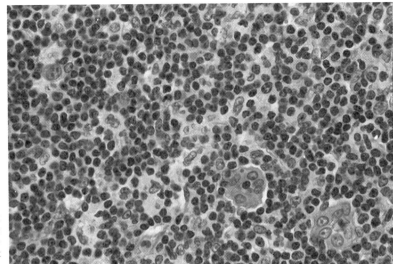

Figure 1–14. Paracortex. Most cells are small lymphocytes; scattered among them are interdigitating reticulum cells with deeply indented, folded nuclei and abundant pale cytoplasm. Two high endothelial venules appear in the right lower corner (H&E stain).

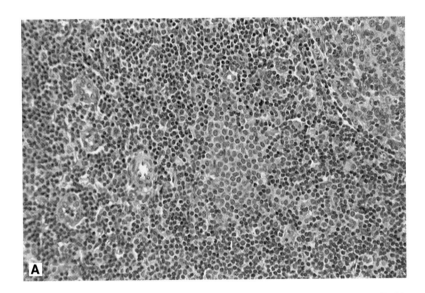

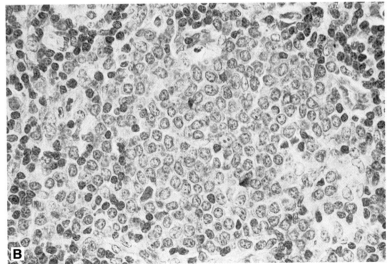

Figure 1–15. Plasmacytoid monocytes. *A,* Within the paracortex is a cluster of cells with more cytoplasm than the surrounding lymphocytes. A germinal center is present in the upper right corner (H&E stain). *B,* Higher power examination shows an aggregate of cells with pale, round nuclei slightly larger than those of small lymphocytes, pale cytoplasm, and ill-defined cell borders (Giemsa stain).

and high endothelial venules (HEV; important in lymphocyte trafficking). IDCs have pale oval to elongate nuclei, sometimes with complex invaginations of the nuclear membrane, and abundant pale cytoplasm. HEVs are lined by endothelial cells with a cuboidal, epithelioid appearance. Small lymphocytes commonly traverse the walls of HEVs. The lymphocytes and some immunoblasts are mature T cells (CD2+, CD3+, CD5+, CD1−, TdT−); other immunoblasts are B cells; helper cells usually outnumber suppressor cells (CD4 > CD8). The IDCs are S-100+ and HLA-DR+ (Fig. 1–14).

Plasmacytoid monocytes (formerly called T-associated plasma cells and plasmacytoid T cells) are sometimes found at the junction of the paracortex and medullary cords, usually in small clusters. They express some but not all monocyte-macrophage-associated antigens and certain T-cell-associated antigens, but no antigens that are T-lineage-specific. They are CD4+, HLA-DR+, CD68+, Ki-M1P+, CD45+ (Fig. 1–15).

MEDULLARY CORDS

The medullary cords are located toward the hilus of the lymph node. Most plasma cells of nodal origin are formed in this area, and most lymph node–derived Ig comes from this area. The medullary cords are occupied by a variable admixture of small lymphocytes, plasmacytoid lymphocytes, immunoblasts, and plasma cells. A few lymphocytes are T cells, but nearly all other cells are of B-lineage and express a variety of classes of polytypic Ig (mainly IgM, IgG, IgA). Plasma cells have cytoplasmic Ig and may not express surface Ig (Fig. 1–16).

SINUSES

The sinuses carry lymph through the lymph node. Afferent lymphatics empty into the subcapsular sinus. Lymph flows through cortical sinuses into medullary sinuses, which drain into efferent lymphatics. Sinuses are occupied by sinus histiocytes and a few small lymphocytes.

References

Berek C: The development of B cells and the B-cell repertoire in the microenvironment of the germinal centre. Immunol Rev 126:5, 1992.

Dorfman RF, Warnke RA: Lymphadenopathy simulating the malignant lymphomas. Hum Pathol 5:519–550, 1974.

Ferry JA, Zukerberg LR, Harris NL: Florid progressive transformation of germinal centers. A syndrome affecting young men, without early progression to nodular lymphocyte predominance Hodgkin's disease. Am J Surg Pathol 16:252–258, 1992.

Harris NL, Demirjian Z: Plasmacytoid T-zone cell proliferation in a patient with chronic myelomonocytic leukemia. Histologic and immunohistologic characterization. Am J Surg Pathol 15(1):87–95, 1991.

Lennert K: Malignant lymphomas other than Hodgkin's disease. New York: Springer-Verlag, 1978.

MacLennan I, Liu Y, Oldfield S, et al: The evolution of B-cell clones. Cur Top Microbiol Immunol 159:37–63, 1990.

Osborne BM, Butler JJ, Gresik MV: Progressive transformation of germinal centers: comparison of 23 pediatric patients to the adult population. Mod Pathol 5:135–140, 1992.

van der Valk P, Meijer CJLM: The histology of reactive lymph nodes. Am J Surg Pathol 11(11):866–882, 1987.

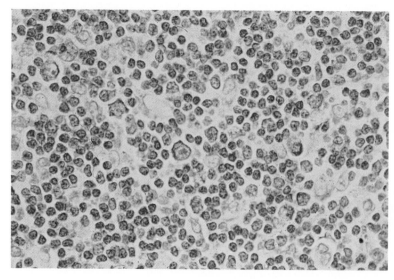

Figure 1–16. Medullary region. In this reactive lymph node, the medulla contains small lymphocytes and scattered immunoblasts. In other cases, blasts may be more or less numerous, and plasma cells may be prominent (Giemsa stain).

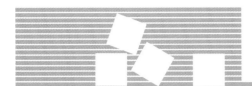

CHAPTER 2

Reactive Lymphoid Hyperplasia

The discussion of reactive lymphoid hyperplasia is categorized mainly by etiology. In reactive hyperplasia of different types, however, hyperplasia of one compartment of the lymph node may predominate, so that reactive hyperplasias may also be classified by pattern, as indicated in Table 2–1.

Table 2–1
REACTIVE LYMPHOID HYPERPLASIA: PREDOMINANT PATTERN BY ETIOLOGY

Follicular Hyperplasia	**Sinusoidal Expansion**
Rheumatoid arthritis	Lymphangiogram effect
Castleman's disease	Sinus histiocytosis with massive lymphadenopathy
HIV infection (early)	Whipple's disease, some cases
Syphilis	**Granulomatous Lymphadenitis**
Bacterial infection (early)	Bacterial infections, including cat scratch disease, lymphogranuloma
Paracortical Hyperplasia	venereum, tularemia, and yersinial lymphadenitis
Dermatopathic lymphadenopathy	Sarcoidosis
Viral infection	Tuberculosis
Postvaccination lymphadenopathy	Fungal infection
Drug-induced hypersensitivity reaction	Whipple's disease, some cases
Kikuchi's disease	Berylliosis
Systemic lupus erythematosus	Lymph nodes draining carcinoma, few cases
Draining region of suppurative inflammation (some cases)	**Mixed Pattern**
Lymph nodes draining carcinoma, few cases	Toxoplasmosis
	Kimura's disease

Viral Infections

INFECTIOUS MONONUCLEOSIS (IM)

Clinical Features

IM is caused by Epstein-Barr virus (EBV) and mainly affects adolescents and young adults, although cases of IM in young children and in adults as old as 80 have been reported. Manifestations of IM include fever, pharyngitis, cervical lymphadenopathy, rash, and atypical lymphocytosis, and a positive heterophile antibody (Monospot) test. More severe cases may have hepatosplenomegaly, generalized lymphadenopathy, hepatic dysfunction, and peripheral cytopenias, and even a hemophagocytic syndrome. In most cases, the illness is self-limited, but rarely splenic rupture, intercurrent infection, Guillain-Barré syndrome, or hemorrhage results in death.

Morphology

The lymph nodal architecture is typically distorted but not effaced by an expanded paracortex containing a polymorphous population of lymphoid cells, including small lymphocytes, intermediate-sized lymphoid cells, immunoblasts, tingible body macrophages, and sometimes plasma cells. The immunoblasts may be atypical, with pleomorphic or lobulated nuclei; Reed-Sternberg (RS)–like cells may be identified. Mitoses are frequent. Individual cell necrosis and larger areas of necrosis are sometimes found. Reactive follicles may be present, but follicular hyperplasia is less prominent than paracortical hyperplasia. At least some sinuses are patent, and frequently they are dilated and contain histiocytes and a polymorphous population of lymphoid cells, including immunoblasts. Lymphoid cells sometimes

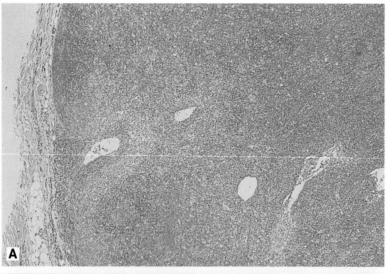

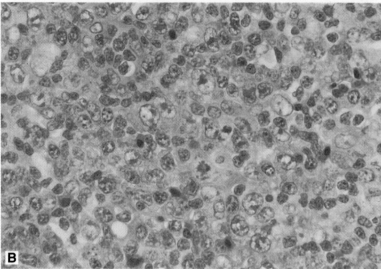

Figure 2–1. Infectious mononucleosis. *A*, Low power view of a lymph node showing marked paracortical expansion with only one reactive follicle at the periphery of the node. Monocytoid B cells are present focally. Sinuses are patent (H&E stain). *B*, High power view of the paracortex shows a spectrum of cells, including small lymphocytes, intermediate-sized transformed cells, and immunoblasts (H&E stain).

infiltrate the capsule and extend into perinodal tissue (Figs. 2–1 and 2–2).

Immunophenotype

The paracortex contains a preponderance of T cells. The CD4:CD8 ratio may be normal or reversed. Most paracortical immunoblasts, however, are B cells (Fig. 2–2*B*). The blasts typically show focal CD30 staining; they are negative for CD15 and EMA. Many RS-like cells in involved tonsillar tissue express EBV latent membrane protein (LMP) (Fig. 2–2*C*), although LMP+ cells are infrequent in lymph nodes and spleen.

Genetic Features

EBV-encoded RNA (EBER) can be detected in immunoblasts in large numbers, almost exclusively in the paracortex.

Differential Diagnosis

Obtaining adequate clinical information is important to make the correct diagnosis, whether the differential diagnosis is lymphoma or other types of reactive hyperplasia.

1. Non-Hodgkin's lymphoma (NHL): When immunoblasts are numerous, NHL must be considered. In favor of IM are lack of architectural effacement, presence of areas readily recognizable as reactive hyperplasia, polymorphous background of lymphoid cells without cleaved cells, and patent sinuses containing lymphoid cells, including blasts. The blasts lack monotypic Ig. In some cases, the possibility of anaplastic large cell lymphoma (ALCL) may be considered. In IM, most blasts are B cells; some are CD30+, but they are typically EMA−. Most ALCLs are T-lineage lymphomas that coexpress EMA. Genotyping studies may be helpful in problematic cases.

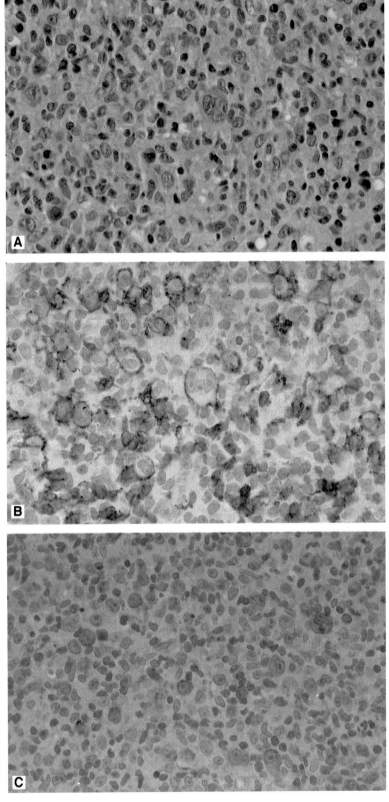

Figure 2–2. Infectious mononucleosis, involving the tonsil of a 6-year-old boy. *A*, Occasional cells that closely resemble Reed-Sternberg cells are visible (H&E stain). *B*, Most of the large cells, including Reed-Sternberg-like cells, are B cells (L26+). *C*, Many of the blasts express Epstein-Barr virus latent membrane protein (*B* and *C*, immunoperoxidase technique on paraffin sections).

2. Hodgkin's disease (HD): The RS-like cells seen in IM do not usually meet strict criteria for identification of RS cells. The polymorphous background of lymphoid cells in the paracortex and the sinuses that is seen in IM excludes HD. Immunoblasts in IM are CD15−.

3. Other types of reactive hyperplasias: Other viral infections, reactions to vaccination, and certain drugs can produce lymphadenopathy with histologic features similar to or indistinguishable from those of IM. In IM, EBER+ immunoblasts are typically present in large numbers, but in other conditions, EBER+ cells are usually lymphocytes present only in small numbers.

   a. Vaccination: Various vaccinations can cause lymphadenopathy. The prototypical example of vaccine-related lymphadenopathy is smallpox (vaccinia) vaccination. Although no longer routinely given, smallpox vaccination has been associated with florid lymphoid hyperplasia often mistaken for lymphoma. Depending on the interval following vaccination, paracortical hyperplasia (short interval) or follicular hyperplasia (longer interval) may predominate. It usually occurs in the region draining the vaccination site, but infrequently may be generalized.

   b. Drug reaction: Various drugs, especially anticonvulsants, may cause lymphadenopathy. Drugs cause hyperplastic lesions with a variety of patterns, but the classic example is the paracortical immunoblastic reaction caused by phenytoin (Dilantin). Eosinophils may be more numerous in lymph nodes (and in the peripheral blood) than in IM. Not all patients with lymphadenopathy who are receiving anticonvulsants have reactive lesions, however. Some have had Hodgkin's disease or NHL. In a few cases, apparently hyperplastic lesions have been followed by the development of lymphoma.

   c. Reaction to gastrointestinal inflammation: In cases of marked acute inflammation in the gastrointestinal tract, such as suppurative appendicitis or intestinal perforation, mesenteric lymph nodes may show a florid immunoblastic reaction (Fig. 2–3).

   d. Lyme disease: Infection by *Borrelia burgdorferi* is often associated with lymphadenopathy, which may be localized or generalized; only rare descriptions of the histologic features of these lymph nodes, however, have been published. In one case, a lymph node showed paracortical hyperplasia with numerous immunoblasts and a microabscess with eosinophils. In a case that we reviewed in a patient suspected of having Lyme disease, we found paracortical immunoblastic hyperplasia and sinuses containing immunoblasts. Spirochetes were not found in either case.

References

Abbondanzo SL, Sato N, Straus SE, Jaffe ES: Acute infectious mononucleosis. CD30 (Ki-1) antigen expression and histologic correlations. (See comments.) Am J Clin Pathol 93(5):698–702, 1990.

Bailey RE: Diagnosis and treatment of infectious mononucleosis. (Review.) Am Fam Physician 49(4):879–888, 1994.

Custer RP, Smith EB: The pathology of infectious mononucleosis. Blood 3:830–857, 1948.

Hartsock RJ, Bellanti JA: Postvaccinial lymphadenitis. GP 39(1):99–105, 1969.

Isaacson PG, Schmid C, Pan L, et al: Epstein-Barr virus latent membrane protein expression by Hodgkin and Reed-Sternberg-like cells in acute infectious mononucleosis. J Pathol 167(3):267–271, 1992.

Mroczek EC, Weisenburger DD, Grierson HL, et al: Fatal infectious mononucleosis and virus-associated hemophagocytic syndrome. Arch Pathol Lab Med 111(6):530–535, 1987.

Niedobitek G, Herbst H, Young LS, et al: Patterns of Epstein-Barr virus infection in non-neoplastic lymphoid tissue. Blood 790:2520–2526, 1992.

Ramakrishnan T, Gloster E, Bonagura VR, et al: Eosinophilic lymphadenitis in Lyme disease. Pediat Infect Dis J 8:180–181, 1989.

Salvador AH, Harrison EGJ, Kyle RA: Lymphadenopathy due to infectious mononucleosis: its confusion with malignant lymphoma. Cancer 27(5):1029–1040, 1971.

Segal GH, Clough JD, Tubbs RR: Autoimmune and iatrogenic causes of lymphadenopathy. (Review.) Sem Oncol 20(6):611–626, 1993.

Segal GH, Kjeldsberg CR, Smith GP, Perkins SL: CD30 antigen expression in florid immunoblastic proliferations. A clinicopathologic study of 14 cases. Am J Clin Pathol 102(3):292–298, 1994.

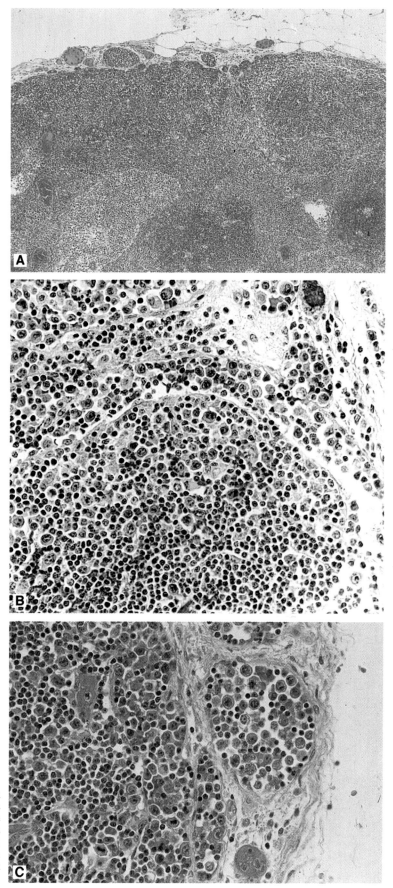

Figure 2–3. Immunoblastic reaction in a mesenteric lymph node in response to a ruptured appendix. *A*, The paracortex is expanded and follicles are not recognizable. Sinuses are dilated (H&E stain). *B*, Numerous large lymphoid cells are present in the paracortex and also in sinuses (H&E stain). *C*, The subcapsular sinus and an adjacent lymphatic contain numerous large transformed lymphoid cells with frequent mitotic figures (H&E stain).

HERPES SIMPLEX LYMPHADENITIS (HSL)

Clinical Features

Infection by herpes simplex virus (type I or II) is an unusual etiology of lymphadenitis, but it can cause localized or generalized adenopathy or involve lymph nodes in the setting of widespread visceral infection. When localized, the lymphadenopathy most often affects inguinal nodes, and it is typically painful. Typical mucocutaneous herpetic lesions are found in most patients, but the lesions may be inconspicuous or they may not appear until after a lymph node biopsy has been performed. Among published cases, nearly half of patients who present with HSL have a history of a hematolymphoid malignancy or develop a malignancy shortly after the diagnosis of HSL. Although a patient with HSL in the setting of disseminated herpes simplex infection has a poor prognosis, HSL is self-limited in most cases.

Morphology

Lymph nodes show discrete areas of necrosis and prominent paracortical hyperplasia with or without follicular hyperplasia. The paracortex may contain numerous immunoblasts. The necrotic areas contain neutrophils, karyorrhectic or amorphous eosinophilic debris, and variable numbers of viral inclusions, ranging from rare to abundant. Most neutrophils are uninucleate, in contrast to the classic multinucleated inclusions found in squamous epithelium. Intact neutrophils are most abundant in early lesions, but may be absent in long-standing lymphadenitis. Histiocytes may surround the necrotic areas, but granulomas are absent. Inflammation may extend into perinodal soft tissue (Fig. 2–4). Similar changes occur in the tonsils in herpetic tonsillitis.

Differential diagnosis

1. Kikuchi's disease: HSL can resemble Kikuchi's disease, particularly in older lesions with few intact neutrophils. Although histiocytes may be prominent in HSL, the histiocytic infiltrate is generally even more pronounced in Kikuchi's disease, and viral inclusions are absent.
2. Systemic lupus erythematosus: Hematoxylin bodies and deposits of basophilic material in the walls of blood vessels are sometimes found in lupus lymphadenopathy, and viral inclusions are absent. Neutrophils are not abundant (see Figs. 2–17 and 2–18).
3. Varicella zoster virus (VZV) rarely causes lymphadenitis; the histologic features are similar to those of HSL. Immunoperoxidase staining for viral antigens and clinical information are helpful in differentiating HSL from VZV.
4. Other infections: The lack of granulomatous inflammation with epithelioid or palisading histiocytes provides evidence against infection caused by mycobacteria, fungi, *Yersinia*, cat scratch bacilli, and *Chlamydia*. Infectious mononucleosis lacks viral inclusions and usually lacks prominent zonal necrosis.
5. Malignant lymphoma: When pronounced paracortical expansion occurs with numerous immunoblasts, the differential diagnosis includes large cell lymphoma. In HSL, the nodal architecture may be distorted, but it is not obliterated, i.e., sinuses remain patent, in contrast to most lymphomas. Discrete foci of necrosis are less common in lymphoma, and HSV inclusions are absent in lymphoma, except in the rare case in which both HSV and lymphoma involve the same site.

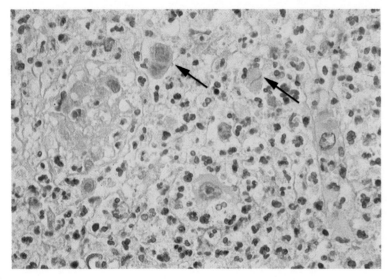

Figure 2–4. Herpes simplex lymphadenitis, from a patient with a history of acute myeloid leukemia awaiting bone marrow transplant. Scattered cells have large eosinophilic nuclear inclusions, often with a ground-glass quality *(arrows)*, in a background of acute inflammation (H&E stain).

References

Epstein JI, Ambinder RF, Kuhajda FP, *et al*: Localized herpes simplex lymphadenitis. Am J Clin Pathol 86(4): 444–448, 1986.

Howat AJ, Campbell AR, Stewart DJ: Generalized lymphadenopathy due to herpes simplex virus type 1. Histopathology 19(6):563–564, 1991.

Miliauskas JR, Leong AS: Localized herpes simplex lymphadenitis: report of three cases and review of the literature. (Review.) Histopathology 19(4):355–360, 1991.

Tamaru J, Mikata A, Horie H, *et al*: Herpes simplex lymphadenitis. Report of two cases with review of the literature. (Review.) Am J Surg Pathol 14(6):571–577, 1990.

Taxy JB, Tillawi I, Goldman PM: Herpes simplex lymphadenitis. An unusual presentation with necrosis and viral particles. Arch Pathol Lab Med 109(11):1043–1044, 1985.

Wat PJ, Strickler JG, Myers JL, Nordstrom MR: Herpes simplex infection causing acute necrotizing tonsillitis. Mayo Clin Proc 69(3):269–271, 1994.

CYTOMEGALOVIRAL LYMPHADENITIS

Clinical Features

Cytomegalovirus (CMV) can cause lymphadenopathy in the setting of a heterophile-negative, infectious mononucleo-sis–like illness. Lymph node enlargement due to CMV infection may also be found in patients who are otherwise asymptomatic. CMV can infect lymphoid tissues in patients who have had Hodgkin's disease, non-Hodgkin's lymphoma, or common variable immunodeficiency, or in patients with a normal immune system. CMV lymphade-nopathy may be localized or generalized.

Morphology

Lymph nodes show florid follicular hyperplasia or paracortical hyperplasia, with interfollicular immunoblasts that range from few to abundant. Monocytoid B cells may also be prominent. Cells with inclusions are usually present focally in relatively small numbers. Occasionally, they are numerous. Neutrophils are often scattered among the infected cells. Inclusions may be found in the paracortex or among monocytoid B cells. The infected cells are sometimes recognizable as endothelial; in other instances, infection of lymphoid cells or histiocytes has been reported (Fig. 2–5).

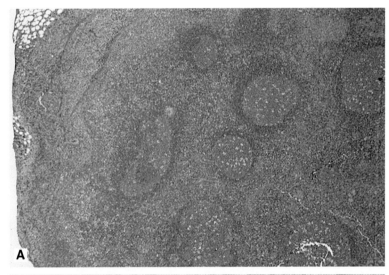

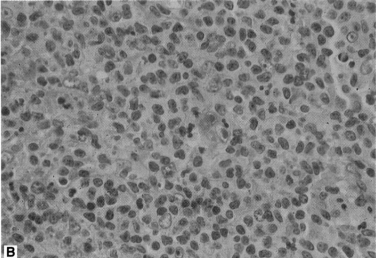

Figure 2–5. Cytomegalovirus (CMV) lymphadenitis. *A,* Low power examination shows florid follicular hyperplasia, with a pale subcapsular band of monocytoid B cells *(left)* (H&E stain). *B,* Centrally, two neighboring cells contain large eosinophilic nuclear inclusions, which resemble the appearance of a Reed-Sternberg cell (H&E stain).

Illustration continued on following page.

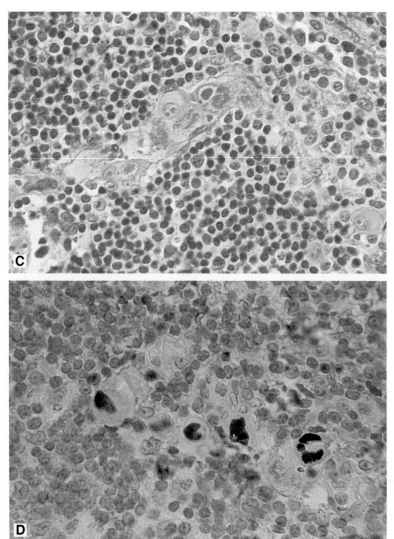

Figure 2–5. *Continued C*, Several endothelial cells contain single large nuclear inclusions and multiple finely granular cytoplasmic inclusions (H&E stain). *D*, The inclusions are positive with antibodies to CMV-associated antigens (immunoperoxidase technique on paraffin section).

Immunophenotype and Genetic Features

CMV-infected cells can be identified in tissue sections using antibodies to CMV-associated antigens (Fig. 2–5D), or using in-situ hybridization with probes for viral DNA. Cells containing inclusions express CD15, usually with a Golgi region or a diffuse cytoplasmic pattern of staining, but without membrane staining. In cases in which lymphoid cells have been reported to be infected, the affected cells appear to be T cells rather than B cells.

Differential Diagnosis

1. Nonspecific reactive hyperplasia: When inclusions are present in small numbers, they may be overlooked.
2. Hodgkin's disease (HD): Cells with nuclear viral inclusions may resemble Reed-Sternberg cells and variants on routinely stained sections; they are reported to express cytoplasmic CD15. CMV lymphadenitis is less likely than Hodgkin's disease to obliterate the nodal architec-

ture. CMV-infected cells often contain granular eosinophilic cytoplasmic inclusions, but the cytoplasm of Reed-Sternberg cells is pale and agranular. Cells with inclusions may be identifiable as endothelial cells, excluding a diagnosis of Hodgkin's disease. Reed-Sternberg cells are more likely to have membrane staining for CD15 than cells with CMV inclusions. Reed-Sternberg cells do not stain with antibodies to CMV.

References

Abramowitz A, Livni N, Morag A, Ravid Z: An immunoperoxidase study of cytomegalovirus mononucleosis. Arch Pathol Lab Med 106(3): 115–118, 1982.

Case Records of the Massachusetts General Hospital, Case 7-1995. N Engl J Med 332:663–671, 1995.

Rushin JM, Riordan GP, Heaton RB, *et al*: Cytomegalovirus-infected cells express Leu-M1 antigen. A potential source of diagnostic error. Am J Pathol 136(5):989–995, 1990.

Younes M, Podesta A, Helie M, Buckley P: Infection of T but not B lymphocytes by cytomegalovirus in lymph node. An immunophenotypic study. Am J Surg Pathol 15(1):75–80, 1991.

Bacterial Infections

CAT SCRATCH DISEASE (CSD)

Clinical Features

Cat scratch disease is the most common cause of chronic, benign lymphadenopathy in the United States, with about 24,000 cases per year. It is due to infection by *Bartonella* (formerly *Rochalimaea*) *henselae*, the same agent that causes bacillary angiomatosis. CSD can affect patients of any age, but 85% are under the age of 18, and more than half are between 3 and 10 years old. A history of exposure to a cat (usually a kitten) can be found in nearly all cases.

Several days after exposure, a papule develops in the skin at the inoculation site; 1 to 2 weeks later, regional lymphadenopathy, most often axillary, develops. The lymphadenopathy usually involves only one node and although more than one lymph node in the same area may be affected, lymphadenopathy hardly ever involves more than one group of nodes. Noncontiguous lymphadenopathy, however, may develop if there is more than one inoculation site or if the inoculation is midline and organisms drain to lymph nodes bilaterally. Two thirds of the patients have fever. Patients may also experience malaise, anorexia, or rarely nausea or abdominal pain. The disease is usually mild and self-limited; some cases remain unrecognized. When the inoculation site is the eye, patients may develop Parinaud's oculoglandular syndrome (granulomatous conjunctivitis and preauricular lymphadenopathy). Severe manifestations, which occur in up to 2% of cases, include encephalopathy and bone, lung, liver, or spleen involvement.

Because the organisms may be difficult to recognize in histologic sections, and because they are difficult to culture, serologic studies may be helpful in establishing a definite diagnosis.

Morphology

The appearance of the infected lymph nodes changes over time. Initially, there is follicular hyperplasia with monocytoid B-cell proliferation. Within aggregates of monocytoid B cells are small foci of necrosis with neutrophils (Fig. 2–6A). These foci are usually close to, or encroach upon, germinal centers, or they may be adjacent to the subcapsular sinus. The paracortex is hyperplastic. Sinuses contain histiocytes, immunoblasts, and neutrophils. With time, the necrotic foci enlarge, extending deeper into the node. They contain pus, fibrin, and cellular debris, and acquire a rim of macrophages. The foci continue to enlarge and coalesce and are surrounded by palisading histiocytes, to produce the classic stellate microabscess or granuloma (Figs. 2–7 and 2–8). The cat scratch bacillus is a small, slender, pleomorphic rod up to 3 μm long, which is best seen with a Warthin-Starry stain. The bacilli are weakly gram-negative, but they are so small that they are close to the limits of light microscopic resolution and thus very difficult to see with a Gram stain. Silver stains, such as the Warthin-Starry stain, appear to coat the bacilli with silver granules, making them larger and easier to recognize. Organisms are most numerous in early lesions (Fig. 2–6B) and virtually absent in the stellate abscesses. Bacilli are present singly, in chains, or in large clumps. They may be found in the walls of blood vessels, in macrophages in necrotic areas, in sinus histiocytes, or in the extracellular space, but they are not found in neutrophils.

Immunophenotype

The granulomas contain a variable mixture of B and T cells in addition to histiocytes.

Differential Diagnosis

A variety of microorganisms may cause necrotizing lymphadenitis that should be considered in the differential diagnosis of CSD. Clinical features, special stains on tissue sections, serologic studies, and culture will establish a definite diagnosis.

1. Lymphadenitis caused by certain bacteria, including *Chlamydia trachomatis* (lymphogranuloma venereum), *Francisella tularensis* (tularemia), *Hemophilus ducreyi* (chancroid), *Yersinia enterocolitica* (pseudotuberculous mesenteric lymphadenitis), *Listeria monocytogenes* (listeriosis), *Pseudomonas mallei* (glanders), and *P. pseudomallei* (melioidosis), shows necrotizing granulomas that may mimic CSD (Fig. 2–9). In nearly all cases, the diseases just listed are associated with significantly greater morbidity than CSD.
2. Infection by pyogenic cocci (e.g., *Staphylococcus, Streptococcus*) causes acute suppurative lymphadenitis with follicular hyperplasia and abscesses that may resemble CSD (Fig. 2–10). The presence of a rim of histiocytes around the abscesses favors CSD.
3. Mycobacteria (*Mycobacterium tuberculosis* and atypical mycobacteria) and fungi can produce lymphadenitis with granulomatous microabscesses similar to those of CSD. This finding is most common in atypical mycobacterial infections of children and in immunocompromised adults. In some late cases of CSD, the necrotic material acquires a pink, amorphous appearance closely resembling the caseation necrosis characteristic of tuberculosis.

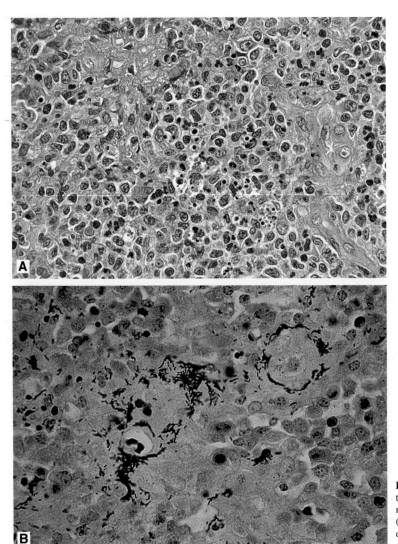

Figure 2–6. Cat scratch disease, early lesion. *A*, A few neutrophils and scant cellular debris are present in an aggregate of monocytoid B cells. Blood vessels show fibrinoid change (H&E stain). *B*, Large numbers of bacteria, many of which encircle small blood vessels, are visible with a Warthin-Starry stain.

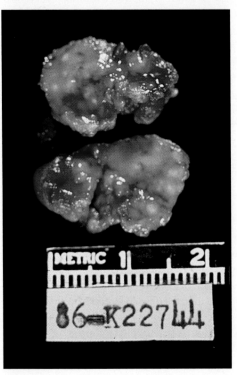

Figure 2–7. Cat scratch disease; axillary lymph node from a 6-year-old boy. Intact areas of the node contain multiple pale nodules, consistent with the presence of granulomas, but much of the node is disrupted by hemorrhage and necrosis.

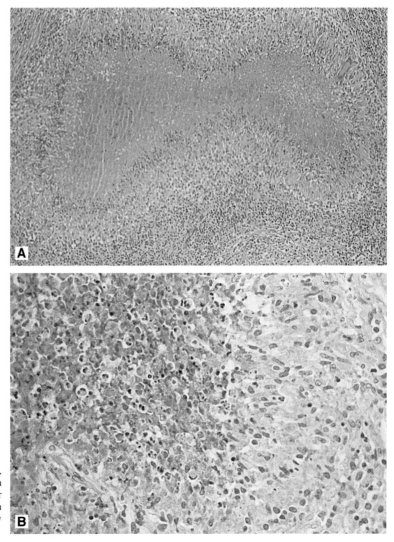

Figure 2–8. Cat scratch disease, fully developed lesion. *A*, Low power view shows a large, irregular granuloma with extensive central necrosis (H&E stain). *B*, A higher power view shows a rim of palisading histiocytes surrounding an area of suppurative necrosis. Microorganisms are not usually identifiable at this stage (H&E stain).

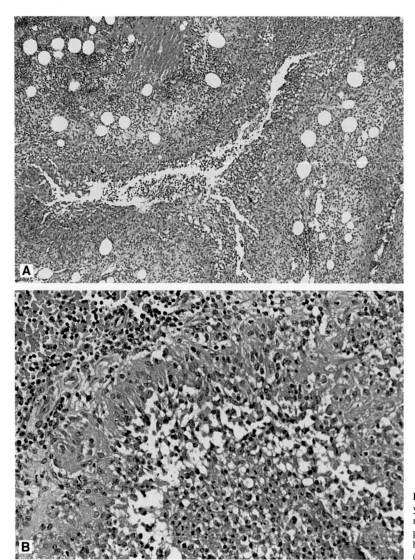

Figure 2–9. Tularemia involving a lymph node from a 7-year-old child. *A*, Low power view shows a stellate microabscess (H&E stain). *B*, Higher power view shows palisading histiocytes and central suppurative necrosis, histologically indistinguishable from cat scratch disease (H&E stain).

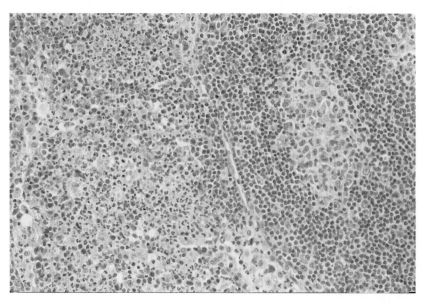

Figure 2–10. Suppurative lymphadenitis in a pericolic lymph node in a patient with peritonitis. The paracortex adjacent to a reactive follicle contains large aggregates of neutrophils, with no evidence of granuloma formation (H&E stain).

References

Adal KA, Cockerell CJ, Petri WA: Cat scratch disease, bacillary angiomatosis and other infections due to Rochalimaea. N Engl J Med 330:1509–1515, 1994.

Bergmans AM, Groothedde JW, Schellekens JF, et al: Etiology of cat scratch disease: comparison of polymerase chain reaction detection of Bartonella (formerly Rochalimaea) and Afipia felis DNA with serology and skin tests. J Inf Dis 171:916–923, 1995.

Case records of the Massachusetts General Hospital. Case 22-1992. A 6½-year-old girl with status epilepticus, cervical lymphadenopathy, pleural effusions, and respiratory distress. (See comments.) N Engl J Med 326(22):1480–1489, 1992.

Facchetti F, Agostini C, Chilosi M, et al: Suppurative granulomatous lymphadenitis. Immunohistochemical evidence for a B-cell-associated granuloma. Am J Surg Pathol 16:955–961, 1992.

Miller-Catchpole R, Variakojis D, Vardiman JW, et al: Cat scratch disease. Identification of bacteria in seven cases of lymphadenitis. Am J Surg Pathol 10:276–281, 1986.

Wear D, Margileth A, Hadfield T, et al: Cat-scratch disease: a bacterial infection. Science 221:1403–1404, 1983.

MYCOBACTERIAL INFECTION

Clinical Features

Approximately one third of the world's population is infected by *Mycobacterium tuberculosis*. Although the proportion of residents of the United States with tuberculosis is much lower than in other parts of the world, the number of cases has increased owing to HIV infection, poor living conditions, homelessness, and higher incidences of drug-resistant strains.

Mycobacterial lymphadenitis may occur in isolation or in conjunction with pulmonary tuberculosis or disseminated infection. Involved nodes usually are slowly enlarging, nontender masses that may be associated with draining sinuses. Any lymph node can be involved, but in patients presenting with peripheral lymphadenopathy, cervical nodes are affected most often. In children, mycobacterial lymphadenitis is much more likely to be due to infection by atypical mycobacteria (*M. scrofulaceum*, *M. kansasii*, or *M. avium* complex).

Morphology

Lymph nodes show multiple, well-formed granulomas composed of epithelioid histiocytes and Langhans-type giant cells; caseation necrosis is present to a variable extent in the centers of the granulomas (Fig. 2–11). Granulomas may consist of loose aggregates of histiocytes in immunosuppressed patients. In children, early granulomas may contain neutrophils and resemble the microabscesses of cat scratch disease (Fig. 2–12*A*). A Ziehl-Neelsen stain is used to identify the organisms, which are usually few in immunocompetent patients (Fig. 2–12*B*). Culture is needed to diagnose cases in which organisms cannot be identified in the biopsy tissue and to distinguish between infections caused by *M. tuberculosis* and atypical mycobacteria.

Immunophenotype

The lymphocytes associated with the granulomas are T cells; B cells are virtually absent.

Differential Diagnosis

1. Sarcoidosis: Cases of mycobacterial lymphadenitis with little or no necrosis resemble sarcoidosis. A Ziehl-Neelsen stain and culture are helpful in establishing a diagnosis; however, the Ziehl-Neelsen stain result is often negative in mycobacterial infection unless there is necrosis.

2. Granulomatous lymphadenitides of infectious etiology (due to fungi, cat scratch bacilli, *Brucella* species, spirochetes, leishmania): Caseation necrosis is more common in mycobacterial infections, although necrosis resembling caseation may be seen with fungal infections and, less often, with other infections. In cases of primary or secondary syphilis, lymph nodes may show non-necrotizing or suppurative granulomas, but they are found in the setting of marked follicular hyperplasia and plasmacytosis.

3. Hodgkin's disease: Hodgkin's disease may be associated with granulomatous inflammation and extensive necrosis. Identification of Reed-Sternberg cells, which tend to be found in greatest numbers at the periphery of necrotic areas, confirms the diagnosis of Hodgkin's disease. The presence of a more polymorphous inflammatory cell infiltrate, containing eosinophils and plasma cells, is more common in Hodgkin's disease.

4. Metastatic carcinoma can be associated with necrotizing or non-necrotizing granulomas in lymph nodes. In the setting of extensive granulomatous inflammation, the carcinoma may be overlooked. Granulomas may also be found in lymph nodes that drain carcinoma but are themselves free of metastases.

References

Dandapat MC, Mishra BM, Dash SP, Kar PK: Peripheral lymph node tuberculosis: a review of 80 cases. Br J Surg 77(8):911–912, 1990.

Facchetti F, Agostini C, Chilosi M, *et al*: Suppurative granulomatous lymphadenitis. Immunohistochemical evidence for a B-cell-associated granuloma. Am J Surg Pathol 16(10):955–961, 1992.

Simon HB: Infections due to mycobacteria. Infect Dis 7:1–25, 1995.

Subrahmanyam M: Role of surgery and chemotherapy for peripheral lymph node tuberculosis. Br J Surg 80(12):1547–1548, 1993.

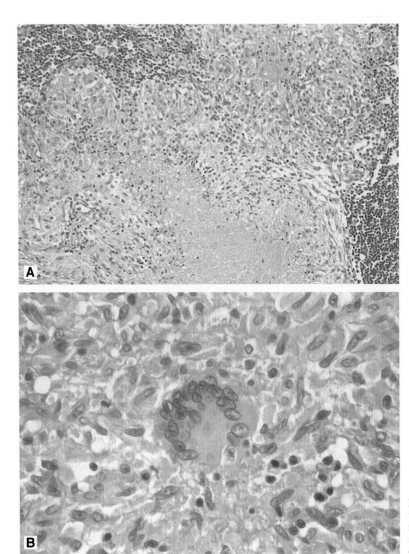

Figure 2–11. Mycobacterial lymphadenitis involving a cervical lymph node in a patient from Africa. *A*, The lymph node shows caseating granulomatous inflammation (H&E stain). *B*, High power view reveals epithelioid histiocytes and occasional Langhans-type giant cells (H&E stain).

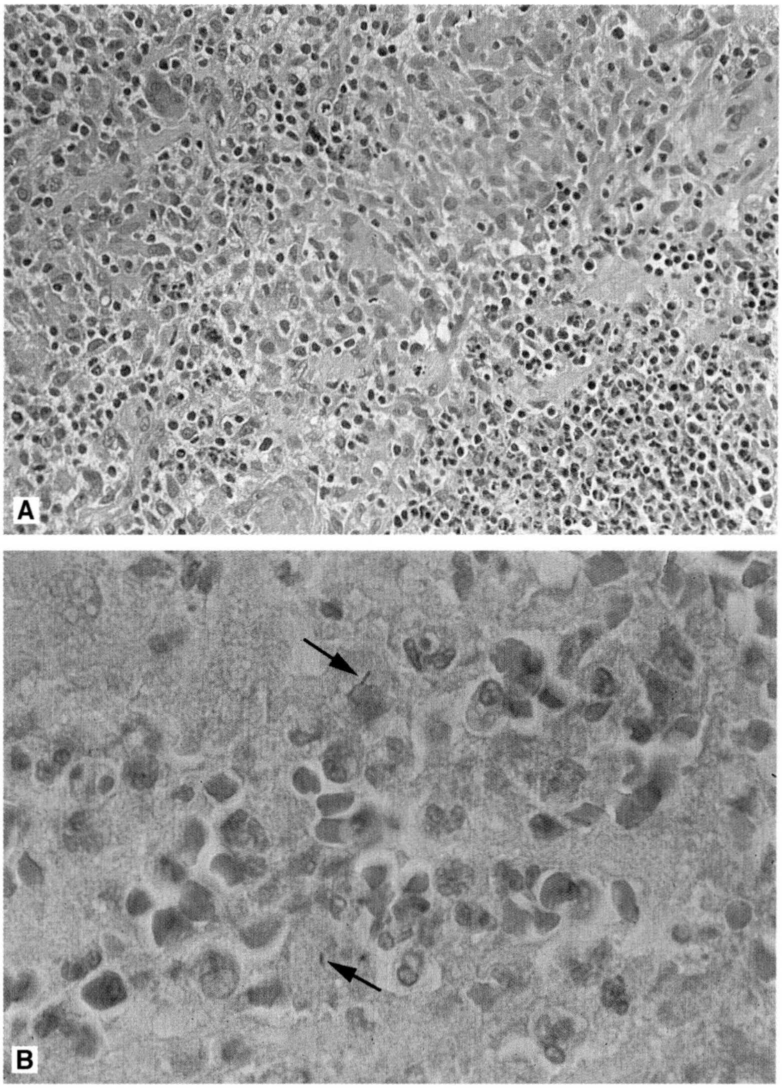

Figure 2–12. Atypical mycobacterial lymphadenitis in a 3-year-old child. *A,* Necrotizing granulomas have neutrophils and suppurative necrosis rather than caseation (H&E stain). *B,* Rare acid-fast bacilli are visible *(arrows)* (Ziehl-Neelsen stain).

Leprosy

Although infection by *Mycobacterium leprae* is uncommon in the United States, it is a major health problem in other parts of the world, with approximately 5.5 million cases of active disease worldwide. Infection by *M. leprae* takes one of two forms—tuberculoid leprosy or lepromatous leprosy—depending on the immunologic status of the host. Intermediate forms between these two extremes exist.

Tuberculoid Leprosy (TL): Mild to moderate enlargement of lymph nodes, which is usually localized, is found in the majority of cases of TL. Involved nodes show non-caseating granulomas, with only rare microorganisms seen on a Fite stain.

Lepromatous Leprosy (LL): Moderate to marked lymphadenopathy, which may be generalized, is found in nearly all cases of LL. Lymph nodes show large aggregates or diffuse infiltrates of histiocytes with abundant, pale, often vacuolated cytoplasm containing numerous bacilli ("lepra cells"). Cortical and medullary sinuses also contain lepra cells.

Differential Diagnosis

TL should be considered in the differential diagnosis of sarcoidosis and other mycobacterial infections. LL is included in the differential diagnosis of storage diseases and other causes of lipid deposition in lymph nodes, such as Whipple's disease. Special stains for microorganisms, culture, and, most importantly, clinical findings are helpful in establishing a diagnosis.

References

Fiallo P, Pesce C, Lenti E, Nunzi E: Short report: erythema nodosum leprosum lymphadenitis. Am J Tropical Med Hygiene 52(4):297–298, 1995.
Simon HB: Infections due to mycobacteria. Infect Dis 7:1–25, 1995.

WHIPPLE'S DISEASE

Clinical Features

Whipple's disease (WD) is a bacterial infection that predominantly affects middle-aged to older men, who usually present with diarrhea, weight loss, abdominal pain, and arthritis. Approximately half of patients have peripheral lymphadenopathy; intra-abdominal nodes may also be enlarged. Lymphadenopathy is occasionally responsible for venous or lymphatic obstruction. The disease can also affect the central nervous system, eyes, heart, lungs and liver. Although symptoms related to GI involvement are generally most prominent, some patients have presented with lymphadenopathy without diarrhea or malabsorption. In some of these unusual cases, the diagnosis was established only at autopsy.

WD responds to broad-spectrum antibiotics. The causative organism has been identified as a previously unrecognized type of actinomycete, *Tropheryma whippelii* gen nov sp nov.

Morphology

The classic findings in lymph nodes in WD include lipogranulomas that have clusters of foamy histiocytes and epithelioid cells and sinuses distended by cystic-appearing, lipid-filled spaces surrounded by foreign body giant cells. The histiocytes have granular, PAS+, diastase-resistant cytoplasm (Figs. 2–13 and 2–14). Electron microscopy reveals that these histiocytes are filled with bacilli. In some cases, however, especially when peripheral lymph nodes have been examined, non-necrotizing granulomas similar to those seen in sarcoidosis can be identified. In such cases, the PAS stain results may be negative or only focally positive, and bacilli may be rare or absent on ultrastructural examination.

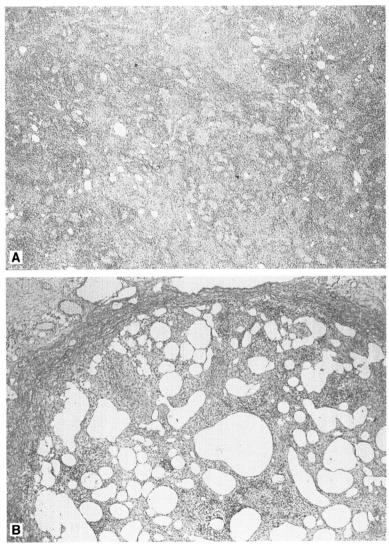

Figure 2–13. Whipple's disease. Affected lymph nodes show marked sinus histiocytosis with lipid vacuoles that range from small *(A)* to large *(B)* (H&E stain).

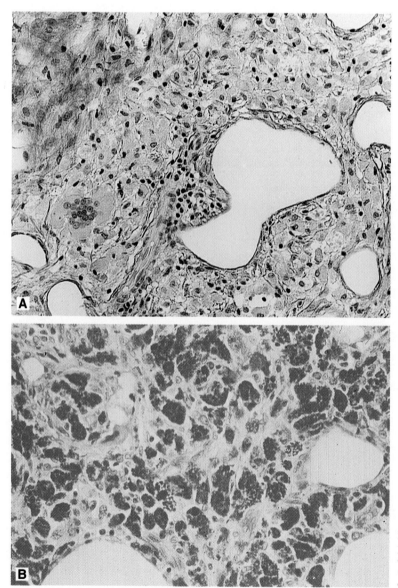

Figure 2–14. Whipple's disease. *A,* High power view shows pools of lipid, numerous histiocytes with finely vacuolated cytoplasm, and occasional multinucleated giant cells (H&E stain). *B,* Histiocytes are distended by PAS-positive material consisting of intact and degenerated bacteria.

Differential Diagnosis

Based on pathologic features, WD has a wide differential diagnosis. Clinical features are highly useful in narrowing the differential possibilities.

1. Lymphangiogram effect: When lymph nodes have a lipogranulomatous appearance, the differential diagnosis includes the effect of lymphangiogram; a PAS stain can exclude this possibility.
2. Sarcoidosis, Crohn's disease, and mycobacterial infections are included in the differential diagnosis when sarcoidal granulomas are found. Special stains for acid-fast bacilli and culture are useful for excluding a mycobacterial infection. Intestinal biopsies are helpful in establishing the diagnosis in cases of Crohn's disease. A PAS stain and electron microscopy may be helpful in differentiating between WD and sarcoidosis, but the findings in some lymph node biopsies in cases of WD are indistinguishable from those in sarcoidosis. If clinical features suggest the possibility of WD, obtaining additional tissue, especially from the small bowel, should be strongly considered.
3. *Mycobacterium avium-intracellulare* (MAI) infection and lepromatous leprosy (LL): When histiocytes with finely granular or vacuolated cytoplasm are prominent, MAI infection (see Fig. 6–17) and LL should be considered. Special stains for microorganisms establish the diagnosis.

References

Ereño C, Lopez JI, Elizalde JM, *et al*: A case of Whipple's disease presenting as supraclavicular lymphadenopathy. A case report. APMIS 101(11): 865–868, 1993.
Relman DA, Schmidt TM, McDermott RP, Falkow S: Identification of the uncultured bacillus of Whipple's disease. N Eng J Med 327:293–301, 1992.
Rodarte JR, Garrison CO, Holley KE, Fontana RS: Whipple's disease simulating sarcoidosis. A case with unique clinical and histologic features. Arch Int Med 129(3):479–482, 1972.
Saleh H, Williams TM, Minda JM, Gupta PK: Whipple's disease involving the mesenteric lymph nodes diagnosed by fine-needle aspiration. Diagn Cytopathol 8(2):177–180, 1992.
Southern JF, Moscicki RA, Magro C, *et al*: Lymphedema, lymphocytic myocarditis, and sarcoidlike granulomatosis. Manifestations of Whipple's disease. JAMA 261(10):1467–1470, 1989.

Fungal Lymphadenitis

Clinical Features

Patients presenting with fungal lymphadenitis are often immunosuppressed because of HIV infection, malignancy (most often, hematolymphoid neoplasia), or iatrogenic immunosuppression; occasionally, patients with normal immunologic function are affected. *Histoplasma capsulatum* and *Cryptococcus neoformans* are the most common fungi causing lymphadenitis. Symptomatic fungal lymphadenitis is uncommonly an isolated finding; patients often have pulmonary involvement or disseminated disease. Patients with normal immunologic function who develop fungal pulmonary infection may also have hilar lymph node involvement. Lymphadenitis in this setting may be asymptomatic; however, histoplasmosis involving mediastinal nodes may be associated with inflammation and severe scarring of the surrounding tissue, producing sclerosing mediastinitis.

Morphology

Infection is associated with granulomatous inflammation, which may be necrotizing. In immunodeficient individuals, granulomas may be poorly formed or absent. Fibrosis and even calcification may develop in old lesions, especially in cases of histoplasmosis.

Cryptococci have the form of yeast, 5 to 10 μm in diameter, and a thick gelatinous capsule that looks like a halo in tissue sections; narrow-based budding may be observed (Fig. 2–15). The capsules are mucicarmine positive. *Histoplasma* are smaller yeasts (2 to 5 μm) with thin but distinct cell walls.

Differential Diagnosis

Similar to that of *Mycobacterium tuberculosis* and atypical mycobacteria.

References

Neubauer MA, Bodensteiner DC: Disseminated histoplasmosis in patients with AIDS. South Med J 85:1166–1170, 1992.
Weinberg GA, Kleiman MB, Grosfeld JL, *et al*: Unusual manifestations of histoplasmosis in childhood. Pediatrics 72:99–105, 1983.
Witt D, McKay D, Schwam L, *et al*: Acquired immune deficiency syndrome presenting as bone marrow and mediastinal cryptococcosis. Am J Med 82:149–150, 1987.

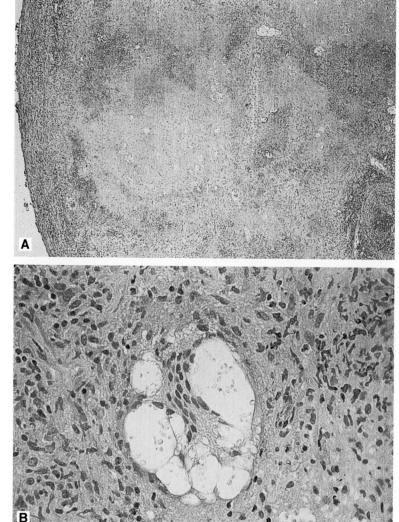

Figure 2–15. Cryptococcal lymphadenitis involving the cervical lymph node of a young woman with no known immunodeficiency. *A*, Large, irregular granulomas replace much of the node (H&E stain). *B*, A multinucleated giant cell engulfs pools of mucoid material containing fungal forms that are barely visible with H&E stain.

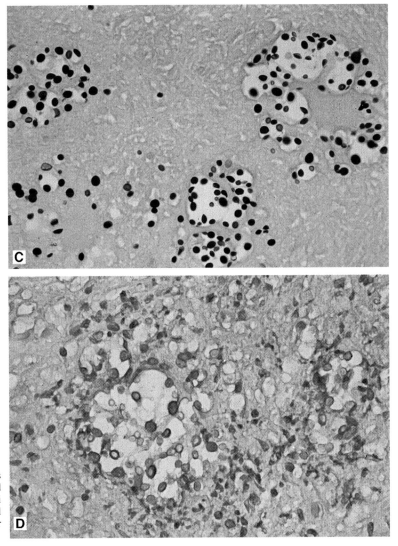

Figure 2–15. *Continued C,* With a silver stain, numerous fungal yeast forms are visible; a few display narrow-based budding (Grocott methenamine silver stain). *D,* The fungi are strongly positive with a mucicarmine stain. This unusual feature is helpful in differentiating cryptococci from other fungi.

Protozoal Lymphadenitis

TOXOPLASMOSIS

Synonym: Piringer-Kuchinka lymphadenitis.

Clinical Features

Although other types of protozoa occasionally cause lymphadenitis, *Toxoplasma gondii* is the only one encountered with any frequency. The most common clinical manifestation of *T. gondii* infection in immunocompetent patients is lymphadenopathy, most often cervical. Patients may be asymptomatic otherwise, or may have malaise, fever, or a sore throat. Atypical lymphocytosis may be seen. The disease is self-limited. Rarely, immunocompetent patients develop serious complications, such as myocarditis or encephalitis, which may be fatal. Immunodeficient patients may develop lymphadenopathy, but are at high risk for severe manifestations, especially encephalitis. Infection during pregnancy may be associated with fetal morbidity or mortality.

Morphology

Lymph nodes show florid follicular hyperplasia with prominent bands of sinusoidal and parasinusoidal monocytoid B cells. The paracortex contains many small, irregular clusters of histiocytes that encroach focally upon germinal centers (Figs. 1–9 and 2–16). The microorganisms are identified in lymph nodes only rarely (Fig. 2–16*E*), even when specimens are studied using the polymerase chain reaction. The diagnosis is normally confirmed using serologic studies.

Differential Diagnosis

Nearly all patients with lymphadenopathy with the foregoing histologic features will have serologic evidence of toxoplasma infection. Other possibilities are discussed next.

1. Leishmanial lymphadenitis: Leishmaniasis can produce lymphadenitis closely resembling that of toxoplasmosis. With *Leishmania* infection, however, microorganisms are usually identifiable in epithelioid histiocytes.
2. Other causes of granulomatous lymphadenitis: Early or partial nodal involvement by cat scratch disease, sarcoidosis, mycobacteria, or primary or secondary syphilis may resemble *Toxoplasma* lymphadenitis, except that in none of these disorders is there such a tendency for epithelioid histiocytes to encroach on lymphoid follicles. Significant areas of necrosis and true granuloma formation are unusual in toxoplasmosis and should lead one to consider other infections.

References

Montoya JG, Remington JS: Studies on the serodiagnosis of toxoplasmic lymphadenitis. Clin Inf Dis 20(4):781–789, 1995.
Weiss LM, Chen Y-Y, Berry GJ, *et al*: Infrequent detection of *Toxoplasma gondii* genome in toxoplasmic lymphadenitis: a polymerase chain reaction study. Hum Pathol 23:154–158, 1992.

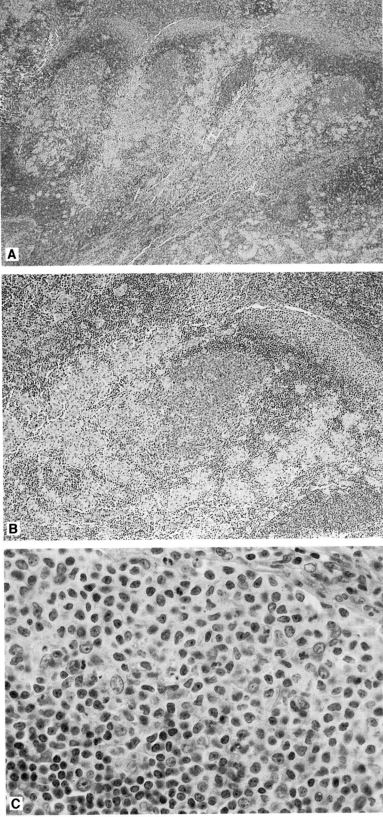

Figure 2–16. Toxoplasma lymphadenitis. *A*, Low power view shows multiple, large, reactive germinal centers, surrounded and focally invaded by clusters of epithelioid histiocytes. A subcapsular band of monocytoid B cells spans nearly the entire width of this figure *(top)* (H&E stain). *B*, At slightly higher power, the paracortex shows multiple small clusters of epithelioid histiocytes encroaching on a germinal center. A pale band of monocytoid B cells also appears over the top of the follicle (H&E stain). *C*, Monocytoid B cells have slightly more irregular nuclei and much more abundant pale cytoplasm than the small lymphocytes at the bottom of the illustration (H&E stain).

Illustration continued on following page.

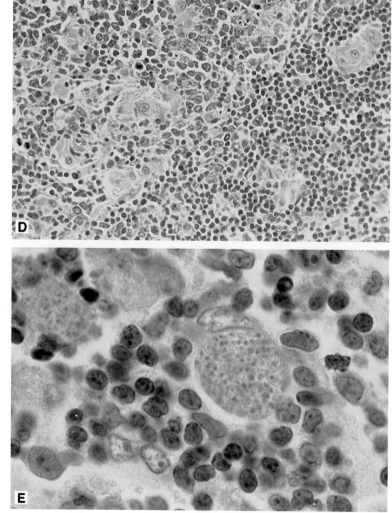

Figure 2–16. *Continued D*, Small clusters of epithelioid histiocytes are present within and adjacent to a reactive follicle (H&E stain). *E*, Encysted parasites, as shown here, are identified in lymph nodes only rarely (H&E stain).

Autoimmune Diseases

Lymphadenopathy is frequently found in association with a variety of autoimmune disorders, including rheumatoid arthritis, juvenile rheumatoid arthritis, systemic lupus erythematosus, primary biliary cirrhosis, mixed connective tissue disease, and others. Lymph node biopsies are not performed routinely in this setting; when they are performed, it is usually to exclude malignancy.

The clinicopathologic features of lymphadenopathy in selected autoimmune disorders are discussed next.

SYSTEMIC LUPUS ERYTHEMATOSUS (SLE)

Clinical Features

Systemic lupus erythematosus (SLE) predominantly affects adolescents and young adults, with a female preponderance. It is characterized by a broad spectrum of clinical manifestations, including arthritis or arthralgias, fever, rash, renal disease, anorexia, nausea and vomiting, serositis, and neurologic manifestations. Up to two thirds of patients have lymphadenopathy (lupus lymphadenitis), which, in decreasing order of frequency, affects cervical, mesenteric, axillary, inguinal, and other node groups. Generalized lymphadenopathy occurs in 12% of cases. Non-Hodgkin's lymphoma and Hodgkin's disease have been reported in patients with SLE, but no definitive increase in the incidence of either of these malignancies has been shown.

Morphology

Lymph nodes may be edematous with areas of hemorrhage. The nodal architecture may be distorted, but it is intact overall. Follicles are hyperplastic or inconspicuous. The paracortex contains foci of necrosis, with a central zone of amorphous eosinophilic debris. Early lesions may show little or no reaction to the necrosis. In established lesions, numerous histiocytes with variable numbers of admixed small and large lymphoid cells surround the necrosis. Granulocytes are sparse or absent. Plasma cells are usually infrequent. Hematoxylin bodies—ill-defined violet structures believed to represent degenerated nuclei that have reacted with antinuclear antibodies—are sometimes found in areas of necrosis, almost exclusively in SLE (Figs. 2–17 and 2–18). Blood vessels in the necrotic foci may show the Azzopardi phenomenon. Periarterial and periarteriolar fibrosis may be seen.

Immunophenotype

Little information is available. In one case, however, the zones of necrosis contained predominantly cells expressing histiocyte-associated antigens and CD3+, CD8+ T-cytotoxic suppressor cells. Outside the necrosis, paracortical cells were predominantly CD4+. Follicles expressed polytypic immunoglobulin.

Differential Diagnosis

1. Kikuchi's disease (see the later section).
2. Malignant lymphoma: Because of overlap in histologic features of lupus lymphadenitis and Kikuchi's disease, criteria similar to those used in the differential diagnosis of lymphoma and Kikuchi's disease can be used to distinguish lymphoma and lupus lymphadenitis (see the later discussion).
3. Infectious lymphadenitis: In cat scratch disease, lymphogranuloma venereum, and *Yersinia* infection, neutrophils are abundant. The character of the necrotic material in tuberculosis is similar to that in lupus lymphadenitis, but epithelioid histiocytes, Langhans-type giant cells and granulomas are not features of the latter.

References

Fox RA, Rosahn PD: The lymph nodes in disseminated lupus erythematosus. Am J Pathol 19:73–79, 1943.

Green JA, Dawson AA, Walker W: Systemic lupus erythematosus and lymphoma. Lancet 2:753–756, 1978.

Ko YH, Lee JD: Fine needle aspiration cytology in lupus lymphadenopathy. A case report. Acta Cytologica 36:748–751, 1992.

Lewis RB, Castor CW, Knisley RE, Bole GG: Frequency of neoplasia in systemic lupus erythematosus and rheumatoid arthritis. Arthr Rheum 19:1256–1260, 1976.

Medeiros LJ, Kaynor B, Harris NL: Lupus lymphadenitis: report of a case with immunohistologic studies on frozen sections. Hum Pathol 20:295–299, 1989.

Segal GH, Clough JD, Tubbs RR: Autoimmune and iatrogenic causes of lymphadenopathy. (Review.) Semin Oncol 20:611–626, 1993.

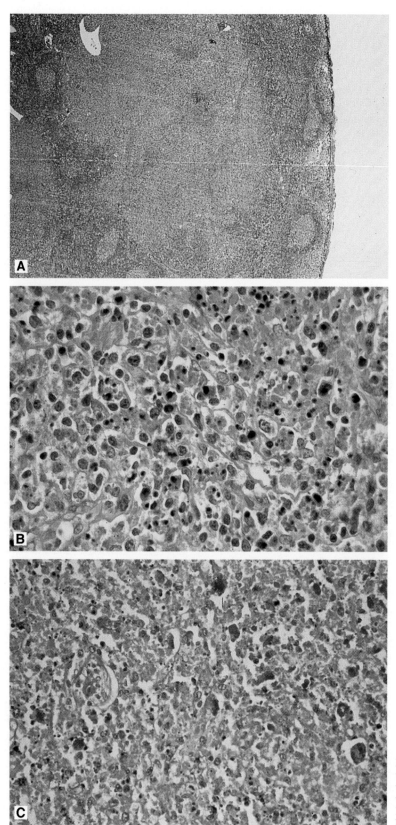

Figure 2–17. Lupus lymphadenitis. *A*, Multiple, small, reactive lymphoid follicles surround a large, pale, necrotic zone in the paracortex (H&E stain). *B*, At higher power, the paracortex shows fibrin, cellular debris, histiocytes, and small and large lymphoid cells (H&E stain). *C*, Multiple bright pink hematoxylin bodies are present (PAS stain).

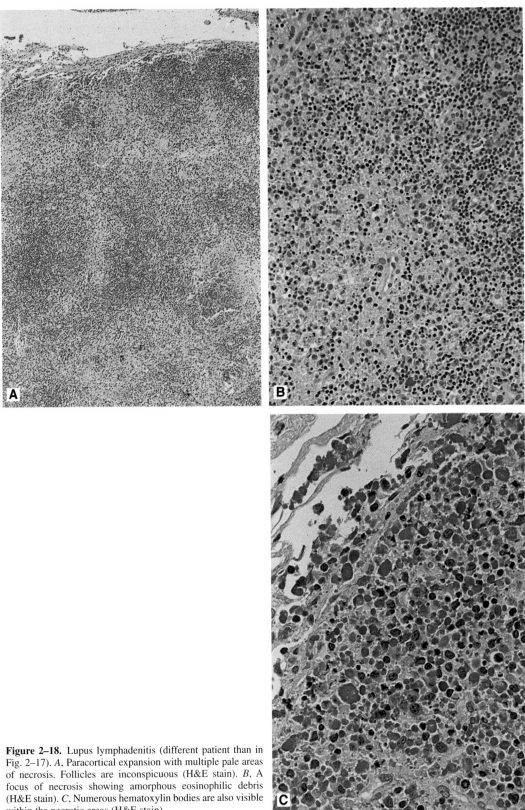

Figure 2–18. Lupus lymphadenitis (different patient than in Fig. 2–17). *A*, Paracortical expansion with multiple pale areas of necrosis. Follicles are inconspicuous (H&E stain). *B*, A focus of necrosis showing amorphous eosinophilic debris (H&E stain). *C*, Numerous hematoxylin bodies are also visible within the necrotic areas (H&E stain).

RHEUMATOID ARTHRITIS (RA)

Clinical Features

Rheumatoid arthritis (RA) is a chronic systemic illness characterized by destructive arthritis and a variety of extra-articular manifestations, including hematologic, cardiovascular, neurologic, and pulmonary abnormalities. Most patients present between the third and seventh decades of life, with a mean in the fourth decade; the M:F ratio is about 1:3. Approximately 75% of patients develop lymphadenopathy owing to reactive hyperplasia at some time during the course of the disease. The lymphadenopathy may be generalized or in the region of an inflamed joint.

Whether RA is associated with an increase in lymphoma, and whether the therapy for RA contributes to an increase in lymphoma, is a matter of debate. Isolated cases of lymphoma arising in RA patients treated with methotrexate have been reported, however, in which the tumors resolved after withdrawal of methotrexate.

Lymphadenopathy is frequent in juvenile RA and occurs in most cases of Still's disease (acute febrile form of juvenile RA). Most cases of Still's disease occur in children, but this disorder also affects adults and is characterized by rheumatoid factor–negative arthritis or arthralgia, fever, sore throat, weight loss, pleuritis, abdominal pain, rash, and abnormal liver function test results.

Morphology and Immunophenotype

Reactive hyperplasia in RA typically shows prominent follicular hyperplasia with sinus histiocytosis. The follicles are present in the cortex and frequently extend into the medulla. Infiltration of the capsule and perinodal fat by lymphocytes is common. Plasmacytosis of the interfollicular region and medulla is common; Russell bodies may be found (Figs. 1–13 and 2–19). Lymph nodes in RA may show sinus neutrophils and stainable iron. In the paracortex, CD4+ T cells predominate, but CD8+ T cells have been found in reactive follicles, an unusual feature.

Hyaline material that stains positive for PAS and negative for Congo red may partially or completely replace lymph nodes; it has been suggested that this is due to long-standing nonspecific inflammation (Fig. 2–19C). Some RA patients develop amyloidosis. In such cases, amyloid may be deposited in lymph nodes. Lymphadenopathy associated with gold therapy has been described; in such cases, gold is present in the form of crystalline material and is associated with a multinucleated giant cell reaction. Patients with Silastic joint prostheses may develop silicone lymphadenopathy.

Patients with lymphadenopathy associated with juvenile RA may have reactive hyperplasia similar to that with RA. Florid immunoblastic proliferation has been described in association with Still's disease. Various types of lymphomas are found in patients with RA with no one type predominating. Most are B-lineage tumors, but a few are T-lineage, including cases of T-large granular lymphocyte leukemia. More than 25% of patients with T-large granular lymphocyte leukemia have RA, however, suggesting that an association exists between these two disorders (see Large Granular Lymphocyte Leukemia, Chapter 4). A few cases with Epstein-Barr virus latent membrane protein (EBV-LMP) expression and Epstein-Barr–encoded RNA-1 (EBER-1) have been reported, leading some investigators to speculate that immunodeficiency plays a role in the development of some cases of lymphoma. EBV+ cases of lymphoma have been heterogeneous, however, including B and T cell lymphomas and Hodgkin's disease.

A question has been raised regarding the involvement of methotrexate in the pathogenesis of some RA-associated lymphomas. Some investigators suggest that the incidence of hematolymphoid neoplasms is not significantly different among patients who do or do not receive methotrexate. Another group found that lymphomas in methotrexate-treated patients tended to have features associated with immunosuppression, including extranodal location, large cell or polymorphous cellular composition, prominent necrosis, and the presence of EBV.

Differential Diagnosis

1. Follicle center lymphoma (FCL): The extensive follicular proliferation characteristic of RA lymph nodes may raise the possibility of FCL. Criteria conventionally used to distinguish FCL and follicular hyperplasia can be used in such instances (see Follicle Center Lymphoma, Chapter 3).
2. Castleman's disease (CD): See the discussion of Castleman's disease later in this chapter.
3. Other causes of follicular hyperplasia: Clinical correlation is required to confirm a diagnosis of lymphadenopathy due to RA. Other causes of lymphadenopathy that may mimic changes seen in RA include syphilis, human immunodeficiency virus infection, and nonspecific follicular hyperplasia.
4. Syphilis: In primary and secondary syphilis, lymph nodes show marked follicular hyperplasia with numerous plasma cells. Unlike nodes in RA, however, they may contain non-necrotizing or suppurative granulomas and show marked capsular and perinodal fibrosis and prominent vascular changes (endarteritis and phlebitis). Spirochetes can be found in blood vessels, germinal centers, and granulomas. The changes characteristic of syphilis are best seen in inguinal nodes. Although secondary syphilis may be associated with diffuse lymphadenopathy, nodes away from the inguinal region may show only nonspecific follicular hyperplasia.

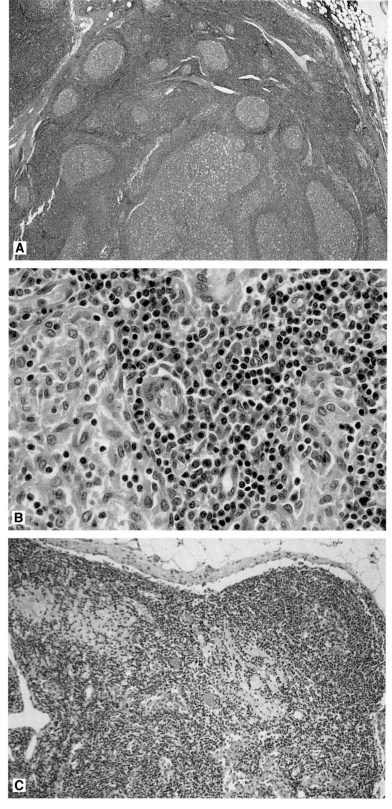

Figure 2–19. Rheumatoid arthritis. *A,* The lymph node shows florid follicular hyperplasia, with multiple lymphoid follicles of variable size and shape that extend close to the hilus (H&E stain). *B,* Plasma cells are abundant in medullary cords *(center);* sinus histiocytes *(right and left)* contain hemo-siderin (H&E stain). *C,* Deposition of hyaline material; the appearance is similar to that commonly found in pelvic lymph nodes, but this lymph node is from the axilla (H&E stain).

References

Banks PM, Witrak GA, Conn DL: Lymphoid neoplasia following connective tissue disease. Mayo Clin Proc 54:104–108, 1979.

Frizzera G: Immunosuppression, autoimmunity and lymphoproliferative disorders. (Editorial.) Hum Pathol 25:627–629, 1994.

Hartsock RJ, Halling LW, King FM: Luetic lymphadenitis: a clinical and histologic study of 20 cases. Am J Clin Pathol 53:304–314, 1970.

Kamel OW, van de Rijn M, LeBrun DP, et al: Lymphoid neoplasms in patients with rheumatoid arthritis and dermatomyositis: frequency of Epstein-Barr virus and other features associated with immunosuppression. (See comments.) Hum Pathol 25(7):638–643, 1994.

Katusic S, Beard CM, Kurland LT, et al: Occurrence of malignant neoplasms in the Rochester, Minnesota, rheumatoid arthritis cohort. Am J Med 78(1A):50–55, 1985.

Kondratowicz GM, Symmons DP, Bacon PA, et al: Rheumatoid lymphadenopathy: a morphological and immunohistochemical study. (See comments.) J Clin Pathol 43:106–113, 1990.

McCluggage WG, Bharucha H: Lymph node hyalinisation in rheumatoid arthritis and systemic sclerosis. J Clin Pathol 47:138–142, 1994.

Moder KG, Tefferi A, Cohen MD, et al: Hematologic malignancies and the use of methotrexate in rheumatoid arthritis: a retrospective study. (Review.) Am J Med 99:276–281, 1995.

Nosanchuk JS, Schnitzer B: Follicular hyperplasia in lymph nodes from patients with rheumatoid arthritis. A clinicopathologic study. Cancer 24:343–354, 1969.

Prior P: Cancer and rheumatoid arthritis: epidemiologic considerations. Am J Med 78(1A):15–21, 1985.

Reichert LJ, Keuning JJ, van Beek M, van Rijthoven AW: Lymph node histology simulating T-cell lymphoma in adult-onset Still's disease. Ann Hematol 65:53–54, 1992.

Rollins SD, Craig JP: Gold-associated lymphadenopathy in a patient with rheumatoid arthritis. Histologic and scanning electron microscopic features. (See comments.) Arch Pathol Lab Med 115:175–177, 1991.

Schlesinger BE, Forsyth CC, White RHR, et al: Observations on the clinical course and treatment of one hundred cases of Still's disease. Arch Dis Child 36:65–76, 1961.

Segal GH, Clough JD, Tubbs RR: Autoimmune and iatrogenic causes of lymphadenopathy. (Review.) Semin Oncol 20(6):611–626, 1993.

Turner DR, Wright DJM: Lymphadenopathy in early syphilis. J Pathol 110:305–308, 1973.

Histiocytic Lesions: Idiopathic, Metabolic, and Iatrogenic

SARCOIDOSIS

Clinical Features

Sarcoidosis is an uncommon disorder of unknown etiology; blacks are affected more often than whites, and women are affected more often than men. Involvement of a wide variety of tissues may occur, but lymph nodes and lung are the most commonly affected. Mediastinal and pulmonary hilar nodes are involved most frequently, but any lymph node may show changes of sarcoidosis. The clinical course is highly variable; some patients are asymptomatic and some develop significant complications, the most common of which is progressive pulmonary fibrosis.

Morphology

Lymph nodes show multiple well-formed granulomas composed of epithelioid histiocytes and multinucleated giant cells, with a few intermixed small lymphocytes and a narrow cuff of small lymphocytes (Fig. 2–20). The granulomas are often confluent, replacing nearly the entire node; when the node is partially involved, the granulomas usually occur in the paracortex. A small amount of fibrin and cellular debris may be seen in the centers of some granulomas, but necrosis is not prominent and caseation is absent. Over time, the granulomas may become hyalinized.

Immunophenotype

Most lymphocytes in and around the granulomas are T cells (mainly CD45RO+ memory T cells). A predominance of T-helper (CD4+) or T-cytotoxic/suppressor (CD8+) cells has been reported in different cases by different investigators, possibly indicating different stages of disease or dissimilarities in the underlying immunologic function of the affected patients.

Differential Diagnosis

Sarcoidosis is a diagnosis of exclusion; its differential diagnosis is broad and includes tuberculosis, fungal infection, tuberculoid leprosy, brucellosis, Whipple's disease, syphilis, and reaction to foreign material. Rarely, Hodgkin's disease or non-Hodgkin's lymphoma is associated with a granulomatous reaction mimicking sarcoidosis (Fig. 2–21). Examination of the intergranulomatous area in these cases reveals Reed-Sternberg cells or atypical lymphoid cells. Patients with Hodgkin's disease may have sarcoidal granulomas in multiple tissues, including liver, spleen, and lymph nodes, without these tissues being involved with Hodgkin's disease (Fig. 2–22). Sarcoidal granulomas may be found in lymph nodes draining tissues involved by carcinoma.

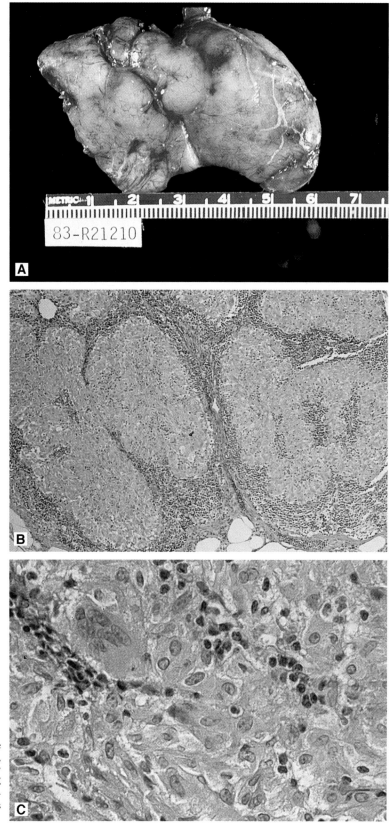

Figure 2–20. Sarcoidosis. *A*, Cross section of a lymph node shows multiple, pale, focally confluent granulomas. *B*, Microscopic examination reveals a lymph node nearly replaced by large, oval, non-necrotizing granulomas (H&E stain). *C*, High power view shows a predominance of epithelioid histiocytes and occasional multinucleated giant cells (H&E stain).

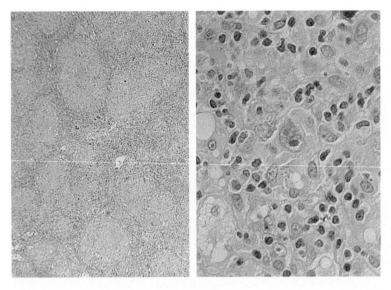

Figure 2–21. Hodgkin's disease mimicking sarcoidosis. Low power view shows numerous non-necrotizing granulomas *(left)*. On high power examination, occasional Reed-Sternberg cells appear intermingled with the histiocytes *(right)* (H&E stain).

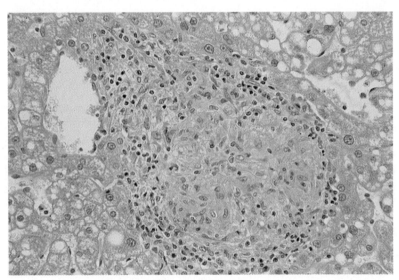

Figure 2–22. Sarcoidal granuloma in the liver of a patient with Hodgkin's disease. The liver was free of Hodgkin's disease (H&E stain).

References

Lenzini L, Tosi P: Histopathological lymph node findings, immunological behavior and radiological thoracic pattern in sarcoidosis. A study of 20 cases. Pathologia Europaea 8:163–171, 1973.

Roncalli M, Servida E: Granulomatous and nongranulomatous lym-phadenitis in sarcoidosis. An immunophenotypic study of seven cases. Pathol Res Prac 185:351–357, 1989.

van den Oord JJ, de Wolf-Peeters C, Facchetti F, Desmet VJ: Cellular composition of hypersensitivity-type granulomas: immunohistochemical analysis of tuberculous and sarcoidal lymphadenitis. Hum Pathol 15:559–565, 1984.

KIKUCHI'S DISEASE (KD)

Synonyms: Histiocytic necrotizing lymphadenitis; Kikuchi's lymphadenitis; Kikuchi-Fujimoto's disease; subacute necrotizing lymphadenitis.

Clinical Features

Kikuchi's disease (KD) appears to be more prevalent among Asian than Western populations. Most patients are young adults, with a preponderance of females. Nearly all patients present with cervical lymphadenopathy, which is usually unilateral and often painful; other nodes are affected occasionally. Infrequently, lymphadenopathy may be generalized. A third to one half of patients have fever at presentation. In addition, 50% have leukopenia; less than 5% have leukocytosis; 25% or more have an atypical lymphocytosis. Occasional patients have a rash. The disease is self-limited and most patients recover without therapy; fewer than 5% develop recurrent lymphadenopathy. A viral cause is suspected but has not been proven.

Morphology

Affected lymph nodes have the following characteristics: prominent paracortical hyperplasia, occasionally with follicular hyperplasia, and one or more variably sized, rounded, irregular or serpiginous, discrete or confluent, eosinophilic areas in the cortex or paracortex which contain histiocytes, lymphocytes, immunoblasts, plasmacytoid monocytes, and karyorrhectic and eosinophilic granular debris. There is a mixture of phagocytic, nonphagocytic, and foamy histiocytes. Phagocytic histiocytes with eccentric sickle-shaped nuclei have been called "crescentic histiocytes"; nonphagocytic histiocytes with eccentric nuclei are called "signet ring histiocytes." Epithelioid histiocytes, plasma cells, and eosinophils appear infrequently, and neutrophils are rare or absent. The infiltrate may extend beyond the capsule into perinodal soft tissue (Figs. 2–23 and 2–24).

KD can be divided into three histologic subtypes, which may represent different stages of the disease: (1) in the proliferative type, the mixture of cells described previously occurs, with karyorrhectic and apoptotic debris, but without coagulative necrosis; (2) in the necrotizing type, coagulative necrosis occurs; and (3) in the xanthomatous type, foamy histiocytes predominate.

Immunophenotype

The histiocytes are lysozyme+, CD68+, and Ki-M1P+. A variable number of T lymphocytes (CD3+, CD43+, CD45RO+) are admixed with the histiocytes, and most are CD8+ (T cytotoxic-suppressor). B cells are virtually absent in the affected areas of the node. The plasmacytoid monocytes are Ki-M1P+, CD68+, and CD4+.

Genetic Features

DNA ploidy studies show a diploid pattern.

Differential Diagnosis

1. Non-Hodgkin's lymphoma (NHL): When immunoblasts are abundant, NHL enters the differential diagnosis. Familiarity with the spectrum of changes found in KD and identification of areas with the polymorphous infiltrate characteristic of KD are essential to rendering the correct diagnosis. KD shows partial nodal involvement more often than NHL. Finding B-lineage antigens on the large lymphoid cells is evidence against KD. Monotypic Ig expression or clonal rearrangement of Ig or T-cell receptor genes excludes KD.
2. Lupus lymphadenitis: Lymphadenitis in patients with systemic lupus erythematosus (SLE) may closely resemble Kikuchi's disease. Finding hematoxylin bodies, neutrophils, plasma cells, or deposition of nuclear material on blood vessels (Azzopardi phenomenon) supports a diagnosis of lupus lymphadenitis over Kikuchi's disease, but these features might not be found in every case of lupus lymphadenitis. Clinical features are sometimes helpful in making a definitive distinction.
3. Metastatic carcinoma: Viewed as isolated cells, some of the histiocytes could mimic signet-ring cell carcinoma; they usually contain cellular debris rather than mucin, however, and express histiocyte-related antigens rather than keratins.

References

Hansmann ML, Kikuchi M, Wacker HH, *et al*: Immunohistochemical monitoring of plasmacytoid cells in lymph node sections of Kikuchi-Fujimoto disease by a new pan-macrophage antibody Ki-M1P. Hum Pathol 23:676–680, 1992.

Kikuchi M, Takeshita M, Eimoto T, *et al*: Histiocytic necrotizing lymphadenitis: clinicopathologic, immunologic, and HLA typing study. *In*: Hanaoka M, Kadin ME, Mikata A, eds. Lymphoid Malignancy: Immunocytology and Cytogenetics. New York: Fields and Wood, 1990; pp 251–257.

Kuo T: Kikuchi's disease (histiocytic necrotizing lymphadenitis). A clinicopathologic study of 79 cases with an analysis of histologic subtypes, immunohistology and DNA ploidy. Am J Surg Pathol 19:798–809, 1995.

Nathwani BN: Kikuchi-Fujimoto disease. Am J Surg Pathol 15:196–197, 1991.

Sumiyoshi Y, Kikuchi M, Takeshita M, *et al*: Immunohistologic studies of Kikuchi's disease. Hum Pathol 24:1114–1119, 1993.

Tsang WYW, Chan JKC, Ng CS: Kikuchi's lymphadenitis. A morphologic analysis of 75 cases with special reference to unusual features. Am J Surg Pathol 18:219–231, 1994.

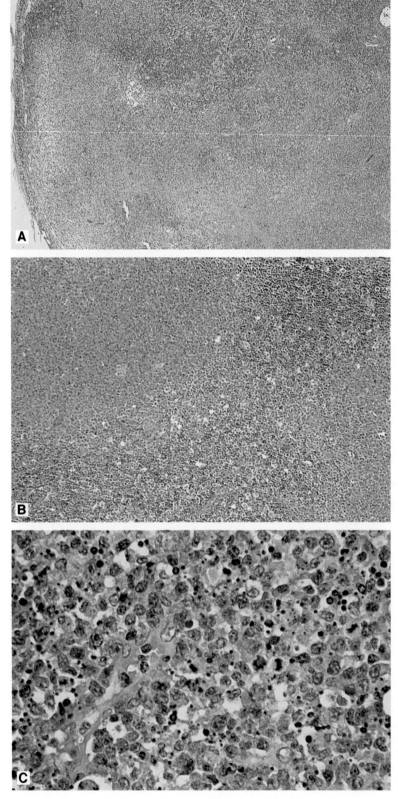

Figure 2–23. Kikuchi's disease. *A*, Large, geographic eosinophilic zones of histiocytes and necrotic debris replace much of the lymph node (H&E stain). *B*, A band of mottled, hyperplastic paracortex separates two necrotic areas (H&E stain). *C*, Numerous large lymphoid cells surround necrotic foci. Mitotic figures are frequent. Scattered histiocytes and abundant apoptotic debris are present, but neutrophils are absent (H&E stain).

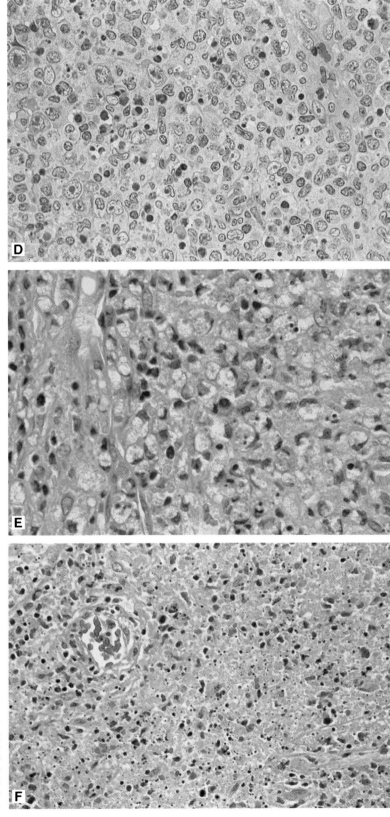

Figure 2–23. *Continued D,* At the periphery of the eosino-philic zone, numerous histiocytes, some with crescent-shaped nuclei, are present, with admixed plasmacytoid monocytes, a few immunoblasts, and apoptotic debris (H&E stain). *E,* signet ring histiocytes form a prominent part of the histiocytic infiltrate (H&E stain). *F,* In the centers of the eosinophilic zones, amorphous pink material and apoptotic debris are present, but there are few intact cells (H&E stain).

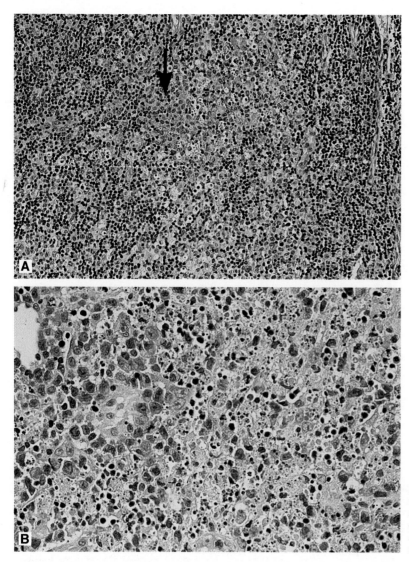

Figure 2–24. Kikuchi's disease. *A,* Low power view shows marked paracortical hyperplasia. The small, irregular aggregate of pale cells in the center are plasmacytoid monocytes *(arrow)* (H&E stain). *B,* Immunoblasts are abundant at the periphery of the necrotic zone in this case (H&E stain).

SINUS HISTIOCYTOSIS WITH MASSIVE LYMPHADENOPATHY (SHML)

Synonym: Rosai-Dorfman disease.

Clinical Features

Sinus histiocytosis with massive lymphadenopathy (SHML) is a disorder of uncertain etiology that mainly affects children and young adults. The classic presentation is massive, painless, bilateral, cervical lymphadenopathy, although other node groups may occasionally be involved, and infrequently generalized lymphadenopathy occurs. In about one third of cases, extranodal sites such as skin, upper respiratory tract, bone, or central nervous system are involved. Patients commonly have fever, leukocytosis, anemia, elevated erythrocyte sedimentation rate, and polyclonal hypergammaglobulinemia. In about 10% of cases, patients have associated immunologic abnormalities, including suscepti-

bility to infection, autoantibody-induced cytopenias, glomerulonephritis, and arthritis.

The clinical course is usually benign, although lymphadenopathy may persist for years. The prognosis is not as good in patients with immunologic dysfunction or multiple sites of involvement. Fourteen deaths in patients with SHML (6.5% of cases in the SHML Registry) have been reported, although in only two cases was death directly attributable to SHML. Most deaths were caused by infection or complications of immunologically mediated diseases.

Morphology

Gross examination shows one or more enlarged lymph nodes, which may be matted together. Sectioning reveals bright yellow tissue. On microscopic examination, cortical and medullary sinuses are greatly dilated by large histiocytes having round to oval vesicular nuclei and often small nucleoli, with abundant, pale, vacuolated cytoplasm and irregular, ill-defined cell borders. The histiocytes contain lymphocytes that appear intact and less often, plasma cells, neutrophils, and erythrocytes, a phenomenon called emperipolesis ("wandering about within"). The intervening lymphoid tissue shows nonspecific changes; medullary cords contain lymphocytes and plasma cells. Eosinophils are virtually absent. The capsule and perinodal soft tissue are often fibrotic, and areas of fibrosis may appear within the node (Fig. 2–25).

SHML may be more difficult to recognize in extranodal sites because the characteristic sinus architecture is not present, and because emperipolesis tends to be less conspicuous. The histiocytes have the same distinctive appearance, however, and emperipolesis is usually identifiable.

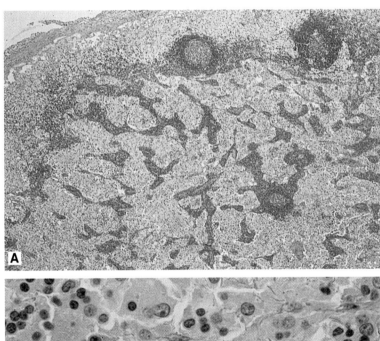

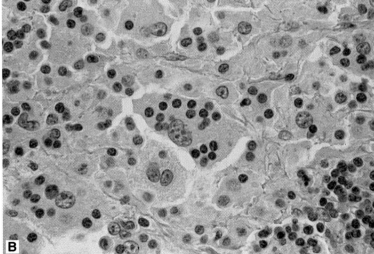

Figure 2–25. Sinus histiocytosis with massive lymphadenopathy. *A,* Sinuses are filled and distended by histiocytes; only a few germinal centers remain, and the paracortex has been compressed into narrow cords (H&E stain). *B,* The histiocytes have abundant, finely granular cytoplasm containing intact-appearing lymphocytes (emperipolesis). The histiocytic nuclei are medium to large and pale; some have distinct red nucleoli (H&E stain).

Immunophenotype

The distinctive histiocytes are positive for S-100, α-1-antitrypsin, α-1-antichymotrypsin, CD11b, CD11c, CD14, CD33, CD68, and activation antigens (CD30, transferrin receptor, interleukin 2 receptor).

Differential Diagnosis

1. Langerhans' cell histiocytosis (histiocytosis X, eosinophilic granuloma): Langerhans' cells have less abundant cytoplasm, more complex nuclear contours, and more distinct cell borders. Emperipolesis is not a feature. Eosinophils may be numerous. Birbeck granules, which are absent in SHML, can be identified using electron microscopy.
2. Nonspecific reactive hyperplasia with sinus histiocytosis: Lymph nodes are not as large, enlargement is not as persistent, and sinuses are not as distended as in SHML. A few sinus histiocytes may show phagocytosis, but emperipolesis is not a feature. Most sinus histiocytes are negative for S-100.
3. Storage disorders: Histiocytes in SHML show emperipolesis and do not contain large amounts of mucopolysaccharides or lipids. Clinical features may be helpful.

References

Foucar E, Rosai J, Dorfman RF: Sinus histiocytosis with massive lymphadenopathy. An analysis of 14 deaths occurring in a patient registry. Cancer 54:1834–1840, 1984.

Montgomery EA, Meis JM, Frizzera G: Rosai-Dorfman disease of soft tissue. Am J Surg Pathol 16:122–129, 1992.

Paulli M, Rosso R, Kindl S, *et al*: Immunophenotypic characterization of the cell infiltrate in five cases of sinus histiocytosis with massive lymphadenopathy (Rosai-Dorfman disease). Hum Pathol 23:647–654, 1992.

Rosai J: Sinus histiocytosis with massive lymphadenopathy. Am J Surg Pathol 15(2):191–192, 1991.

Rosai J, Dorfman RF: Sinus histiocytosis with massive lymphadenopathy. A newly recognized benign clinicopathological entity. Arch Path 87:63–70, 1969.

Sacchi S, Artusi T, Torelli U, Emilia G: Sinus histiocytosis with massive lymphadenopathy. (Review.) Leuk Lymphoma 7:189–194, 1992.

MISCELLANEOUS LYMPHADENOPATHIES WITH HISTIOCYTIC INFILTRATION

Hereditary storage diseases, such as Niemann-Pick disease and Gaucher's disease, may be associated with nodal infiltration by histiocytes distended with storage products. The appearance of the histiocytes is similar to their appearance in other tissues.

Lymphangiograms, most commonly performed for the staging of Hodgkin's disease, produce lipogranulomas, with sinusoidal distension by foamy histiocytes, multinucleated giant cells, and large and small vacuoles of contrast material. Eosinophils may be found in the medullary cords.

Lymphangiograms affect nodes along the iliac arteries and the aorta, but not nodes in the portal circulation. Lipogranulomas commonly exist in lymph nodes related to the portal circulation in the absence of a history of lymphangiogram and probably result from deposition of lipids related to the diet and to bile metabolites (Fig. 2–26).

Hyperlipidemia is a rare cause of lymphadenopathy. Severe hyperlipidemia has been associated with droplets of lipid in nodal sinuses and large numbers of lipid-laden macrophages.

Prosthetic joint replacements tend to deteriorate over time; occasionally, this process is associated with a reaction to foreign material in regional lymph nodes. The histiocytic reaction may be confined to distended sinuses or may extend to involve the paracortex. Prosthetic devices containing metal, polyethylene, and cement (polymethylmethacrylate) are associated with sheets of histiocytes with granular eosinophilic cytoplasm; metal and refractile foreign material are visible (Figs. 2–27 and 2–28). Reaction to Silastic joint prostheses (silicone lymphadenopathy) consists of granulomas with multinucleated giant cells containing pale yellow, refractile particles of silicone.

Mammary prostheses (bag-gel prostheses or silicone injection) may also result in adenopathy. Silicone lymphadenopathy in this setting tends to show diffuse infiltrates of histiocytes with marked cytoplasmic vacuolization and extracellular deposits of pale foreign material forming prominent cystic spaces.

Prostatic carcinoma treated with androgen ablative therapy is reported to be associated with a xanthomatous reaction in lymph nodes harboring metastatic carcinoma.

References

Albores-Saavedra J, Vuitch F, Delgado R, *et al*: Sinus histiocytosis of pelvic lymph nodes after hip replacement. A histiocytic proliferation induced by cobalt-chromium and titanium. Am J Surg Pathol 18:83–90, 1994.

Debuch H, Wiedemann HR: Lymph node excision as a simple diagnostic aid in rare lipidoses. Eur J Pediatr 129:99–101, 1978.

Dorfman RF, Warnke RA: Lymphadenopathy simulating the malignant lymphomas. Hum Pathol 5:519–550, 1974.

Elleder M, Jirasek A, Smid F, *et al*: An unusual case of phospholipidosis. Virch Arch A, Pathol Anat Histol 377:329–338, 1978.

Leaf DA, Illingworth DR, Connor WE: Lymphadenopathy associated with severe hypertriglyceridemia. (*See* comments.) JAMA 264:727–728, 1990.

O'Connell JX, Rosenberg AE: Histiocytic lymphadenitis associated with a large joint prosthesis. Am J Clin Pathol 99:314–316, 1993.

Rivero MA, Schwartz DS, Mies C: Silicone lymphadenopathy involving intramammary lymph nodes: a new complication of silicone mammaplasty. Am J Roentgen 162:1089–1090, 1994.

Rogers LA, Longtine JA, Garnick MB, Pinkus GS: Silicone lymphadenopathy in a long distance runner: complication of a silastic prosthesis. Hum Pathol 19:1237–1239, 1988.

Schned AR, Gormley EA: Florid xanthomatous pelvic lymph node reaction to metastatic prostatic adenocarcinoma. A sequela of preoperative androgen deprivation therapy. Arch Pathol Lab Med 120:96–100, 1996.

Segal GH, Clough JD, Tubbs RR: Autoimmune and iatrogenic causes of lymphadenopathy. (Review.) Semin Oncol 20:611–626, 1993.

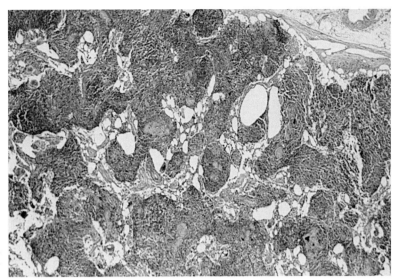

Figure 2–26. Lymphangiogram effect. This lymph node, obtained during staging laparotomy for Hodgkin's disease, shows sinus histiocytosis with lipogranulomas (H&E stain).

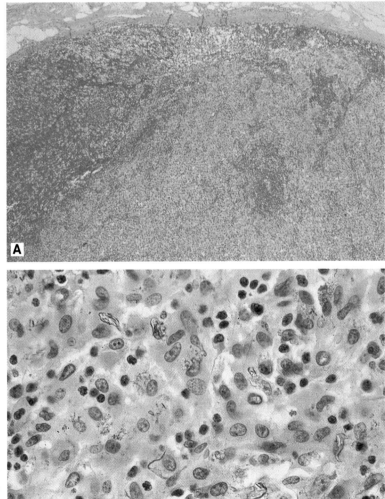

Figure 2–27. Histiocytic reaction to Teflon from a prosthetic device. *A*, Low power view shows sheets of histiocytes in a preauricular lymph node from a patient who had a temporomandibular joint prosthesis (H&E stain). *B*, Higher power examination shows histiocytes containing irregular fragments of a yellow-green refractile material that is consistent with Teflon (H&E stain).

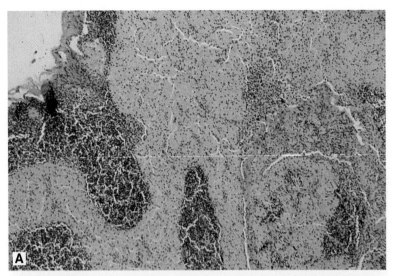

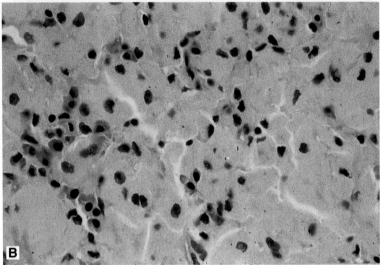

Figure 2–28. Histiocytic reaction to metal from a prosthetic device. *A,* Sheets of histiocytes fill and expand the sinuses, compressing normal lymphoid tissue. The low power appearance is reminiscent of sinus histiocytosis with massive lymphadenopathy (*compare with* Fig. 2–25) (H&E stain). *B,* High power view shows histiocytes with abundant, granular, eosinophilic cytoplasm containing tiny black shards of metal (H&E stain).

Miscellaneous

CASTLEMAN'S DISEASE (CD)

Synonyms: Giant lymph node hyperplasia; angiofollicular lymphoid hyperplasia.

Classification: Subtypes of Castleman's disease (CD), based on morphology, are the hyaline-vascular and plasma cell variants. The former comprises 80 to 90% of cases; the latter comprises about 10 to 20% of cases. Cases with features intermediate between the two types ("transitional" or "mixed" type) may be seen occasionally.

Hyaline-Vascular Variant (HVCD)

Clinical Features

Hyaline-vascular variant (HVCD) affects patients of any age, but most are young adults. Females may be affected slightly more often than males. Patients present with lymphadenopathy in a single site in nearly all cases; in the remainder, the lesion involves an extranodal site. Rarely, more than one site is involved. The mediastinum is affected most often (Fig. 2–29*A*), followed by nodes in the neck, the

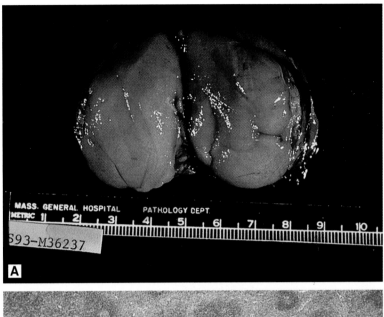

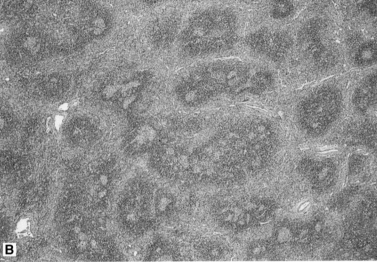

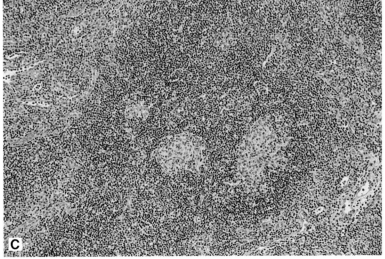

Figure 2–29. Castleman's disease, hyaline-vascular type. *A,* Mediastinal mass from a young woman. The lesion is a well-circumscribed, deep tan-orange mass. *B,* Low power view shows a proliferation of lymphoid follicles of different sizes and shapes throughout the node. The follicles consist mainly of mantle zone lymphocytes with variable numbers of small germinal centers within each mantle (H&E stain). *C,* One follicle shows a predominant population of small mantle zone lymphocytes and several small irregular germinal centers (H&E stain).

Illustration continued on following page.

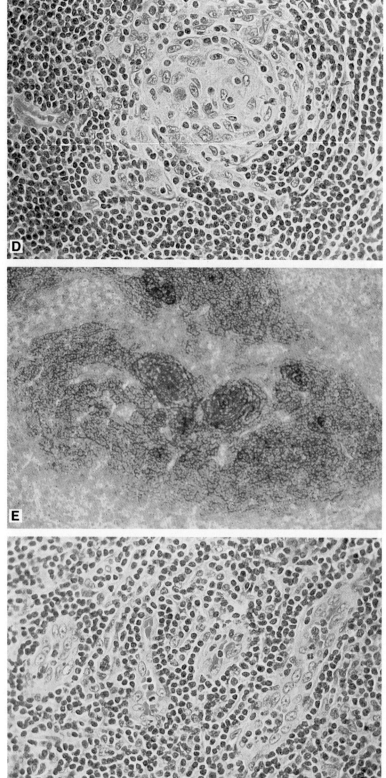

Figure 2–29. *Continued D,* A single germinal center is pierced by a small blood vessel. The germinal center is depleted of lymphoid cells, with a predominance of follicular dendritic cells. The surrounding mantle zone cells line up in an orderly array, best seen on the right (H&E stain). *E,* With antibody to CD21, which stains follicular dendritic cells, dendritic staining is demonstrated throughout this follicle. The staining is more coarse in the several small germinal centers than in the mantle zone (immunoperoxidase technique on frozen sections). *F,* The interfollicular area shows a predominance of small lymphocytes and high endothelial venules (H&E stain).

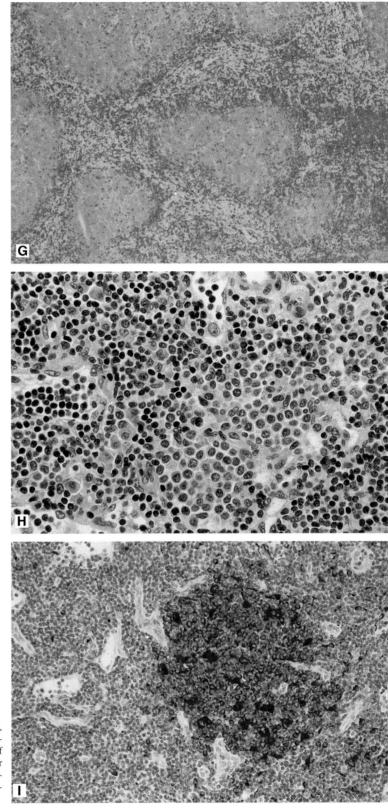

Figure 2–29. *Continued G,* T cells, with antibody to CD3, show a positive reaction in the interfollicular area (immunoperoxidase technique on frozen sections). *H,* An aggregate of plasmacytoid monocytes is also visible in the interfollicular area (H&E stain). *I,* The plasmacytoid monocytes are highlighted with an anti-CD68 antibody (immunoperoxidase technique on paraffin section).

abdomen, and other sites. Systemic symptoms are usually absent. HVCD almost never recurs after excision. The etiology is uncertain, but it may be related to a developmental abnormality of the follicles, possibly caused by abnormal or dysplastic follicular dendritic cells.

Morphology

HVCD is characterized by lymphoid follicles with small, hyalinized germinal centers and broad mantle zones. Each follicle may contain one or more germinal centers; some follicles contain no recognizable germinal centers. The germinal centers contain an increased proportion of follicular dendritic cells (FDCs) and endothelial cells and relatively few B cells. Mantle zone lymphocytes are arranged in concentric rings ("onion skin" pattern) around the germinal center. Large, bizarre, dystrophic cells with scant cytoplasm, thought to be abnormal FDCs, may be found in the follicles. Follicles are often radially penetrated by a blood vessel ("lollipop follicle"). The interfollicular region shows increased numbers of high endothelial venules and of small vessels with flat endothelium and hyalinized walls and sometimes clusters of plasmacytoid monocytes. Plasma cells may be present singly or in small clusters, but sheets of plasma cells are absent. Epithelioid histiocytes, granulomas, eosinophils, and immunoblasts are inconspicuous or absent. In some cases, patent sinuses may appear in residual normal lymphoid tissue at the periphery of the lesion, but in general they are absent. Fibrosis is common peripherally and also in bands running through the lesion (Fig. 2–29).

Immunophenotype

Follicles contain B cells expressing polytypic immunoglobulin and FDCs (CD21+) (Fig. 2–29*E*). T cells (CD3+, CD45RO+) are present in smaller than normal numbers in follicles and interfollicular area (Fig. 2–29*G*). Many interfollicular blood vessels are Factor 8+, CD34+, HECA-452+, and MECA-79+, which are consistent with high endothelial venules. The interfollicular area also contains CD68+ plasmacytoid monocytes (Fig. 2–29*H* and *I*) and S-100+ interdigitating reticulum cells. FDCs have aberrant expression of adhesion molecules.

Genetic Features

Immunoglobulin heavy chain and T-cell receptor genes are germline in nearly all cases, although in a few cases classified as HVCD, immunoglobulin gene rearrangements have been found.

Plasma Cell Variant (PCCD)

Clinical Features

Plasma cell variant (PCCD) occurs in two forms: localized and multicentric (or systemic). In the localized form, PCCD affects a single anatomic site, usually the mediastinal or intra-abdominal lymph nodes. Patients of any age can be affected, but most are young adults. They may be asymptomatic, but systemic symptoms, including fever, weight loss, and fatigue, are common, and many have anemia, elevated erythrocyte sedimentation rate, and hyperglobulinemia. Following excision of the mass, the symptoms and laboratory abnormalities disappear and patients do well.

In the multicentric form, most patients are middle-aged to older adults. Patients present with peripheral lymphadenopathy and with constitutional symptoms that tend to be more severe than those in localized PCCD. Most also have hepatosplenomegaly, many have mediastinal and intra-abdominal adenopathy, and some have neurologic findings or renal disease. Some have POEMS syndrome (polyneuropathy, organomegaly, endocrinopathy, monoclonal gammopathy, and skin changes). (POEMS syndrome is discussed in more detail in Chapter 3, under Plasmacytoma/Plasma Cell Myeloma.) The immunologic function of many patients is abnormal, and they develop severe infections and have an increased incidence of neoplasms of the type associated with immunodeficiency (e.g., Kaposi's sarcoma and lymphoma). The clinical course varies: some patients have relatively mild but persistent disease; some have episodic remissions and exacerbations; and some have rapidly progressive fatal disease. The mortality rate is greater than 50%, and only a fraction of living patients are asymptomatic. The causes of death include progressive PCCD, infection, renal failure, neurologic disease, and other malignancies.

Morphology

Changes are similar in localized and multicentric PCCD. Sheets of mature plasma cells occur in the interfollicular area, sometimes with Russell bodies, in addition to small blood vessels. The follicles may be hyperplastic follicles of the usual type or hyaline-vascular follicles or a mixture of the two types (Figs. 2–30 and 2–31). In some areas, sinuses may be obliterated, but they are patent at least focally. In some cases (which may represent an early stage of disease), immunoblasts and high endothelial venules are present in large numbers in addition to plasma cells in the interfollicular region. In late stages of disease, the appearance may resemble HVCD.

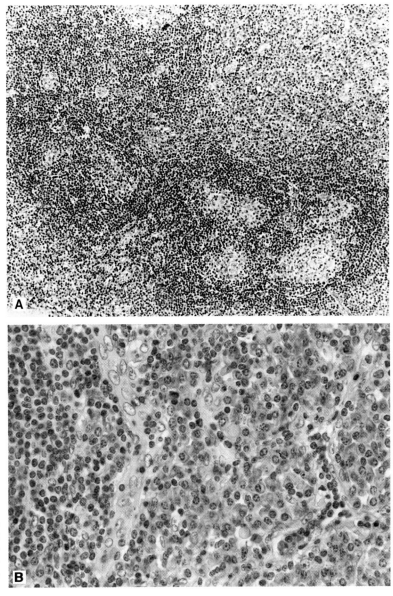

Figure 2–30. Castleman's disease, plasma cell type, localized, in a mesenteric lymph node of an adolescent girl. *A*, An abnormal follicle has multiple germinal centers and an interfollicular region with numerous plasma cells (H&E stain). *B*, The interfollicular area contains sheets of plasma cells, some with Russell bodies (H&E stain).

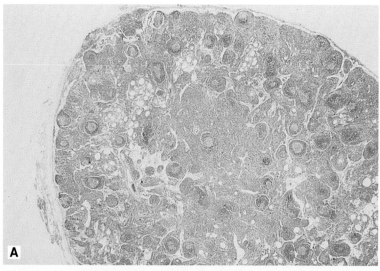

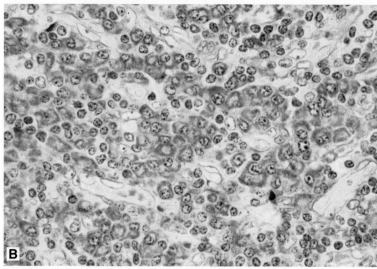

Figure 2–31. Castleman's disease, plasma cell type, multicentric. *A*, At low power, the interfollicular area is pink because of the presence of sheets of plasma cells. Follicles are relatively small, but most lack the distinctive features of those found in hyaline-vascular Castleman's disease. This patient had POEMS (polyneuropathy, organomegaly, endocrinopathy, M protein, skin changes) syndrome (H&E stain). *B*, High power view shows numerous mature plasma cells in addition to increased numbers of small blood vessels (Giemsa stain).

Immunophenotype

Plasma cells in approximately 50% of cases express monotypic immunoglobulin, which is nearly always IgGλ or IgAλ (Fig. 2–31*C* and *D*). In the remainder of cases, plasma cells express polytypic immunoglobulin.

Genetic Features

The reported frequency of immunoglobulin gene rearrangement varies greatly, ranging from a small minority to a majority. In a few cases, clonal T-cell receptor gene rearrangement has been described. Surprisingly, the finding of monotypic immunoglobulin or of clonal rearrangements

does not correlate well with distribution of disease (localized or multicentric) or with prognosis.

The Kaposi's sarcoma–associated herpes-virus–like DNA sequences have been found in 100% of cases classified as multicentric PCCD in HIV-positive patients, and in many cases of multicentric PCCD in HIV-negative patients. The Kaposi's sarcoma–associated herpes virus is discussed in more detail in Chapter 3, under Primary Effusion Lymphoma.

Differential Diagnosis

Castleman's disease is a diagnosis of exclusion. A wide variety of specific diseases may be associated with morphologic features resembling those of Castleman's disease, and these

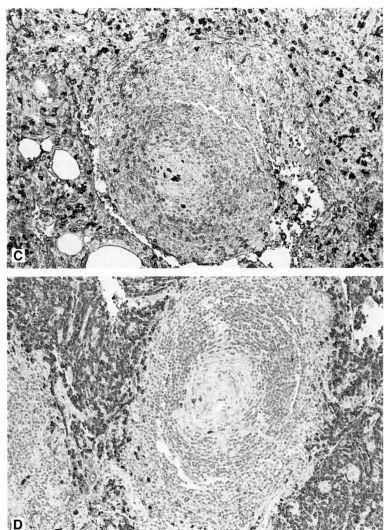

Figure 2–31. *Continued C* and *D,* In this case, the plasma cells are monotypic. Only scattered κ+ cells are present *(C),* while λ+ cells form sheets *(D)* (immunoperoxidase technique on paraffin sections).

should be ruled out before making a diagnosis of Castleman's disease.

1. Differential Diagnosis of HVCD
   a. Mantle cell lymphoma (MCL): Because HVCD is characterized by prominent mantle zones, MCL with a mantle zone pattern should be considered in the differential diagnosis of HVCD. Residual follicle centers in mantle cell lymphoma do not show hyaline-vascular features, and the interfollicular region lacks the distinctive appearance seen in HVCD. Immunophenotyping is definitive in difficult cases.
   b. Follicle center lymphoma (FCL): Some cases of FCL have sclerotic neoplastic follicles. When early nodal involvement occurs in such cases (i.e., the architecture is not effaced), the appearance may resemble HVCD. In FCL, mantle zones should not be prominent, and the interfollicular area should not be hypervascular. Immunophenotyping is definitive in difficult cases.
   c. Thymoma: In the first reports of Castleman's disease, the resemblance of hyaline-vascular follicles to Hassall's corpuscles was noted. HVCD and thymoma, however, do not otherwise resemble one another; Castleman's disease arises in lymph nodes rather than the thymus, and patients with thymomas are usually older than those with HVCD.
   d. Angioimmunoblastic T-cell lymphoma (AIL-TCL): AIL-TCL may contain aggregates of FDCs that resemble the FDC-rich germinal centers of hyaline-vascular follicles, but they are usually present at the

periphery of the node, and they usually have little or no mantle zone. The interfollicular region may have a striking increase in small blood vessels, but the interfollicular lymphoid cells usually have appreciable cytologic atypia and may have an abnormal T-cell immunophenotype. Lymphadenopathy may not be localized, and patients often have systemic symptoms.

2. Differential Diagnosis of PCCD

   a. Rheumatoid arthritis (RA): Lymphadenopathy in patients with RA has features that overlap those of PCCD. Clinical correlation is helpful in distinguishing between the two.

   b. Syphilis: Affected lymph nodes, particularly those in the inguinal region, are associated with distinctive pathologic findings. Lymphadenitis with follicular hyperplasia and numerous plasma cells is seen. Unlike PCCD, luetic lymphadenitis may show sarcoidal or necrotizing granulomas and inflamed vessels. Spirochetes are found easily in primary syphilis and may be found in secondary syphilis. In primary syphilis, lymphadenopathy is localized to nodes draining the chancre, and in secondary syphilis, lymphadenopathy is disseminated.

   c. Plasmacytoma: Nodal plasmacytomas are rare, and proliferation of lymphoid follicles is not a feature. The presence of polytypic plasma cells excludes plasmacytoma, but they are often seen in PCCD. Finding monotypic κ+ plasma cells is unusual in PCCD, although there may be cases in which the distinction is a matter of terminology.

   d. Lymphoplasmacytic lymphoma (LPL): LPL often partially involves nodes and may produce an interfollicular infiltrate of lymphocytes and plasma cells, with sparing of follicles that resembles PCCD. The demonstration of an interfollicular population of B lymphocytes provides evidence against PCCD. Unlike PCCD, LPL usually expresses monotypic IgM and does not preferentially express λ light chain.

3. Differential Diagnosis of both HVCD and PCCD

   a. Hodgkin's disease (HD): Rare cases of HD are associated with changes reminiscent of HVCD or PCCD. The HD may appear in the interfollicular area of the tissue with the CD-like changes, or the HD may occupy an area adjacent to the CD-like area (Fig. 2–32).

   b. Human immunodeficiency virus (HIV) infection: HIV-infected patients may develop lymphadenopathy with increased numbers of plasma cells, prominent vascularity, or interfollicular lymphoid depletion. The changes may closely resemble CD. It is a matter of debate whether a diagnosis of CD should be made in this setting, or whether the findings should be interpreted as changes mimicking CD due to HIV infection, or Kaposi's sarcoma–associated herpesvirus as discussed previously. Because of the association of Kaposi's sarcoma with CD-like changes, especially in the HIV-positive population, lymph nodes with these features should be examined carefully to rule out Kaposi's sarcoma.

   c. Miscellaneous: One or more features of CD may be found in lymph nodes showing reactive hyperplasia that is otherwise nonspecific. Such cases should not be interpreted as CD.

References

Abdel-Reheim FA, Koss W, Rappaport ES, Arber DA: Coexistence of Hodgkin's disease and giant lymph node hyperplasia of the plasma-cell type (Castleman's disease). Arch Pathol Lab Med 120:91–96, 1996.

Castleman B, Iverson L, Menendez VP: Localized mediastinal lymph node hyperplasia resembling thymoma. Cancer 9:822, 1956.

Danon AD, Krishnan J, Frizzera G: Morpho-immunophenotypic diversity of Castleman's disease, hyaline-vascular type: with emphasis on a stroma-rich variant and a new pathogenetic hypothesis. Virchows Archiv A Pathol Anat 423:369–382, 1993.

Frizzera G: Castleman's disease and related disorders. (Review.) Semin Diagn Pathol 5:346–364, 1988.

Keller AR, Hochholzer L, Castleman B: Hyaline-vascular and plasma-cell types of giant lymph node hyperplasia of the mediastinum and other locations. Cancer 29:670–683, 1972.

Menke DM, Tiemann M, Camoriano JK, et al: Diagnosis of Castleman's disease by identification of an immunophenotypically aberrant population of mantle zone B lymphocytes in paraffin-embedded lymph node biopsies. Am J Clin Pathol 105:268–276, 1996.

Molinie V, Diebold J: Hodgkin's disease associated with localized or multicentric Castleman's disease. Arch Pathol Lab Med 119:201, 1984.

Ohyashiki JH, Ohyashiki K, Kawakubo K, et al: Molecular genetic, cytogenetic, and immunophenotypic analyses in Castleman's disease of the plasma cell type. Am J Clin Pathol 101:290–295, 1994.

Peterson BA, Frizzera G: Multicentric Castleman's disease. Semin Oncol 20:636–647, 1993.

Radaszkiewicz T, Hansmann M-L, Lennert K: Monoclonality and polyclonality of plasma cells in Castleman's disease of the plasma cell variant. Histopathology 14:11–24, 1989.

Ruco LP, Gearing AJH, Pigott R, et al: Expression of ECAM-1, VCAM-1 and ELAM-1 in angiofollicular lymph node hyperplasia (Castleman's disease): evidence for dysplasia of follicular dendritic reticulum cells. Histopathology 19:523–528, 1991.

Soulier J, Grollet L, Oksenhendler E, et al: Kaposi's sarcoma-associated herpesvirus-like DNA sequences in multicentric Castleman's disease. Blood 84:1276–1280, 1995.

Soulier J, Grollet L, Oksenhendler E, et al: Molecular analysis of clonality in Castleman's disease. Blood 86:1131–1138, 1995.

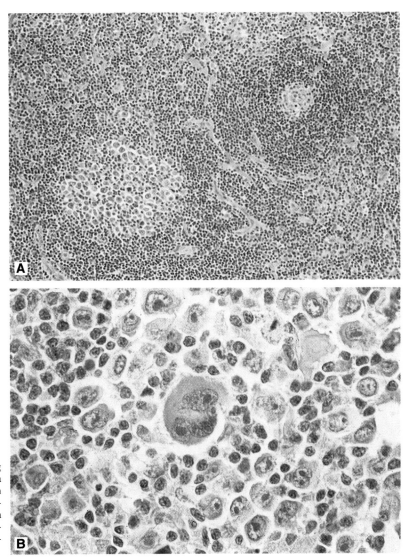

Figure 2–32. Hodgkin's disease with changes resembling Castleman's disease. *A,* The upper right corner shows a hyaline-vascular follicle. In the lower left corner is an aggregate of large cells that could be mistaken for a follicle on low power examination. The interfollicular area appears hypervascular (H&E stain). *B,* High power examination of the aggregate of large cells shows Reed-Sternberg cells and variants (H&E stain).

KIMURA'S DISEASE

Clinical Features

Kimura's disease is a chronic inflammatory disorder that mainly affects the area of the head and neck; it is associated with one or more lesions in subcutaneous tissue and salivary glands and lymphadenopathy. Kimura's disease affects patients from childhood to middle age; most patients are adults, with a male preponderance. The disease is more common among Asian populations. Patients may have peripheral eosinophilia and elevated serum IgE levels. Lesions may persist or recur over a period of months or years. The etiology of Kimura's disease is uncertain, but it may represent an aberrant immune reaction to an unknown stimulus.

Morphology

Lesions in soft tissue are poorly circumscribed and consist of a dense infiltrate of lymphocytes, eosinophils, mast cells, and plasma cells along with many small vessels and dense fibrosis. Numerous reactive follicles are present; their germinal centers may be vascularized or may be invaded and disrupted by eosinophils. Polykaryocytes may be present, most often in the follicles. Involved lymph nodes show follicular hyperplasia with increased numbers of eosinophils in the paracortex, sinusoids, perinodal soft tissue, and within follicles, sometimes with the formation of eosinophilic microabscesses. The number of paracortical postcapillary venules is increased. Distinguishing an inflamed, fibrotic lymph node from a lesion primarily involving soft tissue may be difficult on microscopic examination (Fig. 2–33).

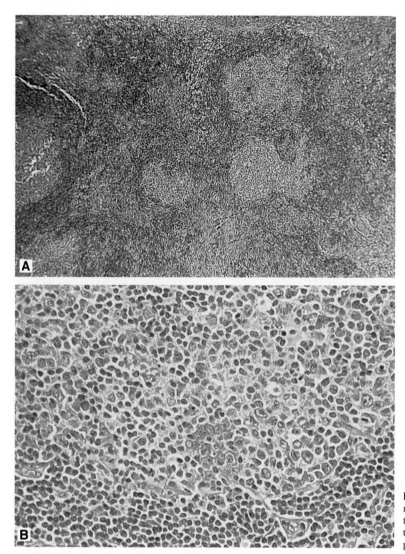

Figure 2–33. Kimura's disease. *A*, This lymph node shows marked follicular hyperplasia with patchy sclerosis within the node; sclerosis also extends irregularly into adjacent soft tissue (H&E stain). *B*, The germinal center contains a large polykaryocyte just below the center (H&E stain).

Immunophenotype

Kimura's disease has the distinctive finding of IgE-positive dendritic networks in germinal centers (Fig. 2–33D).

Differential Diagnosis

1. Angiolymphoid hyperplasia with eosinophilia (ALHE) (epithelioid hemangioma): Both ALHE and Kimura's

disease tend to produce lesions with prominent blood vessels and eosinophils in the region of the head and neck. ALHE is associated with larger numbers of smaller lesions that are better circumscribed and more superficially located (i.e., in the dermis) than Kimura's disease. Lymphoid follicles and fibrosis are not always seen in ALHE. ALHE is not associated with lymphadenopathy or salivary gland involvement. The most distinctive feature of ALHE is prominent epithelioid, or histiocytoid,

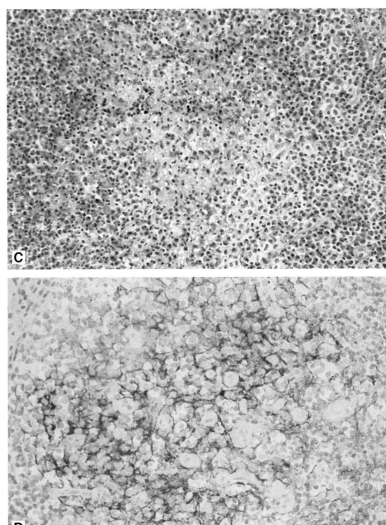

Figure 2–33. *Continued C*, An interfollicular focus of necrosis has numerous eosinophils (H&E stain). *D*, A follicle shows a dendritic pattern of staining for IgE (immunoperoxidase technique on paraffin section).

endothelial cells, which are not seen in Kimura's disease (Fig. 2–34).

2. Measles: The clinical and pathologic features of Kimura's disease are not suggestive of measles, except for the presence of polykaryocytes (Warthin-Finkeldey giant cells), which traditionally have been associated with measles infection. Polykaryocytes, however, are a nonspecific finding, and they can be seen in a variety of hyperplastic and neoplastic lymphoid proliferations.

References

Googe PB, Harris NL, Mihm MC, Jr.: Kimura's disease and angiolymphoid hyperplasia with eosinophilia: two distinct histopathological entities. J Cutan Pathol 14:263–271, 1987.

Hui PK, Chan JKC, Ng CS, *et al*: Lymphadenopathy of Kimura's disease. Am J Surg Pathol 13:177–186, 1989.

Kuo T-T, Shih L-Y, Chan H-L: Kimura's disease. Involvement of regional lymph nodes and distinction from angiolymphoid hyperplasia with eosinophilia. Am J Surg Pathol 12:843–854, 1988.

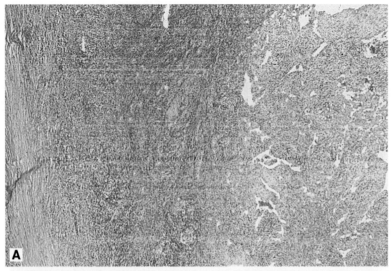

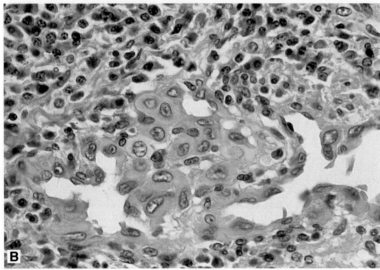

Figure 2–34. Angiolymphoid hyperplasia with eosinophilia (ALHE). *A*, This soft tissue nodule consists of a central vascular area *(right)*, surrounded by a rim of lymphoid tissue. The interface with the surrounding tissue is smooth (H&E stain). *B*, High power examination shows endothelial cells with a distinctive "epithelioid" or "histiocytoid" appearance (H&E stain).

DERMATOPATHIC LYMPHADENOPATHY (DL)

Synonym: Lipomelanotic reticulosis (older terminology).

Clinical Features

Dermatopathic lymphadenopathy (DL) is found in patients with a variety of chronic dermatoses or with mycosis fungoides (MF). The affected lymph nodes drain the abnormal skin. In some cases, patients do not have appreciable skin disease.

Morphology

Lymph nodes show marked expansion of the paracortex, with formation of large, pale nodules containing lympho-cytes, occasional immunoblasts, and numerous histiocytes with abundant pale cytoplasm including interdigitating dendritic cells (IDC), Langerhans' cells, and phagocytic histiocytes containing melanin, lipid, and occasionally iron. Small numbers of lymphocytes with irregular nuclei, reminiscent of the cerebriform cells that are characteristic of MF, may be found, even in patients with no evidence of lymphoma. Follicular hyperplasia and sinus histiocytosis may be present, although follicles may be inconspicuous (Fig. 2–35).

Immunophenotype

The paracortical T cells are predominantly T-helper cells, with a CD4:CD8 ratio that is, on average, higher than that of nonspecific lymphoid hyperplasia. The IDCs and Langerhans' cells are S-100+, CD1+, and HLA-DR+. The phago-

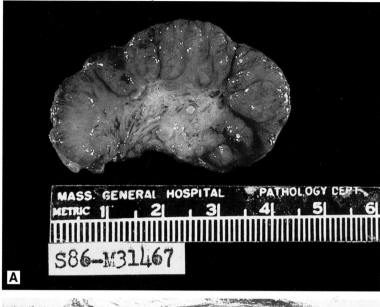

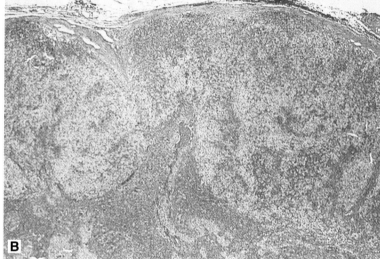

Figure 2–35. Dermatopathic lymphadenopathy. *A*, The lymph node shows a lobulated expansion of the paracortex, which is tan-yellow. The intact hilus is white and fibrotic. *B*, The paracortex is markedly expanded, predominantly by histiocytes with abundant pale cytoplasm. Follicular hyperplasia is inconspicuous (H&E stain).

Illustration continued on following page.

cytic histiocytes are lysozyme+. B cells express polyclonal immunoglobulin. Findings in patients with and without MF are similar.

Genetic Features

Most cases of DL in patients with MF show clonal T-cell receptor gene rearrangements, suggesting that nodal involvement by MF is frequent and may be subtle and difficult to appreciate on routine sections.

Differential Diagnosis

1. Early nodal involvement by MF: In some cases of MF, usually late in the course of the disease, nodal involvement by lymphoma is obvious with distortion or obliteration of the normal architecture by atypical lymphoid cells that may be cerebriform or may resemble immunoblasts or Reed-Sternberg cells. Many patients with MF, however, have lymph nodes showing only changes of DL on routine sections. Genotyping, cytogenetics, electron microscopy, and DNA cytophotometry

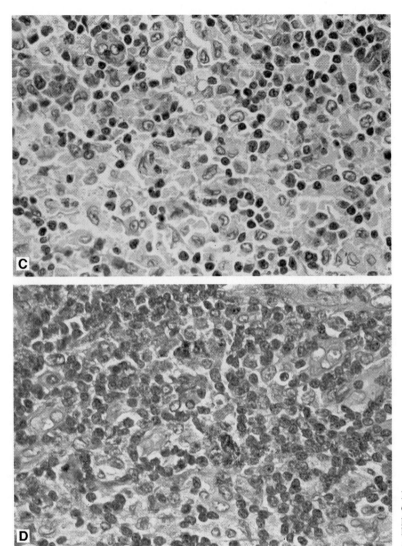

Figure 2–35. *Continued C*, A high power view of the paracortex shows histiocytes that have oval, pale nuclei with complex nuclear folding and indentation, consistent with Langerhans' cells and interdigitating dendritic cells (H&E stain). *D*, Abundant melanin is visible in some areas (H&E stain).

may be used to identify subtle lymphomatous involvement; however, going to such lengths may not be worthwhile, because some studies have reported an adverse prognosis associated with palpable lymph nodes regardless of histology.

References

Burke J, Khalil S, Rappaport H: Dermatopathic lymphadenopathy. An immunophenotypic comparison of cases associated and unassociated with mycosis fungoides. Am J Pathol 123:256–263, 1986.

Herrera GA: Light microscopic, S-100 immunostaining, and ultrastructural analysis of dermatopathic lymphadenopathy, with or without associated mycosis fungoides. Am J Clin Pathol 87:187–195, 1987.

Scheffer E, Meijer CJLM, Van Vloten WA: Dermatopathic lymphadenopathy and lymph node involvement in mycosis fungoides. Cancer 45:137–148, 1980.

Weiss L, Hu E, Wood G, Moulds C, *et al*: Clonal rearrangements of T cell receptor genes in mycosis fungoides and dermatopathic lymphadenopathy. N Engl J Med 313:539–544, 1985.

Weiss LM, Wood GS, Warnke RA: Immunophenotypic differences between dermatopathic lymphadenopathy and lymph node involvement in mycosis fungoides. Am J Pathol 120:179–185, 1985.

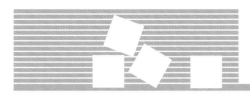

Introduction to Chapters 3 and 4
Non-Hodgkin's Lymphomas

In this Atlas, lymphomas are classified using the Revised European-American Lymphoma (R.E.A.L.) Classification. The corresponding diagnosis in other classifications is given for lymphomas in each category in the text that follows. In addition, R.E.A.L. diagnostic categories are shown in comparison to the corresponding diagnostic categories in the Kiel Classification and the Working Formulation for B-cell neoplasms in Table 3–1 and for T-cell neoplasms in Table 4–1 (see Chapter 4). Several disorders not included as separate entities in the R.E.A.L. Classification—immunoproliferative small intestinal disease, T-cell-rich B-cell lymphoma, intravascular large B-cell lymphoma, primary effusion lymphoma, and lymphomatoid granulomatosis—are discussed in Chapters 3 and 4 for completeness, because

Table 3–1

COMPARISON OF B-CELL NEOPLASMS IN THE REVISED EUROPEAN-AMERICAN LYMPHOMA (R.E.A.L.) CLASSIFICATION WITH THE KIEL CLASSIFICATION AND THE WORKING FORMULATION

Kiel Classification	R.E.A.L. Classification	Working Formulation
B-lymphoblastic	Precursor B-lymphoblastic lymphoma/ leukemia	Lymphoblastic
B-lymphocytic, CLL	B-cell chronic lymphocytic leukemia/ small lymphocytic lymphoma	*Small lymphocytic, consistent with CLL*
B-lymphocytic, prolymphocytic leukemia		Small lymphocytic, plasmacytoid
Lymphoplasmacytoid immunocytoma		
Lymphoplasmacytic immunocytoma	Lymphoplasmacytic lymphoma	*Small lymphocytic, plasmacytoid*
		Diffuse, mixed small and large cell
Centrocytic	Mantle cell lymphoma	Small lymphocytic
Centroblastic, centrocytoid subtype		*Diffuse, small cleaved cell*
		Follicular, small cleaved cell
		Diffuse, mixed small and large cell
		Diffuse, large cleaved cell
Centroblastic-centrocytic, follicular	Follicle center lymphoma, follicular	
	Grade I	*Follicular, predominantly small cleaved cell*
	Grade II	*Follicular, mixed small and large cell*
Centroblastic, follicular	Grade III	Follicular, predominantly large cell
Centroblastic-centrocytic, diffuse	Follicle center lymphoma, diffuse, small cell (provisional entity)	Diffuse, small cleaved cell
		Diffuse, mixed small and large cell
	Extranodal marginal zone B-cell lymphoma (low grade B-cell lymphoma of MALT type)	*Small lymphocytic*
		Diffuse, small cleaved cell
		Diffuse, mixed small and large cell
Monocytoid, including marginal zone	Nodal marginal zone B-cell lymphoma (provisional entity)	*Small lymphocytic*
Immunocytoma		Diffuse, small cleaved cell
		Diffuse, mixed small and large cell
		Unclassifiable
	Splenic marginal zone B-cell lymphoma (provisional entity)	*Small lymphocytic*
		Diffuse, small cleaved cell
Hairy cell leukemia	Hairy cell leukemia	
Plasmacytic	Plasmacytoma/myeloma	Extramedullary plasmacytoma
Centroblastic (monomorphic, polymorphic and multilobated subtypes)	Diffuse large B-cell lymphoma	*Diffuse, large cell*
		Large cell immunoblastic
		Diffuse, mixed small and large cell
B-immunoblastic		
B-large cell anaplastic (Ki-1+)		
—*	Primary mediastinal large B-cell lymphoma	*Diffuse, large cell*
		Large cell immunoblastic
Burkitt's lymphoma	Burkitt's lymphoma	Small noncleaved cell, Burkitt's
?Burkitt's lymphoma with cytoplasmic immunoglobulin	High grade B-cell lymphoma, Burkitt-like (provisional)	*Small noncleaved cell, non-Burkitt's*
?Some cases of centroblastic and immunoblastic		Diffuse, large cell
		Large cell immunoblastic

When more than one Kiel or Working Formulation category is listed, those in *Italic* type constitute the majority of the cases.

* Not listed in classification, but discussed as rare or ambiguous type.

Modified from Table 2 in Harris NL, Jaffe ES, Stein H, *et al*: A revised European-American Classification of lymphoid neoplasms: a proposal from the International Lymphoma Study Group. Blood 84:1361–1392, 1994.

Table 3–2
CLUSTER DESIGNATION OF LEUKOCYTE-ASSOCIATED MOLECULES

CD	Common Name(s)	Monoclonal Antibodies	Distribution
1 a	T6, gp49	Leu6, T6, OKT6	Cortical thymocytes, Langerhans' cells
2	T11, SER, LFA-2	Leu5b, T11, OKT11	Pan-T, thymocytes, NK cells
3	T3 e	Leu4, T3, OKT3, UCHT1	Pan-T, T specific, thymocytes
3	T3 z	TIA-2	Pan-T, thymocytes, NK cells
4	T4, GP59	Leu3a, T4, OKT4/4a	T-helper cells (MHC Class II restricted), thymocytes, monocytes
5	T1, Tp67	Leu1, T1, OKT1	T cells, thymocytes, some B cells, (B-CLL, MCL)*
6	T12	T12, OKT17, TU33	Pan-T, medullary thymocytes, B cells
7	3A1	Leu9, 3A1, RT7 1, TU14	Prethymocytes, most circulating T cells, NK subset, (ALL)
8	T8	Leu2a, T8, OKT8a	T cytotoxic-suppressor (MHC Class I restricted), NK subset, thymocytes, SCS
9	BA-2, p24	CLB-thromb/8, BA-2, J2	Monocytes, pre-B, platelets, activated T cells
10	CALLA	Anti-CALLA, J5, OKB-cALLa	Pre-B, granulocytes, fibroblasts, (ALL)
11 a	LFA, L integrin	LFA-1, 2H8	Leukocytes, thymocytes
11 b	MAC1, Mo1, CR3, M integrin	Leu15, Mo1, OKM1	Granulocytes, monocytes, NK cells
11 c	p150/95, X integrin	LeuM5	Monocytes, granulocytes, activated CD8+ T cells, NK, B subset, (HCL)
15	X Hapten, LNFP III	LeuM1, MY1	Granulocytes, monocytes, activated T cells, (RS cells)
16	IgG FcR IIIA/FcR IIIB	Leu11, OK-NK	NK cells, granulocytes, macrophages
18	LFA b chain; LEUCAM	LFA-1b, 60.3, MHM23	Leukocytes
19	B4	Leu12, B4, OKpanB	Pre-B, pan-B, activated B
20	B1, Bp35	Leu16, B1, L26	B cells
21	CR2, EBV-R	Anti-CR2, B2, OKB7	B cells, C3d red cells, FDC
22	Bgp135	Leu14, OKB22, TO15, B3	Pan-B, in cytoplasm of early and mature cells
23	Blast-2	Leu20, B6, Blast-2	Activated B, FDC, (CLL)
24	BA-1; HSA/heat stable antigen	OKB2, BA1, HB8, HB9	Pan-B, granulocytes, monocytes
25	IL2R	Anti-IL2R, OKT26a, Tac	Activated T cells, B cells, monocytes, thymocytes, basophils, eosinophils, (HCL)
27	p55(dimer)	OKT18A, S152, VIT14	T cells, thymocytes, plasma cells (cytoplasmic)
28	gp44	9.3, KOLT 2, 15E8	T subset (cytotoxic precursors), plasma cells
29	VLA b-1, platelet GPIIa	4B4, K20	Leukocytes; weak on granulocytes, not on RBC
30	Ki-1 antigen	BERH2	Activated T and B cells, (RS cells)
40	gp50	G28-5, S2C6	B and T cells, monocytes, IDC, some epithelium
43	gp95, sialophorin	Leu22, G10-2, G19-1	T cells, B subset, NK, monocytes, plasma and myeloid cells
44	HCAM, Hermes, Pgp-1	Leu44, A3D8, 1-173	Leukocytes, red cells
45	LCA/T200	HLe-1, LCA	Leukocyte common antigen, all leukocytes except plasma cells
45 RA	LCA-RA	Leu18, 2H4	Suppressor-inducer CD4+, suppressor CD8+, monocytes, NK, B cells
45 RB	LCA-RB	PD17/26/16	T subset, B cells, monocytes, granulocytes
45 RO	LCA-RO	UCHL1, A7, OPD4	Helper-inducer CD4+, cytotoxic CD8+, thymocytes, granulocytes, monocytes
56	NCAM, NKH-1	Leu19, NKH-1A	Pan-NK, activated T cells
57	HNK-1	Leu7, L183, L186	T cell and NK cell subset
70	Ki-24	Ki-24, HNE 51, HNC 142	Activated B and T cells, (RS cells)
75 w	CDw75	LN1, HH2, EBU-141	Mature B cells
80	B7-1/BB1	B7-1/BB1	Activated B cells, macrophages
86	B7-2, FUN-1, BU63	BU63, FUN-1	B cells, NK cells, monocytes, (lymphomas, RS cells)
95	APO-1, FAS	7C11, APO-1, IPO-4	T cells, B cells, thymocytes, liver, heart, (various malignant cell lines)
100	BB18, A8, semaphorin	BB18, BD16, A8	T cells, germinal center B cells, NK cells, granulocytes, monocytes, platelets
103	HML-1	2G5.1, F3F7, LF61, B-Ly7	Intraepithelial mucosal lymphocytes (HCL)

* Neoplasms or neoplastic cells are in parentheses
(Information in this table is available through the courtesy of Dr. F. Preffer.)

Abbreviations

ALL	Acute Lymphoblastic Leukemia	LNFP	Lacto-N-Fucose Pentosyl III
CALLA	Common Acute Lymphoblastic Leukemia Antigen	MCL	Mantle Cell Lymphoma
CLL	Chronic Lymphocytic Leukemia	MHC	Major Histocompatibility Complex
EBV	Epstein-Barr Virus	NCAM	Neural Cell Adhesion Molecule
FDC	Follicular Dendritic Cells	NK	Natural Killer
HCAM	Homing Cell Adhesion Molecule	R	Receptor
HCL	Hairy Cell Leukemia	RBC	Red Blood Cells
HML	Human Mucosal Lymphocyte	RS cells	Reed-Sternberg Cells
ICAM	Intercellular Adhesion Molecule	SCS	Sinusoidal Cells in Spleen
IDC	Interdigitating Dendritic Cells	SER	Sheep Erythrocyte Receptor
LCA	Leukocyte Common Antigen	VLA	Very Late Antigen
LFA	Lymphocyte Function–Associated		

Table 3–3
ABBREVIATIONS

CD	cluster designation
Ig	immunoglobulin
sIg	surface immunoglobulin
cIg	cytoplasmic immunoglobulin
cMu	cytoplasmic mu heavy chain
TCR	T-cell receptor
MoAb	monoclonal antibody
EBV	Epstein-Barr virus
EBV LMP	EBV latent membrane protein
EBER	EBV-encoded RNA
EMA	epithelial membrane antigen
FDC	follicular dendritic cell
IDC	interdigitating dendritic cell
ISH	in situ hybridization
PCR	polymerase chain reaction
SBH	Southern blot hybridization
CNS	central nervous system
GI	gastrointestinal
+	> 90% of cases positive
+/−	> 50% of cases positive
−/+	< 50% of cases positive
−	< 10% of cases positive

they have distinctive clinical and pathologic features. A list of cluster designations (CD) of leukocyte-associated molecules, many of which are referred to in Chapters 3 and 4, is included in Table 3–2 and frequently used abbreviations appear in Table 3–3.

References

Chan JKC, Banks PM, Cleary ML, *et al*: A revised European-American classification of lymphoid neoplasms proposed by the International Lymphoma Study Group. A summary version. Am J Clin Pathol 103:543–560, 1995.

Harris NL, Jaffe ES, Stein H, *et al*: A revised European-American classification of lymphoid neoplasms: a proposal from the International Lymphoma Study Group. Blood 84:1361–1392, 1994.

CHAPTER 3

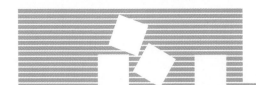

Non-Hodgkin's Lymphomas:
B-Cell Neoplasms

The clinical and pathologic features of B-cell neoplasms are summarized in Table 3–4. Lymphomas derived from B lymphoid cells are believed to correspond to neoplastic transformation of B cells at particular stages of differentiation (Fig. 3–1). This chapter begins with a discussion of lymphoma of precursor B-cell origin and then proceeds to lymphomas derived from more mature, "peripheral" B cells.

Table 3–4

B-CELL NEOPLASMS

Category	Neoplastic Cells	Unusual Immunophenotype	Genetic Features	Patients Affected	Sites Affected	Usual Behavior
1. Precursor B-lymphoblastic lymphoma/leukemia	B-lymphoblasts	TdT+, CD19+, CD79a+, CD10+/−, HLA-Dr+, sIg−	IgH-R, TCR-G or R, unmutated IgV	Children > adults	Bone marrow, blood; less often skin, bone, lymph nodes	Aggressive; usually curable
2. B-chronic lymphocytic leukemia	Small lymphocytes, prolymphocytes, paraimmunoblasts	Faint sIgM(D)+, CD19+, CD20+, CD5+, CD23+	IgH-R, IgL-R, trisomy 12 in a minority, 13q abnormalities, unmutated IgV	Older adults M>F	Bone marrow, blood, lymph nodes	Indolent, not curable
3. Lymphoplasmacytic lymphoma/immunocytoma	Small lymphocytes, plasmacytoid lymphocytes, plasma cells	s and cIgM+, CD19+, CD20+, CD5−, CD10−	IgH-R, IgL-R, some mutations of IgV	Older adults M>F	Bone marrow, lymph nodes, blood	Indolent, not curable (Waldenström's macroglobulinemia)
4. Mantle cell lymphoma	Small irregular lymphoid cells (mantle cells)	sIgMD+, λ>κ, CD19+, CD20+, CD5+, CD23−, cyclin D1+	IgH-R, IgL-R, t(11;14) (bc1-1), unmutated IgV	Older adults M>F	Lymph nodes, spleen, Waldeyer's ring, GI tract, marrow, blood	Moderately aggressive, not curable
5. Follicle center lymphoma	Centrocytes and centroblasts	sIg+, CD19+, CD20+, CD10+/−, CD5−	IgH-R, IgL-R, t(14;18) (bc1-2), ongoing mutations of IgV	Adults M=F	Lymph nodes, marrow, spleen, rarely extranodal sites	Indolent, not curable
6. Marginal zone B-cell lymphoma						
a. Extranodal	Small lymphocytes, marginal zone B cells, monocytoid B cells, few blasts, plasma cells	sIgM+, cIgM+/−, CD19+, CD20+, CD5−, CD10−, CD23−	IgH-R, IgL-R, trisomy 3 common, on-going mutations of IgV	Adults M=F	GI tract, lung, salivary glands, thyroid, orbit, other extranodal sites	Indolent; often curable if localized
b. Nodal	Same	Same	IgH-R, IgL-R	Same	Lymph nodes	Indolent; sometimes curable
7. Splenic marginal zone lymphoma	Mantle and marginal zone B cells, few blasts, +/−plasma cells, +/−villous lymphocytes	sIgM+, D+/−, cIg−/+, CD43−	IgH-R, IgL-R	Older adults	Spleen, marrow, blood (villous lymphocytes), liver, abdominal nodes	Indolent; good response to splenectomy
8. Hairy cell leukemia	Hairy cells	sIg+, CD19+, CD20+, CD5−, CD10−, CD23−, CD11c+, CD25+	IgH-R, IgL-R, mutated IgV	Adults	Spleen, marrow, blood	Indolent
9. Plasmacytoma/myeloma	Plasma cells, +/−plasmablasts	sIg−, cIg+ (G or A), CD19−, CD20−, CD45−/+	IgH and IgL-R or deleted, mutated IgV	Adults	Marrow, bone, less often other extranodal sites	Moderately aggressive, incurable
10. Diffuse large B-cell lymphoma	Centroblasts, immunoblasts, large centrocytes, multilobated cells, occasionally anaplastic large cells	sIg+ (or sIg−), CD19+, CD20+, CD45+, CD10−/+	IgH-R, IgL-R, bc1-6-R in a minority, bc1-2-R in a minority	Adults>children	Lymph nodes and extranodal sites (CNS, bone, GI)	Aggressive, potentially curable
a. Primary mediastinal large B-cell lymphoma	Same	Same	IgH-R, IgL-R	Adults F>M	Thymus	Same
11. Burkitt's lymphoma	Medium-sized blast cells	sIgM+, CD19+, CD20+, CD10+, CD5−, CD23−	IgH-R, IgL-R; t(8;14), t(8;22), or t(2;8)(c-myc); mutated IgV	Children>adults	Facial bones, GI, ovaries, other extranodal sites, lymph nodes	Highly aggressive; potentially curable
12. High grade B-cell lymphoma, Burkitt-like	Blast cells, more pleomorphic than classic Burkitt's	sIg+, cIg+/−, B-antigen+, CD5−, usually CD10−	IgH-R, IgL-R, bc1-2-R in 30%, c-myc-R is rare	Adults>children	Lymph nodes>extranodal sites	Highly aggressive, worse prognosis than Burkitt's

Abbreviations: IgH, Ig heavy chain genes; IgL, Ig light chain genes; R, rearranged; G, germline; TCR, T-cell receptor genes; IgV, Ig variable region genes; M, males; F, females.

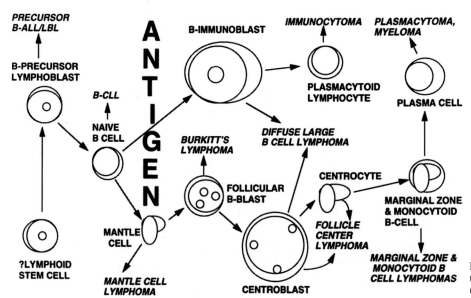

Figure 3–1. B-cell differentiation with postulated neoplastic counterparts (*in italics*). (*Compare with Fig. 1–1.*)

Precursor B-Cell Neoplasm

PRECURSOR B-LYMPHOBLASTIC LYMPHOMA/LEUKEMIA

Synonyms: Rappaport: lymphoblastic (formerly diffuse poorly differentiated lymphocytic); Kiel: lymphoblastic, B-cell type; Lukes-Collins: undefined cell; Working Formulation: lymphoblastic; French-American-British (FAB) classification: acute lymphoblastic leukemia (ALL), L1 and L2.

Clinical Features

Approximately 80% of acute lymphoblastic leukemia (ALL) cases but less than 20% of lymphoblastic lymphoma (LBL) cases are B-precursor type. Children are affected more often than adults. Most patients present with acute leukemia with bone marrow and peripheral blood involvement; a small proportion presents with solid tumors, most often in skin, bone, or lymph nodes, with or without bone marrow or peripheral blood involvement. By convention, a patient with one or more mass lesions with greater than 25% lymphoblasts in the marrow is considered to have ALL. The disease is highly aggressive but frequently curable with available therapy.

Morphology

Lymphoblasts are slightly larger than small lymphocytes but smaller than the cells of large B-cell lymphoma, having round or convoluted nuclei, fine chromatin, inconspicuous nucleoli, and scant, faintly basophilic cytoplasm. B-LBL has a diffuse pattern with frequent mitoses. Tingible body macrophages may be present, resulting in a starry-sky pattern (Fig. 3–2). Among patients with a leukemic presentation, marrow involvement is almost always diffuse and extensive, with only small numbers of residual hematopoietic elements.

Immunophenotype

Tumor cells are typically TdT+, CD19+, CD79a+, CD22+, CD20−/+, CD10+/−, HLA-DR+, sIg−, cMu−/+, CD34+/−, with expression of CD13 or CD33 in some cases. Antibodies to CD79a (mb-1: IgM-associated protein) are useful in identifying the infrequent CD19− cases and can be useful in paraffin sections. CD45 may be weak or undetectable in paraffin sections.

Genetic Features

Ig heavy chain genes are usually rearranged; Ig light chain genes may be rearranged. TCR genes are usually germline but may be rearranged. Cytogenetic abnormalities are variable. Some common recurring abnormalities are described; they are not specific for B-LBL or B-ALL, and certain ones may be found in T-LBL or T-ALL, in myeloid leukemias, or in mixed lineage leukemias. Hyperdiploidy with more than 50 chromosomes is associated with a favorable prognosis.

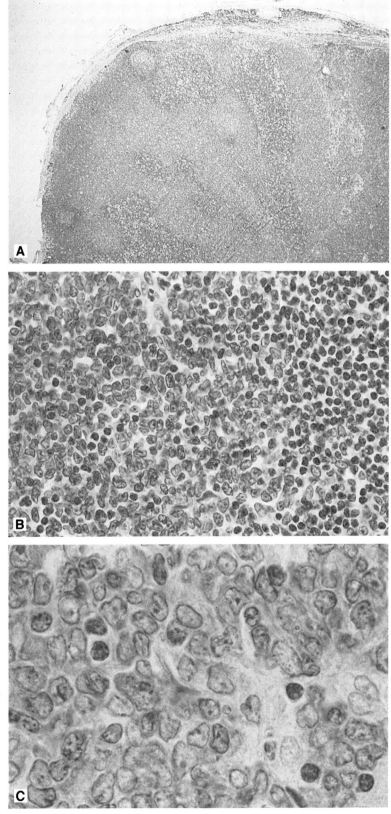

Figure 3–2. Precursor B-cell lymphoma. *A,* An infiltrate of primitive cells, which are pale violet, replaces much of the node. Focally, dark bands of residual paracortex and a few small follicles remain (H&E stain). *B,* Higher power view shows B-precursor cells with nuclei that are slightly larger and more irregular, and chromatin that is more finely dispersed than that of the adjacent small lymphocytes (*right*) (H&E stain). *C,* The neoplastic cells have oval, angulated, or indented nuclei, occasionally small nucleoli, and scant cytoplasm (Giemsa stain).

Hyperdiploidy with 47 to 50 chromosomes and normal diploidy are associated with an intermediate prognosis. Hypodiploidy is associated with an intermediate to poor prognosis. Pseudodiploidy (cases with 46 chromosomes but with structural abnormalities), Philadelphia chromosome (t(9;22)(q34;q11)), t(1;19)(q23;p13), and t(4;11)(p21;q23) are associated with a poor outcome.

Postulated Normal Counterpart

Bone-marrow-derived precursor B cell.

Differential Diagnosis

1. T-lymphoblastic lymphoma (T-LBL): Histologic features cannot be used to predict B- or T-lineage, and immunophenotyping is required to distinguish between B- and T-LBL. Clinical features may be helpful in differentiation, such as the frequent association of T-LBL, but not B-LBL, with a mediastinal mass.
2. Mantle cell lymphoma (MCL): The morphology of LBL and the blastoid variant of MCL overlaps. MCL occurs almost exclusively in adults, however, and although bone marrow involvement is frequent, it is often focal and neoplastic cells are found only occasionally in the peripheral blood. Immunophenotyping provides a definitive diagnosis (B-LBL: TdT+, sIg−; MCL: sIg+, TdT−).
3. Acute myeloid leukemia (AML)/granulocytic sarcoma (GS): Cases of AML or GS composed of cells with little appreciable myeloid differentiation may mimic LBL. Examination of touch preparations or aspirate smears can be helpful in identifying granules or Auer rods in AML/GS. Enzyme histochemical stains or immunologic studies confirm the diagnosis (B-LBL: CD19+, CD22+, CD10+, CD79a+; AML: myeloperoxidase+, lysozyme+, CD13+, CD33+, CAE+).
4. Chronic lymphocytic leukemia (CLL): In some cases of LBL, the tumor cells are close to the size of a small lymphocyte and have chromatin that is relatively condensed. When the patient is an adult, the differential diagnosis includes CLL. The presence of pseudofollicles supports a diagnosis of CLL. The presence of appreciable numbers of mitotic figures in the absence of pseudofollicles should raise the possibility of LBL. Immunophenotyping provides a definitive diagnosis (CLL: sIg+, TdT−, CD10−; B-LBL: sIg−, TdT+, CD10+).
5. Hematogones: Hematogones (lymphoid precursor cells) are normally found in the bone marrow of young children. In a variety of conditions, including marrow regeneration following chemotherapy, their numbers may increase. This effect is most striking in children but is occasionally seen in adults. The morphology and immunophenotype of hematogones and neoplastic lymphoblasts overlap somewhat, and occasionally, distinguishing between ALL and hematogones is difficult. At the time of primary diagnosis of ALL, however, particularly in children, the normal marrow elements are virtually replaced by the leukemic infiltrate. Even when hematogones are abundant, they are sprinkled evenly among hematopoietic precursors in sections of the bone marrow biopsy specimen. Unlike lymphoblasts, hematogones have round nuclei that often have a small, peripherally located notch, smudged chromatin, and inconspicuous or absent nucleoli. Their immunophenotype reflects a range of maturational stages; some are CD19+, CD20−, CD10+, and TdT+ like lymphoblasts, but others are CD19+, CD20+, CD10−, and TdT−, indicating a more mature stage. They lack cytogenetic abnormalities (Fig. 3–3).

References

Borowitz M, Croker B, Metzgar R: Lymphoblastic lymphoma with the phenotype of common acute lymphoblastic leukemia. Am J Clin Pathol 79:387–391, 1983.

Brunning RD, McKenna RW: Atlas of tumor pathology: tumors of the bone marrow. Washington, D.C.: Armed Forces Institute of Pathology, 1994.

Korsmeyer S, Arnold A, Bakhshi A, et al: Immunoglobulin gene rearrangement and cell surface antigen expression in acute lymphocytic leukemias of T-cell and B-cell precursor origins. J Clin Invest 71:301–313, 1983.

Mason D, Cordell J, Tse A, et al: The IgM-associated protein mb-1 as a marker of normal and neoplastic B-cells. J Immunol 147(8):2474–2482, 1991.

Nathwani B, Kim H, Rappaport H: Malignant lymphoma, lymphoblastic. Cancer 38:964–983, 1976.

Sander C, Medeiros L, Abruzzo L, et al: Lymphoblastic lymphoma presenting in cutaneous sites: a clinicopathologic analysis of six cases. J Am Acad Dermatol 25:1023–1031, 1991.

Sixth International Workshop on Chromosomes in Leukemia, London, England, May 11–18, 1987: Selected papers. Cancer Genet Cytogenet 40:171–216, 1989.

Tawa A, Hozumi N, Minden M, et al: Rearrangements of the T-cell receptor β chain gene in non-T-cell, non-B-cell acute lymphoblastic leukemia in childhood. N Engl J Med 313:1033–1037, 1985.

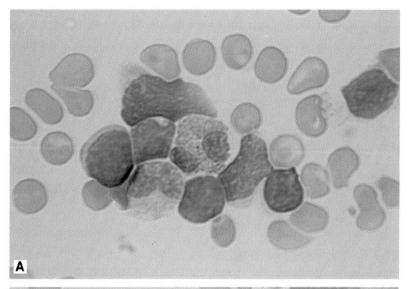

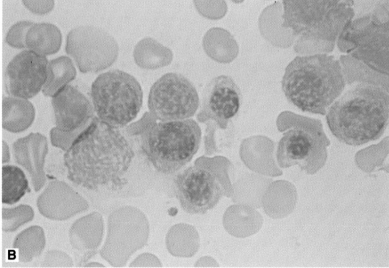

Figure 3–3. Specimens from a 1-year-old girl with anemia due to transient erythroblastopenia. *A,* At presentation, the patient had markedly decreased numbers of erythroid precursors, increased numbers of hematogones, and normal myeloid maturation. This figure shows several hematogones; they are slightly larger than normal lymphocytes and have smudgy chromatin, scant cytoplasm, and inconspicuous or absent nucleoli. The lymphoid cell at the lower right has slightly more condensed chromatin and may be a mature cell, rather than a hematogone. On initial examination of this smear, the patient's disorder was interpreted as acute lymphoblastic leukemia (Wright-Giemsa stain). *B,* One week later, the child had marked erythroid hyperplasia and hematogones were not conspicuous (Wright-Giemsa stain).

Peripheral B-Cell Neoplasms

B-CELL CHRONIC LYMPHOCYTIC LEUKEMIA (B-CLL)/SMALL LYMPHOCYTIC LYMPHOMA (B-SLL)

Synonyms: Rappaport: well-differentiated lymphocytic, diffuse; Kiel: B-CLL; immunocytoma, lymphoplasmacytoid type; Lukes-Collins: small lymphocyte B, B-CLL; Working Formulation: small lymphocytic, consistent with CLL.

Clinical Features

B-CLL is the most common adult leukemia in North America and Western Europe; it is much less prevalent in Asia and Africa. Most cases of B-CLL occur in older adults, with a male : female ratio of 2 : 1. Patients present with constitutional symptoms, fatigue, susceptibility to infections, or occasionally autoimmune hemolytic anemia. Occasionally, B-CLL is an incidental finding in lymph nodes or other tissues removed for unrelated reasons. Most patients have bone marrow and peripheral blood involvement at presentation, with or without lymphadenopathy or hepatosplenomegaly. Occasionally, patients present primarily with lymphadenopathy, but most of them have marrow and blood involvement found during the staging process or develop involvement shortly thereafter. Rare nonleukemic cases have been described. B-CLL commonly involves multiple lymph nodes, spleen, and liver; a variety of extranodal sites may also be involved. Some patients have a small M-component. The clinical course is indolent, but this disease is not usually curable with available therapy.

Transformation to large B-cell lymphoma (Richter's syndrome) occurs in approximately 5% of cases. Patients with this complication present with acute onset of fever and rapidly enlarging asymmetric lymphadenopathy. The large cell lymphoma may be identified while it is still localized, usually in lymph nodes or bone marrow, or occasionally in an extranodal site, but it usually disseminates rapidly. Involvement of spleen, liver, and gastrointestinal tract is common. B-CLL that has undergone transformation is typically unresponsive to treatment, and most patients die in a few months. A small number of patients have had transformation of B-CLL to a lymphoma with features of Hodgkin's disease. Prolymphocytic transformation occurs occasionally and is usually accompanied by progressive disease that responds poorly to treatment.

Morphology

Criteria suggested for a diagnosis of CLL include absolute lymphocyte count greater than 10×10^9/L sustained for at least 4 weeks in the peripheral blood *and* greater than 30% replacement of the marrow cellularity. In the presence of smaller numbers of blood and bone marrow lymphocytes, a diagnosis of B-CLL can be made if the results of immunophenotyping are consistent with B-CLL. Fewer than 10% of peripheral blood lymphoid cells are prolymphocytes (Fig. 3–4A). Patients with more than 10% but less than 55% prolymphocytes are said to have chronic lymphocytic leukemia/prolymphocytic leukemia (CLL/PLL). Patients with a history of CLL who have more than 55% prolymphocytes have prolymphocytic transformation.

Lymph nodes involved by B-CLL typically show a characteristic diffuse infiltrate with scattered, vaguely delineated pale areas, creating a pseudofollicular pattern. The predominant cell is a small lymphocyte, which is the same size as or slightly larger than a normal lymphocyte, with clumped chromatin, a round or infrequently irregular nucleus, and often a small nucleolus. Variable numbers of larger lymphoid cells—prolymphocytes and paraimmunoblasts—are also present. Usually, they are clustered in pseudofollicles (growth centers, proliferation centers), which results in a pseudofollicular pattern (Fig. 3–4, B and C). Less often, they are distributed evenly throughout the node. Prolymphocytes are intermediate-sized cells with round nuclei, moderately clumped chromatin, a single prominent nucleolus, and a moderate amount of pale cytoplasm. Paraimmunoblasts are large cells that resemble immunoblasts, except that their cytoplasm is pale rather than deep blue with a Giemsa stain. Increased numbers of large cells may be associated with a more aggressive course.

Bone marrow involvement appears as nodular, interstitial, or diffuse infiltrates of small lymphoid cells or a mixture of these patterns. Occasionally, pseudofollicles may be recognizable. Even when marrow involvement is extensive, hematopoietic elements immediately adjacent to bony trabeculae may be spared. Diffuse marrow involvement is associated with a worse prognosis (Fig. 3–4, D and E).

Occasional cases with the characteristic morphology and immunophenotype of B-CLL have plasmacytoid differentiation, with cIg and often a small M component. These cases correspond to the "lymphoplasmacyt*oid*" immunocytoma of the Kiel Classification; they have a prognosis similar to or possibly slightly worse than those without this feature.

Specimens from cases with Richter's transformation have the appearance of a diffuse, large B-cell lymphoma. They are usually relatively monomorphous, being composed of immunoblasts or centroblasts (Fig. 3–5), but sometimes the tumor cells have a bizarre anaplastic appearance (Fig. 3–6). Occasionally one sees a transition between B-CLL and diffuse large-cell lymphoma, and the appearance may suggest an outgrowth of sheets of paraimmunoblasts.

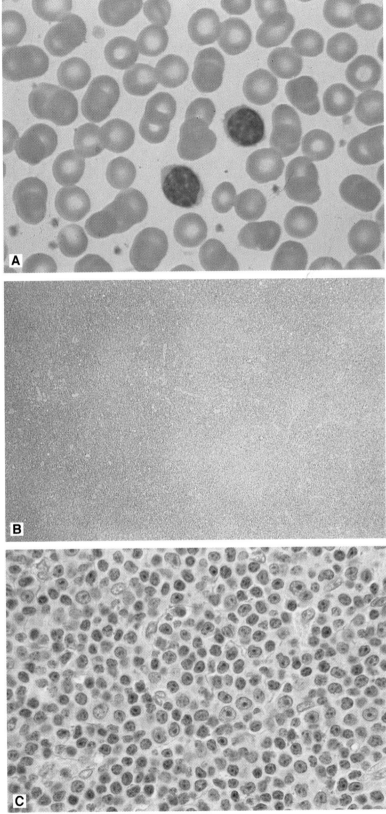

Figure 3–4. B-cell chronic lymphocytic leukemia (B-CLL). *A*, The peripheral blood shows lymphocytosis with small, mature lymphocytes (Wright-Giemsa stain). *B*, Low power view of a lymph node shows a diffuse infiltrate of small lymphocytes with occasional, poorly delineated, pale pseudofollicles (H&E stain). *C*, High power examination of a pseudofollicle shows small lymphocytes admixed with many prolymphocytes and occasional paraimmunoblasts (H&E stain).

Illustration continued on following page.

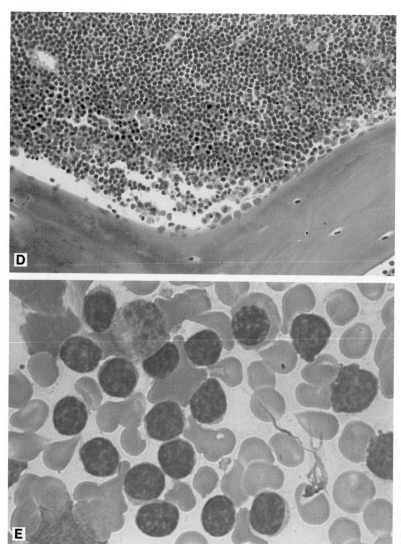

Figure 3–4. *Continued D,* The bone marrow shows a dense, diffuse infiltrate of small lymphocytes. A few normal precursors remain immediately adjacent to the bony trabecula (H&E stain). *E,* The smear from bone marrow aspirate shows a striking increase in small lymphocytes (Wright-Giemsa stain).

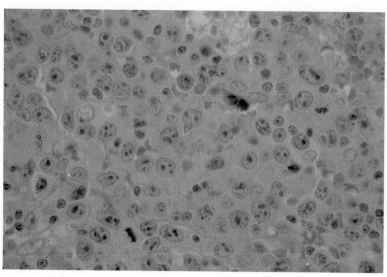

Figure 3–5. B-cell chronic lymphocytic leukemia with an area of large cell transformation shows sheets of immunoblasts (Giemsa stain).

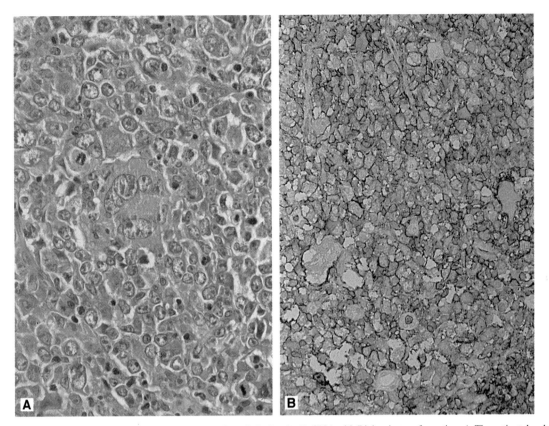

Figure 3–6. Older woman with a history of B-cell chronic lymphocytic leukemia (B-CLL) with Richter's transformation. *A,* The patient developed a large polypoid mass within the uterine cavity. Examination revealed a high grade malignant tumor composed of bizarre, pleomorphic cells (H&E stain). *B,* The tumor cells are CD45+ (shown here) and CD20+, supporting the interpretation of transformation of B-CLL (immunoperoxidase technique on paraffin section).

Rarely, otherwise typically appearing cases of B-CLL contain large cells resembling Reed-Sternberg (RS) cells both morphologically and immunophenotypically (CD15+, CD30+, L26+/−). In most of these cases, the RS-like cells are infected with Epstein-Barr virus (EBV) and express EBV latent membrane protein (LMP) (Fig. 3–7). Some of these patients develop a Richter's-like transformation that resembles Hodgkin's disease. It has been suggested that EBV is involved in the transformation of the CLL in such cases (Fig. 3–8).

Immunophenotype

Neoplastic cells express faint sIgM+, sIgD+/−, B-cell-associated antigen+ (CD19+, CD20+, CD79a+) (often faint), CD22−/+, CD5+, CD23+, CD43+, CD11c−/+ (faint), and CD10−. A minority of cases have cytoplasmic Ig, which is consistent with plasmacytic differentiation.

Genetics

Ig heavy and light chain genes are clonally rearranged. The variable region of the heavy chain gene shows little or no somatic mutation, corresponding to a "naive" B cell (one not previously exposed to antigen). Approximately half of all cases have cytogenetic abnormalities. Trisomy 12 and abnormalities of 13q and 14q are the most frequent chromosomal abnormalities. Translocation t(14;19), involving the putative oncogene bcl-3 on chromosome 19, occurs rarely and may be found in association with trisomy 12. Trisomy 12 may be present in a higher proportion of cases that develop Richter's syndrome. Trisomy 12 is also associated with atypical morphology, i.e., cases with a high proportion of prolymphocytes (>10% but < 55%) in the peripheral blood (CLL/PLL) and with atypical immunophenotypic features, including bright CD20 expression, bright surface light chain expression, and absence of CD23. Abnormalities of 13q often involve deletions in the area of 13q12−13q14; several tumor suppressor genes in this portion of 13q may be involved in the development or progression of CLL. These include RB1 (the retinoblastoma gene), DBM (deleted in B-cell malignancy), and BRCA2 (breast cancer susceptibility gene). One group has demonstrated frequent deletions of BRCA2 in B-CLL and suggests that loss of BRCA2 may be involved in the pathogenesis of a substantial number of cases of B-CLL.

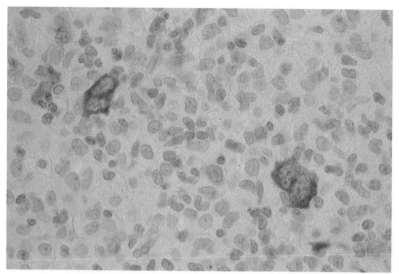

Figure 3–7. B-cell chronic lymphocytic leukemia with large cells reminiscent of Reed-Sternberg cells, expressing Epstein-Barr virus latent membrane protein (immunoperoxidase technique on paraffin section).

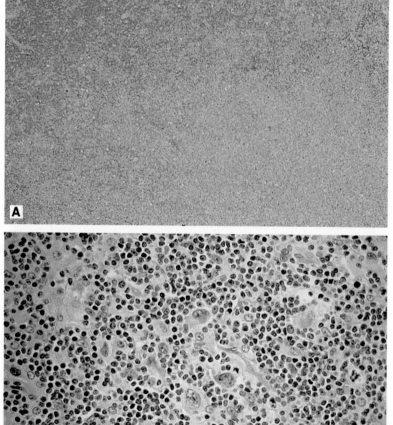

Figure 3–8. B-cell chronic lymphocytic leukemia (B-CLL) with Hodgkin's disease–like transformation. *A,* Low power view shows a dark area of residual B-CLL and a pale area with Hodgkin's disease–like transformation (H&E stain). *B,* In the area with CLL, scattered large cells have the appearance of Reed-Sternberg cell variants (H&E stain).

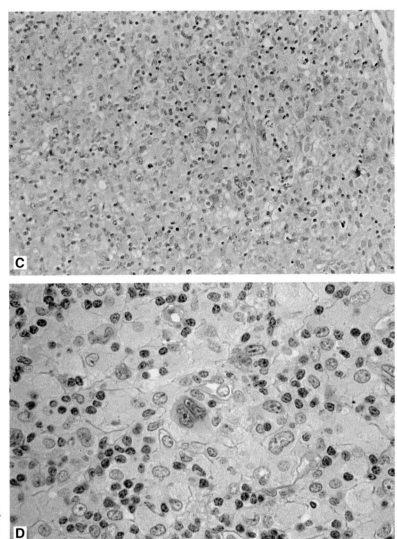

Figure 3–8. *Continued C,* In the Hodgkin's disease–like area, large atypical cells are scattered in a background of lymphocytes and histiocytes (H&E stain). *D,* Binucleate Reed-Sternberg cells are present occasionally (H&E stain).

Analysis of cases of Richter's transformation has caused some debate concerning the origin of the large cell lymphoma. Although some studies suggested that the large cell lymphoma represents a second primary tumor in some cases, other studies support a clonal relationship between the B-CLL and the large cell lymphoma in most instances.

Postulated Normal Counterpart

Recirculating naive CD5+, CD23+ peripheral B cell.

Differential Diagnosis

1. Mantle cell lymphoma (MCL): When nuclear irregularity is prominent in cases of B-CLL, a diagnosis of MCL may be considered. The presence of pseudofollicles, prolymphocytes, and paraimmunoblasts excludes MCL.

MCLs are nearly always CD23−, whereas B-CLL is CD23+. B-CLL is almost always negative for cyclin D1.
2. Follicle center lymphoma (FCL): When the pseudofollicular pattern is prominent, FCL may enter the differential diagnosis. True neoplastic follicles are almost always better circumscribed than pseudofollicles, and the cells of FCL are usually more prominently cleaved. FCLs are CD5−, CD10+/−. Bcl-2 expression is not helpful in distinguishing the two because it is found in both B-CLL and FCL.
3. B-cell prolymphocytic leukemia (B-PLL): Patients with de novo B-PLL present with splenomegaly and an extremely high white blood cell count. More than 55% of cells in the peripheral blood are prolymphocytes. The prognosis is poor. Prolymphocytic transformation of B-CLL may be considered in the differential diagnosis of B-PLL. In favor of de novo B-PLL are the clinical features, lack of a prior history of B-CLL, strong sIg

expression, CD22 expression, and absence of CD5. Immunophenotypic features, however, may not provide definitive distinction; for example, loss of CD5 has been described during prolymphocytic transformation of B-CLL.

4. T-cell chronic lymphocytic leukemia (T-CLL): T-CLL is not associated with the formation of pseudofollicles and often shows increased vascularity in involved lymph nodes. Immunophenotyping is required for a definitive diagnosis.

5. Non-neoplastic lymphoid aggregates: Non-neoplastic lymphoid aggregates are commonly found in the bone marrow of older adults, and may raise the suspicion of CLL with a nodular pattern. In favor of a diagnosis of CLL are the relatively large size and number of poorly circumscribed aggregates that infiltrate the surrounding hematopoietic marrow.

References

Ben-Ezra J, Burke J, Swartz W, *et al*: Small lymphocytic lymphoma: a clinicopathologic analysis of 268 cases. Blood 73:579–587, 1989.

Bennett J, Catovsky D, Daniel M-T, *et al*: Proposals for the classification of chronic (mature) B and T lymphoid leukemias. J Clin Pathol 42:567–584, 1989.

Brecher M, Banks P: Hodgkin's disease variant of Richter's syndrome: report of eight cases. Am J Clin Pathol 93:333–339, 1990.

Brittinger G, Bartels H, Common H, *et al*: Clinical and prognostic relevance of the Kiel classification of non-Hodgkin lymphomas: results of a prospective multicenter study by the Kiel Lymphoma Study Group. Hematol Oncol 2:269–306, 1984.

Brynes RK, McCourty A, Sun NCJ, Koo CH: Trisomy 12 in Richter's transformation of chronic lymphocytic leukemia. Am J Clin Pathol 104:199–203, 1995.

Faguet GB: Chronic lymphocytic leukemia: an updated review. J Clin Oncol 12:1974–1990, 1994.

Finn WG, Thangavelu M, Yelavarthi KK, *et al*: Karyotype correlates with peripheral blood morphology and immunophenotype in chronic lymphocytic leukemia. Am J Clin Pathol 105:458–467, 1996.

Garcia-Marco JA, Caldas C, Price CM, *et al*: Frequent somatic deletion of the 13q12.3 locus encompassing BRCA2 in chronic lymphocytic leukemia. Blood 88(5):1568–1575, 1996.

Harris N, Bhan A: B-cell neoplasms of the lymphocytic, lymphoplasmacytoid, and plasma cell types: immunohistologic analysis and clinical correlation. Hum Pathol 16:829–837, 1985.

Kipps T: The CD5 B cell. Adv Immunol 47:117–185, 1989.

Lennert K, Tamm I, Wacker H-H: Histopathology and immunocytochemistry of lymph node biopsies in chronic lymphocytic leukemia and immunocytoma. Leuk Lymphoma (Suppl):157–160, 1991.

O'Brien S, del Giglio A, Keating M: Advances in biology and treatment of B-cell chronic lymphocytic leukemia. Blood 85:307–318, 1995.

Richter M: Generalized reticular cell sarcoma of lymph nodes associated with lymphocytic leukemia. Am J Pathol 4:285–292, 1928.

Zukerberg L, Medeiros L, Ferry J, Harris N: Diffuse low-grade B-cell lymphomas: four clinically distinct subtypes defined by a combination of morphologic and immunophenotypic features. Am J Clin Pathol 100:373–385, 1993.

LYMPHOPLASMACYTIC LYMPHOMA (LPL)/IMMUNOCYTOMA

Synonyms: Rappaport: well-differentiated lymphocytic, plasmacytoid; diffuse mixed lymphocytic and histiocytic; Kiel: immunocytoma, lymphoplasmacytic type; Lukes-Collins: plasmacytic-lymphocytic; Working Formulation: small lymphocytic, plasmacytoid; diffuse mixed small and large cell, plasmacytoid.

Clinical Features

LPL/immunocytoma is a rare disorder that predominantly affects older adults. The bone marrow, lymph nodes, and spleen are frequently involved. Other extranodal sites and peripheral blood are involved less often. Most patients have a monoclonal serum paraprotein of IgM type. Most patients with Waldenström's macroglobulinemia have LPL. The course is indolent. LPL usually is not curable with available treatment. Transformation to large cell lymphoma may occur.

Morphology

The tumor consists of small lymphocytes, plasmacytoid lymphocytes (cells with abundant basophilic cytoplasm, but lymphocyte-like nuclei), and plasma cells, and by definition, lacks features of B-CLL, mantle cell, follicle center, or marginal zone lymphomas. In lymph nodes, the growth pattern may be diffuse with obliteration of the underlying nodal architecture, or the infiltrate may be interfollicular with sparing of the sinuses. Plasmacytoid lymphocytes and plasma cells may be intermingled with small lymphocytes or may form relatively discrete zones. Dutcher bodies—intranuclear protrusions of Ig-containing cytoplasm that stain positively with a PAS stain—may be found in the neoplastic cells. In some cases, cytoplasmic immunoglobulin is abundant in plasma cells, and they may acquire the shape of signet-ring cells (Figs. 3–9 and 3–10).

In the bone marrow, LPL may produce poorly circumscribed aggregates or diffuse infiltrates of small lymphoid cells, plasmacytoid lymphocytes, and plasma cells. Involvement ranges from focal and rather subtle to extensive. The neoplastic population can usually be identified on smears from aspirates (Fig. 3–11).

When large cell transformation occurs, the neoplastic cells usually have the appearance of centroblasts or immunoblasts (Fig. 3–12).

Immunophenotype

Tumor cells are sIg+, cIg+ (some cells) usually of IgM type, usually without IgD. They have B-cell-associated antigens CD19+, CD20+, CD22+, CD79a+, CD5−, CD10−, CD43+/−, CD25−/+, or CD11c−/+.

Genetic Features

Ig heavy and light chain genes are clonally rearranged. Ig genes show somatic mutation, indicating a post-antigen-stimulated stage.

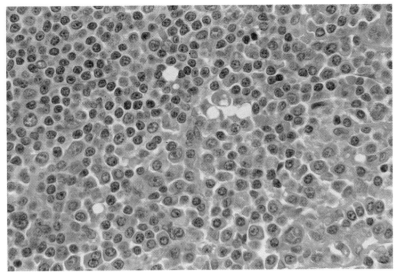

Figure 3–9. This lymphoplasmacytic lymphoma consists of a mixture of small lymphocytes and plasma cells (H&E stain).

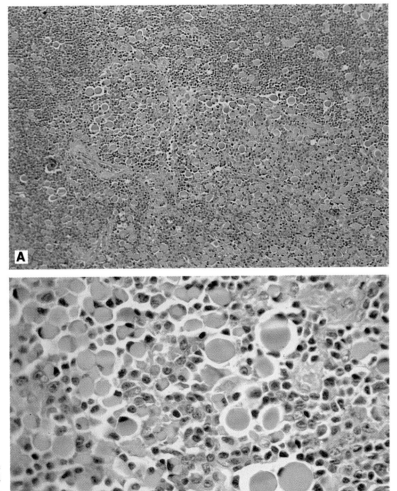

Figure 3–10. Lymphoplasmacytic lymphoma. *A,* This case shows a broad eosinophilic zone of plasma cells (H&E stain). *B,* Higher power examination shows that the cytoplasm of the plasma cells is distended by immunoglobulin, giving it a hyaline pink appearance. The plasma cells resemble signet ring cells, except that their cytoplasm is not clear (H&E stain).

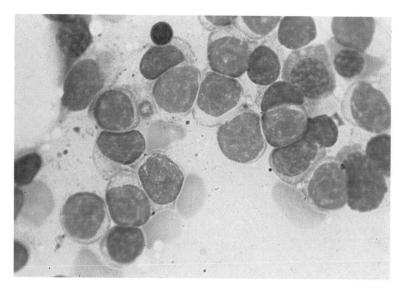

Figure 3–11. Lymphoplasmacytic lymphoma associated with Waldenström's macroglobulinemia. A smear of bone marrow aspirate shows numerous plasmacytoid lymphocytes (Wright-Giemsa stain).

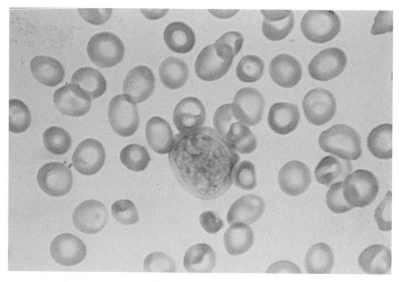

Figure 3–12. Large cell transformation of lymphoplasmacytic lymphoma. Large lymphoid cells are found in the peripheral blood in this case (Wright-Giemsa stain).

Postulated Normal Counterpart

CD5− peripheral B lymphocyte stimulated to differentiate into a plasma cell.

Differential Diagnosis

1. Other low grade B-cell lymphomas (B-cell chronic lymphocytic leukemia [B-CLL], follicle center lymphoma [FCL], and marginal zone cell lymphoma) may occasionally exhibit plasmacytic differentiation or may be associated with a serum paraprotein and enter the differential diagnosis of LPL. If the specimen demonstrates specific histologic features of any of the foregoing entities, LPL is excluded. CD5 expression (found in B-CLL) or CD10 expression (often found in FCL) tends to rule out LPL. In contrast to LPL, marginal zone lymphomas contain a component of marginal zone cells, but the distinction between the two can be difficult. Unlike LPL, mantle cell lymphomas have scant cytoplasm, express CD5, and do not show plasmacytic differentiation.

2. Plasma cell myeloma: Cases of LPL with predominant bone marrow involvement may be included in the differential diagnosis of myeloma. Lack of a lymphocytic component and IgG, IgA, or light chain only expression (in contrast to IgM) favor myeloma over LPL.

3. Castleman's disease: *See* Castleman's Disease, Chapter 2.

References

Harris N, Bhan A: B-cell neoplasms of the lymphocytic, lymphoplasmacytoid, and plasma cell types: immunohistologic analysis and clinical correlation. Hum Pathol 16:829–837, 1985.

Lennert K, Tamm I, Wacker H-H: Histopathology and immunocytochemistry of lymph node biopsies in chronic lymphocytic leukemia and immunocytoma. Leuk Lymphoma (Suppl):157–160, 1991.

Stein H, Lennert K, Feller A, Mason D: Immunohistological analysis of human lymphoma: correlation of histological and immunological categories. Adv Cancer Res 42:67–147, 1984.

Zukerberg L, Medeiros L, Ferry J, Harris N: Diffuse low-grade B-cell lymphomas: four clinically distinct subtypes defined by a combination of morphologic and immunophenotypic features. Am J Clin Pathol 100:373–385, 1993.

MANTLE CELL LYMPHOMA (MCL)

Synonyms: Rappaport: intermediate lymphocytic or poorly differentiated lymphocytic, diffuse or nodular; Kiel: centrocytic (mantle cell) lymphoma; Lukes-Collins: small cleaved follicular center cell; Working Formulation: small cleaved cell, diffuse or nodular; rarely diffuse mixed or large cleaved cell; other: mantle zone lymphoma.

Clinical Features

Mantle cell lymphoma (MCL) accounts for about 5% to 6% of adult non-Hodgkin's lymphoma in the United States and Europe. It occurs in older adults, affecting men more often than women. It is usually widespread at the time of diagnosis. The sites most commonly involved are lymph nodes, spleen, Waldeyer's ring, bone marrow, blood, and the gastrointestinal tract (multiple lymphomatous polyposis). It is a moderately aggressive lymphoma that seems incurable with available treatment. The median length of survival ranges from 3 to 5 years. Survival may be longer in cases in which the lymphoma has a nodular or a mantle zone pattern rather than a diffuse pattern, but is shorter in cases of the blastoid variant. Transformation from MCL of the usual type to the blastoid variant occurs, although transformation to a large cell lymphoma composed of centroblast or immunoblast-like cells is not a feature of MCL.

Morphology

Mantle cell lymphoma (MCL) usually has a diffuse or vaguely nodular pattern (Fig. 3–13). In many cases the tumor involves the mantle zones of some reactive follicles; less commonly, a mantle zone pattern occurs throughout the involved tissue (Fig. 3–14). MCL is typically composed exclusively of small to medium-sized lymphoid cells, usually slightly larger than normal lymphocytes, with more dispersed chromatin, scant pale cytoplasm, and inconspicuous nucleoli. The nuclei are usually irregular (Fig. 3–15). In some cases, however, the cells are nearly round and in others they may be very small and resemble normal lymphocytes. Large transformed cells with basophilic cytoplasm (centroblast or immunoblast-like cells) are rare or absent. A small proportion of cases have larger nuclei with more dispersed chromatin and a high proliferation fraction reminiscent of lymphoblastic lymphoma; the term "blastoid variant" has been applied to these cases (Fig. 3–16). Many cases contain individually scattered epithelioid histiocytes, creating a starry-sky appearance at low magnification (see Fig. 3–13).

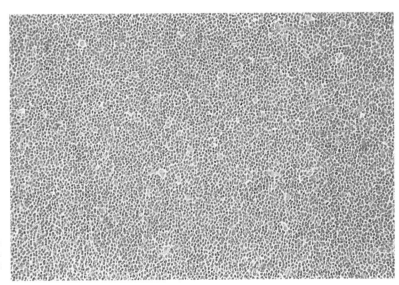

Figure 3–13. Mantle cell lymphoma, diffuse pattern. This case had a diffuse infiltrate of small lymphoid cells with single pale histiocytes scattered among the neoplastic cells (H&E stain).

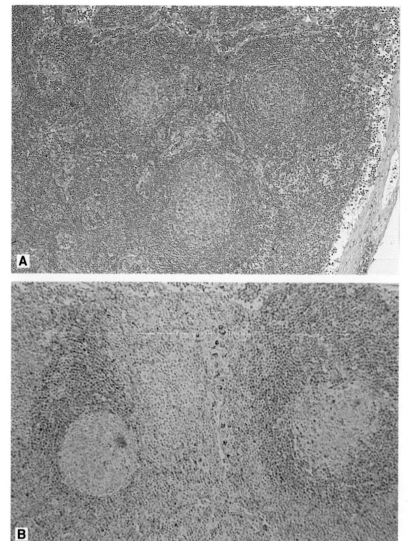

Figure 3–14. Mantle cell lymphoma, mantle zone pattern. *A,* Neoplastic cells are confined more or less to the mantles of follicles with residual reactive germinal centers (H&E stain). *B,* Neoplastic cells in mantle zones are highlighted with an antibody to cyclin D1 (immunoperoxidase technique on paraffin section).

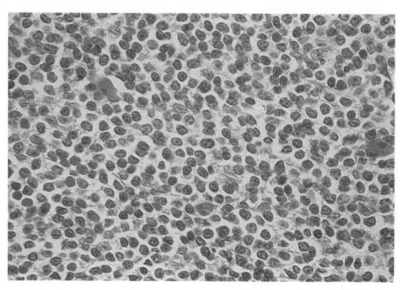

Figure 3–15. Mantle cell lymphoma. The lymphoma is composed of a monotonous population of lymphoid cells that are marginally larger than normal lymphocytes, with slightly more irregular nuclei and slightly more open chromatin. Cytoplasm is scant (H&E stain).

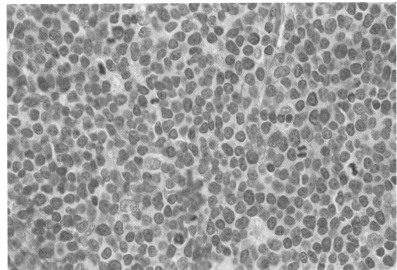

Figure 3–16. Mantle cell lymphoma (MCL), blastoid variant. Neoplastic cells are slightly larger than in the usual case of MCL. The chromatin is finely dispersed and the mitotic rate is high (H&E stain).

When the gastrointestinal (GI) tract is involved by MCL, it is frequently in the form of multiple lymphomatous polyposis (MLP). MLP can occur anywhere in the GI tract, but the colon is involved most often. On gross examination, the normal mucosa is replaced by innumerable smooth-surfaced polyps, usually ranging from a few millimeters to 2 cm in greatest dimension; larger polyps are seen occasionally. On microscopic examination, the lamina propria is filled and expanded by multiple nodules of mantle cells. Some nodules may contain residual reactive germinal centers. In some cases, the nodularity is less apparent and the infiltrate appears diffuse. The regional lymph nodes are usually involved by MCL in patients with MLP. Other types of lymphoma rarely take the form of MLP, but this pattern of involvement is usually due to MCL (Fig. 3–17).

Bone marrow involvement appears most often in the form of infiltrative interstitial collections or nodular aggregates of small irregular lymphoid cells that are more often intertrabecular than paratrabecular. Less frequently, marrow involvement is diffuse (Fig. 3–18). The neoplastic cells are usually recognizable on the aspirate smear when the core biopsy specimen shows lymphoma. In aspirate smears and in the peripheral blood, MCL has the appearance of small to intermediate-sized lymphoid cells (7 to 10 μm) with round, slightly irregular or cleaved nuclei, condensed chromatin, sometimes one to two small inconspicuous nucleoli, and scant cytoplasm. MCL in the spleen is usually confined to the white pulp (Fig. 3–19).

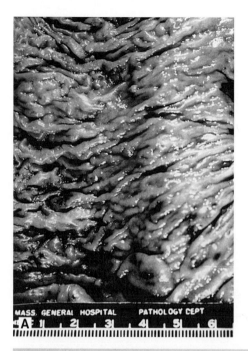

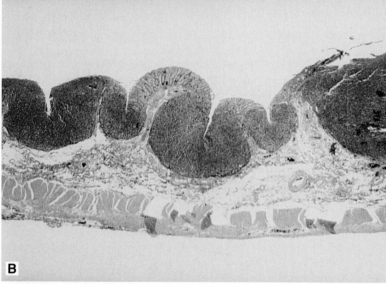

Figure 3–17. Multiple lymphomatous polyposis. *A,* The mucosa of the colon shows extensive, finely nodular thickening. *B,* The lamina propria shows a dense infiltrate of neoplastic mantle cells (H&E stain).

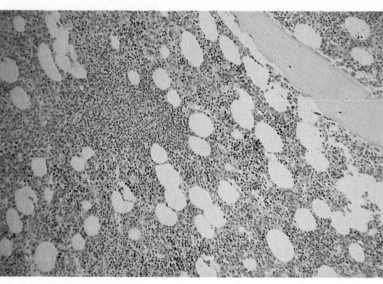

Figure 3–18. Mantle cell lymphoma, bone marrow involvement. This specimen shows two poorly circumscribed, nonparatrabecular lymphoid aggregates (larger one, *upper left*; smaller one, *lower right*) (Giemsa stain).

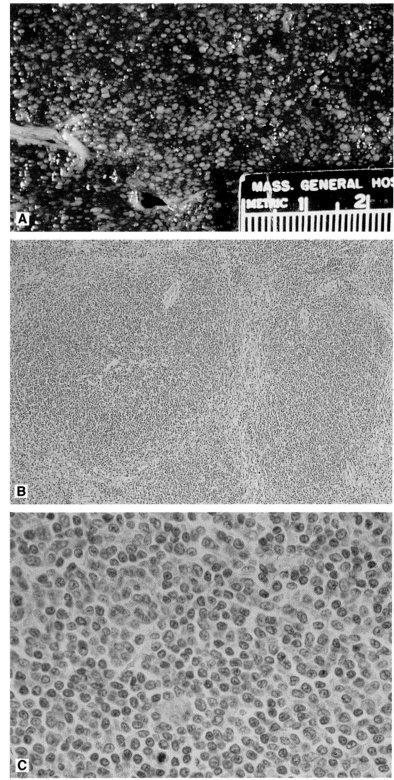

Figure 3–19 Mantle cell lymphoma involving the spleen. *A,* The spleen is greatly enlarged. Gross inspection shows prominent white pulp. *B,* On microscopic examination, mantle cells have replaced the normal white pulp elements, producing multiple large, crowded nodules (Giemsa stain). *C,* The mantle cells are small, slightly irregular lymphoid cells. Large transformed cells are absent (Giemsa stain).

Immunophenotype

Tumor cells are sIgM+, IgD+, λ > κ, with B-cell-associated antigen (CD19+, CD20+, CD22+), CD5+, CD10−, CD23−, CD43+, CD11c−, and nuclear cyclin D1+. A prominent, disorganized meshwork of follicular dendritic cells (FDC) may be demonstrated using antibodies to CD21 or CD23. Among reactive and neoplastic lymphoid proliferations, nuclear cyclin D1 expression is unique to MCL with rare exceptions (Fig. 3–14*B*).

Genetic Features

Ig heavy and light chain genes are clonally rearranged, with little or no somatic mutation, which is consistent with derivation from a pregerminal center stage B-cell. In most cases, a chromosomal translocation t(11;14) involves the Ig heavy chain locus and the bcl-1 locus on the long arm of chromosome 11. This translocation is associated with overexpression of the cyclin D1 (PRAD1) gene and with high levels of cyclin D1 mRNA and protein.

Postulated Normal Counterpart

CD5+, CD23− pre-antigen stimulation peripheral B cell of inner follicle mantle.

Differential Diagnosis

1. B-cell chronic lymphocytic leukemia (B-CLL): The presence of prolymphocytes and paraimmunoblasts excludes MCL. Unlike MCL, B-CLL typically expresses CD23 and is almost always negative for cyclin D1.
2. Follicle center lymphoma (FCL): FCL is characteristically composed of a mixture of small cleaved cells (frequently more irregular than the cells of MCL) and large noncleaved cells (centroblasts); the latter are not found in MCL. FCL is CD5−, cyclin D1−, and CD43−.
3. Marginal zone cell lymphoma: Unlike MCL, marginal zone cell lymphoma is composed of CD5− cells, which typically have abundant cytoplasm, frequent plasmacytic differentiation, and occasional admixed blast cells. Cyclin D1 expression is absent. D heavy chain expression is much more common in MCL.

    When MCL has prominent splenic involvement, splenic marginal zone cell lymphoma (SMZL) may be included in the differential diagnosis. In addition to the differential features just described for marginal zone cell lymphoma in general, the following may be helpful in the differential diagnosis with SMZL: Even when MCL is associated with prominent splenomegaly, it usually also produces peripheral lymphadenopathy, in contrast to SMZL. Both lymphomas have white pulp involvement, but red pulp involvement is typically inconspicuous in MCL and may be prominent in SMZL.
4. Lymphoblastic lymphoma: See the earlier discussion of precursor B-lymphoblastic lymphoma/leukemia.

References

de Boer CJ, van Krieken JH, Kluin-Nelemans HC, *et al*: Cyclin D1 messenger RNA overexpression as a marker for mantle cell lymphoma. Oncogene 10:1833–1840, 1995.

Harris N, Nadler L, Bhan A: Immunohistologic characterization of two malignant lymphomas of germinal center type (centroblastic/centrocytic and centrocytic) with monoclonal antibodies: follicular and diffuse lymphomas of small cleaved cell types are related but distinct entities. Am J Pathol 117:262–272, 1984.

Hummel M, Tamaru J, Kalvelage B, Stein H: Mantle cell (previously centrocytic) lymphomas express VH genes with no or very little somatic mutations like the physiologic cells of the follicle mantle. Blood 84:403–407, 1994.

Inghirami G, Foitl D, Sabichi A, *et al*: Autoantibody-associated cross-reactive idiotype-bearing human B lymphocytes: distribution and characterization, including IgVH gene and CD5 antigen expression. Blood 78:1503–1515, 1991.

Lardelli P, Bookman M, Sundeen J, *et al*: Lymphocytic lymphoma of intermediate differentiation. Morphologic and immunophenotypic spectrum and clinical correlations. Am J Surg Pathol 14:752–763, 1990.

Lennert K, Feller A: Histopathology of Non-Hodgkin's Lymphomas. New York: Springer-Verlag, 1992.

Medeiros L, van Krieken J, Jaffe E, Raffeld M: Association of bcl-1 rearrangements with lymphocytic lymphoma of intermediate differentiation. Blood 76:2086–2090, 1990.

Norton AJ, Matthews J, Pappa V, *et al*: Mantle cell lymphoma: natural history defined in a serially biopsied population over a 20-year period. Ann Oncol 6:249–256, 1995.

Pittaluga S, Wlodarska I, Stul MS, *et al*: Mantle cell lymphoma: a clinicopathologic study of 55 cases. Histopathology 26:17–24, 1995.

Rosenberg C, Wong E, Petty E, *et al*: Overexpression of PRAD1, a candidate BCL1 breakpoint region oncogene, in centrocytic lymphomas. Proc Natl Acad Sci USA 88:9638–9642, 1991.

Segal GH, Masih AS, Fox AC, *et al*: CD5− expressing B-cell non-Hodgkin's lymphomas with bcl-1 gene rearrangement have a relatively homogeneous immunophenotype and are associated with an overall poor prognosis. Blood 85(6):1570–1579, 1995.

Swerdlow SH, Zukerberg LR, Yang W-I, *et al*: The morphologic spectrum of non-Hodgkin's lymphomas with BCL/1 cyclin D1 gene rearrangements. Am J Surg Pathol 20(5):627–640, 1996.

Wasman J, Rosenthal NS, Farhi DC: Mantle cell lymphoma. Morphologic findings in bone marrow involvement. Am J Clin Pathol 106:196–200, 1996.

Zucca E, Roggero E, Pinotti G, *et al*: Patterns of survival in mantle cell lymphoma. Ann Oncol 63:257–262, 1995.

Zukerberg LR, Yang W-I, Arnold A, Harris NL: Cyclin D1 expression in non-Hodgkin's lymphomas. Detection by immunohistochemistry. Am J Clin Pathol 103:756–760, 1995.

FOLLICLE CENTER LYMPHOMA (FCL)

Follicle Center Lymphoma, Follicular (FCL-F): (Provisional Cytologic Grades—I [Predominantly Small Cell], II [Mixed Small and Large Cell], III [Predominantly Large Cell])

Synonyms: Rappaport: nodular poorly differentiated lymphocytic, mixed lymphocytic-histiocytic, or histiocytic; Kiel: centroblastic/centrocytic follicular; follicular centroblastic; Lukes-Collins: small cleaved, large cleaved, or large noncleaved, follicular center cell; Working Formulation: follicular, small cleaved, mixed, or large cell.

Follicle Center Lymphoma, Diffuse (FCL-D) (Provisional Subtype; Predominantly Small Cell)

Synonyms: Rappaport: diffuse poorly differentiated lymphocytic; Kiel: centroblastic/centrocytic, diffuse; Lukes-Collins: diffuse small cleaved follicular center cell; Working Formulation: diffuse small cleaved cell, diffuse mixed.

The overwhelming majority of cases of follicle center lymphoma (FCL) have a follicular architecture, at least focally. Rarely, lymphomas with the cellular composition and immunophenotype of FCL are entirely diffuse; it may be assumed that they represent the diffuse counterpart of a follicle center lymphoma. Such lymphomas are designated follicle center lymphoma, diffuse (FCL-D). FCL with follicular and diffuse patterns are considered together in the following discussion.

Clinical Features

FCL is the most common adult non-Hodgkin's lymphoma in the United States (40% of cases); the incidence is apparently lower elsewhere. FCL predominantly affects adults, with males and females equally affected. Most patients have widespread disease at diagnosis. Lymph nodes are most commonly involved, but FCL may also involve spleen, bone marrow, and occasionally peripheral blood; rarely, extranodal sites such as the gastrointestinal tract or skin are involved. The clinical course is generally indolent. FCL usually is not curable with available treatment, although some data suggest that a subset of patients may be cured with aggressive therapy. A better prognosis is associated with a predominant follicular pattern. Both the number of centroblasts and the size of the centrocytes also appear to correlate with prognosis. Transformation to diffuse large B-cell lymphoma occurs more frequently with FCL than with other low grade lymphomas.

Morphology

FCL-F is composed of a mixture of follicle center cells, usually a majority of centrocytes (cleaved follicle center cells) and a minority of centroblasts (large noncleaved follicle center cells). The pattern is at least partially follicular, but diffuse areas may be present. Neoplastic follicles usually fill the node from capsule to hilus; frequently, abnormal follicles invade the capsule and perinodal soft tissue, with splitting and reduplication of the capsule. Follicles are often crowded, and mantle zones may be attenuated or absent. Sclerosis is common in diffuse areas (Fig. 3–20).

The proportion of centroblasts and the size of the centrocytes vary among cases. Follicle center lymphoma cannot be sharply divided into distinct subtypes but rather shows a continuous gradation in the number of large cells. In the United States, follicular lymphomas have been separated into three categories: predominantly small, mixed small and large, and predominantly large cell. Because this terminology implies distinct tumor types, the use of the terms FCL-F, Grade I, Grade II, and Grade III is suggested in the R.E.A.L. Classification. Methods of grading vary among institutions. At the Massachusetts General Hospital, the criteria proposed by Mann and Berard are used to grade FCLs, i.e., 0 to 5 large cells/hpf = Grade I/predominantly small cleaved; 6 to 15 large cells/hpf = Grade II/mixed; 16 or more large cells/hpf = Grade III/predominantly large cell (Fig. 3–20 *C, D,* and *E*).

Rarely, FCL has a component of cells resembling signet-ring cells caused by cytoplasmic accumulation of Ig (Fig. 3–21). An unusual variant of follicle center lymphoma, known as the floral variant, is characterized by a proliferation of follicles with prominent mantle zones that invaginate into the follicle center, dividing the follicle center into multiple lobules that impart an appearance reminiscent of a flower's petals. This variant is especially likely to cause problems in the differential diagnosis with follicular hyperplasia. Neoplastic follicles of this type may mimic follicles with follicle lysis (Fig. 3–22; *compare with* Fig. 1–13).

Bone marrow involvement typically takes the form of paratrabecular lymphoid aggregates (Fig. 3–23). In the spleen, FCL predominantly involves the white pulp, although small aggregates of neoplastic cells may be found in the red pulp. Nodules of FCL in the spleen may closely mimic normal white pulp. A nodular pattern of involvement of the spleen by lymphoma is not diagnostic of FCL; a variety of lymphomas involve white pulp, producing a nodular but not a true follicular pattern.

High grade transformation takes the form of a diffuse large B-cell lymphoma (Fig. 3–24).

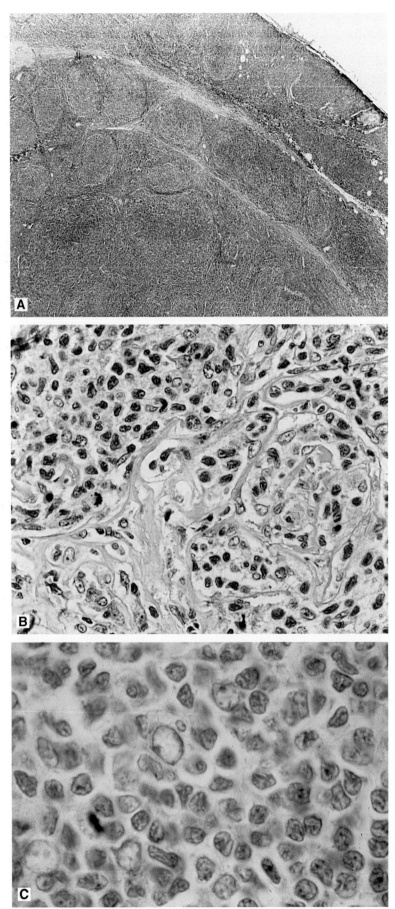

Figure 3–20. Follicle center lymphoma (FCL). *A,* Follicle center lymphoma, follicular pattern. Neoplastic follicles invade the capsule of the lymph node, where they are associated with splitting and reduplication of the capsule (H&E stain). *B,* FCL, diffuse pattern. Diffuse areas of FCLs, as in this case, are often associated with sclerosis, so that neoplastic cells are divided into irregular nests (H&E stain). (*A* and *B,* from Harris NL, Ferry JA: Follicular lymphomas and related disorders. *In:* Knowles DM, ed. Neoplastic hematopathology. Baltimore: Williams & Wilkins, 1992; 645–674.) *C,* Grade I FCL. Centrocytes (small cleaved cells) predominate, with only rare centroblasts (large non-cleaved cells) appearing (Giemsa stain).

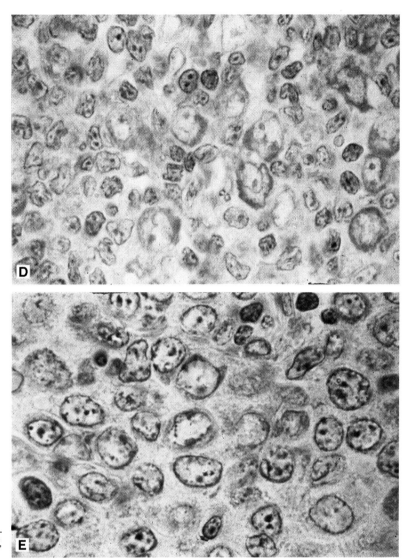

Figure 3–20. *Continued D,* Grade II FCL. There is a mixture of centrocytes and centroblasts (Giemsa stain). *E,* Grade III FCL. Centroblasts predominate (Giemsa stain).

Immunophenotype

The tumor cells are usually sIg+ (IgM > IgG > IgA, with or without IgD), B-cell-associated antigen+ (CD19+, CD20+, CD22+, CD79a+), CD10+/−, CD5−, CD23−/+, CD43−, CD11c−, and bcl-2 protein+. Tightly organized meshworks of FDC are present in follicular areas.

Genetic Features

Ig heavy and light chain genes are clonally rearranged. They also show a high rate of somatic mutation and a high rate of intraclonal variability, which is consistent with ongoing mutation analogous to non-neoplastic follicle center cells. In 70% to 95% of cases, cytogenetic studies reveal a (14;18)(q32;q21) translocation. This t(14;18) results in rearrangement of the bcl-2 gene, which causes expression of an "anti-apoptosis" gene that normally is switched off at the translational level in follicle center cells.

Postulated Normal Counterpart

Follicle center B cells, both centrocytes (small cleaved follicle center cells) and centroblasts (large noncleaved follicle center cells).

Differential Diagnosis

1. Reactive lymphoid hyperplasia (RLH): Cases of RLH with a prominent component of follicular hyperplasia may be difficult to distinguish from FCL. Reactive follicles typically vary in size and shape, have discrete mantle zones, are not crowded, do not extend outside the lymph node, and are composed of lymphoid cells of various types with frequent mitoses and admixed tingible body macrophages. In contrast, neoplastic follicles tend to be crowded and uniform in size, to fill the node from the hilus to the capsule, often extending into perinodal tissue, to lack well formed mantle zones, and to be com-

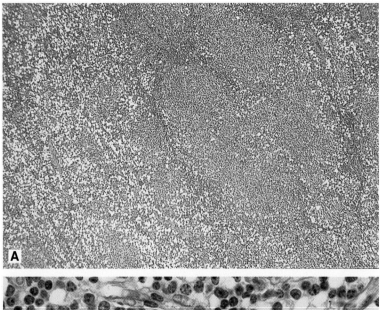

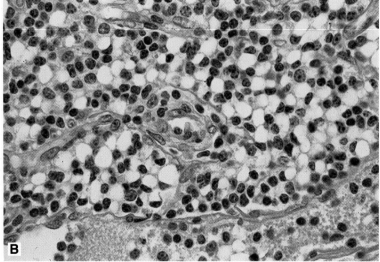

Figure 3–21. Follicle center lymphoma, signet ring variant. *A,* At low power, the nodal architecture is obliterated by a proliferation of poorly circumscribed follicles surrounded by a predominantly diffuse infiltrate of cells with clear cytoplasm (H&E stain). *B,* At high power, these neoplastic B cells resemble signet ring cells (H&E stain).

posed of a relatively monomorphous population of cells, with few mitoses and rare or absent tingible body macrophages. In FCL, follicle center cells are often present outside follicles. Neoplastic follicles only rarely show "polarization."

Frozen section immunohistochemistry demonstrates polytypic Ig in reactive follicles, whereas neoplastic follicles express monotypic Ig, or rarely, are negative for Ig. When only paraffin-embedded tissue is available, staining for bcl-2 protein can be definitive. Neoplastic follicles are almost always bcl-2+, whereas B cells in reactive follicle centers are bcl-2−. T cells in reactive follicles, which may be numerous, express bcl-2 protein. Thus, bcl-2 protein expression should be interpreted only in conjunction with B- and T-cell markers. In addition, primary follicles or other lymphoid nodules without germinal centers will be bcl-2+; therefore, this antigen is useful only in distinguishing reactive follicle centers from FCL.

2. Mantle cell lymphomas (MCL) have a nodular or a diffuse pattern, and thus may enter the differential diagnosis of FCL-F and FCL-D. The presence of blast cells excludes MCL. In contrast to FCL, MCL is CD5+, cyclin D1+. Both FCL and MCL express bcl-2 protein, which thus is not useful in differential diagnosis.
3. Marginal zone B-cell lymphomas with prominent follicular colonization can mimic FCL-F, and those without follicular colonization can mimic FCL-D. In contrast to FCL, marginal zone B-cell lymphomas are CD10− and often have neoplastic cells with abundant pale cytoplasm, plasmacytic differentiation, and in certain extranodal sites, lymphoepithelial lesions. Although bcl-2 can be useful in distinguishing reactive follicle centers in marginal zone B-cell lymphoma from FCL, colonized follicles may be bcl-2+ and mimic FCL.

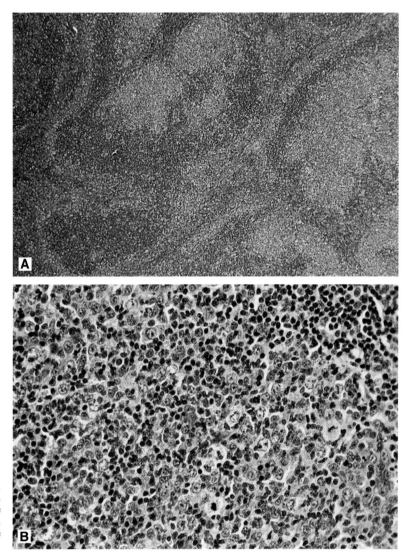

Figure 3–22. Follicle center lymphoma, floral variant. *A,* At low power, multiple large follicles fill the lymph node. Slender bands of mantle cells invade the neoplastic follicle center, producing a lobated or floral pattern (H&E stain). *B,* The high power view shows a mixture of small and large follicle center cells (H&E stain).

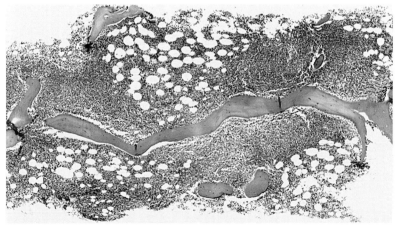

Figure 3–23. Bone marrow involvement in follicle center lymphoma (FCL). Bone marrow involvement in cases of FCL most often has a paratrabecular pattern, as seen in this case, in which the lymphoma is unusually extensive (H&E stain). (From Harris NL, Ferry JA: Follicular lymphomas and related disorders. *In:* Knowles DM, ed. Neoplastic hematopathology. Baltimore: Williams & Wilkins, 1992; 645–674.)

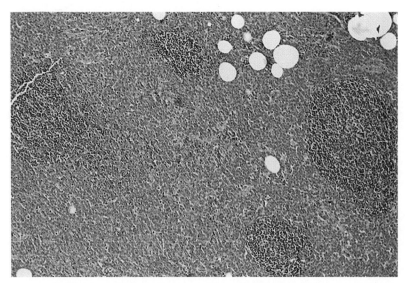

Figure 3–24. Follicle center lymphoma with large cell transformation. A low grade component remains in the form of a few dark neoplastic follicles, but most of the node is occupied by a diffuse proliferation of large lymphoid cells (H&E stain).

References

Bartlett NL, Rizeq M, Dorfmann RF, *et al*: Follicular large-cell lymphoma: intermediate or low grade? J Clin Oncol 12:1349–1357, 1994.

Besa PC, McLaughlin PW, Cox JD, Fuller LM: Long term assessment of patterns of treatment failure and survival in patients with stage I or II follicular lymphomas. Cancer 75:2361–2367, 1995.

Goates JJ, Kamel OW, LeBrun DP, *et al*: Floral variant of follicular lymphoma. Immunological and molecular studies support a neoplastic process. Am J Surg Pathol 18(1):37–47, 1994.

Harris N, Nadler L, Bhan A: Immunohistologic characterization of two malignant lymphomas of germinal center type (centroblastic/centrocytic and centrocytic) with monoclonal antibodies: follicular and diffuse lymphomas of small cleaved cell types are related but distinct entities. Am J Pathol 117:262–272, 1984.

Lennert K: Malignant Lymphomas Other Than Hodgkin's Disease. New York, Springer-Verlag, 1978.

Lennert K, Feller A: Histopathology of Non-Hodgkin's Lymphomas. New York: Springer-Verlag, 1992.

Mann R, Berard C: Criteria for the cytologic subclassification of follicular lymphomas: a proposed alternative method. Hematol Oncol 1:187–192, 1982.

Martin AR, Weisenburger DD, Chan WC, *et al*: Prognostic value of cellular proliferation and histologic grade in follicular lymphoma. Blood 85:3671–3678, 1995.

Nathwani B, Metter G, Miller T, *et al*: What should be the morphologic criteria for the subdivision of follicular lymphomas? Blood 68:837–845, 1986.

Pezzella F, Tse A, Cordell J, *et al*: Expression of the bcl-2 oncogene protein is not specific for the 14-18 chromosomal translocation. Am J Pathol 137:225–232, 1990.

van Krieken JHJM. Histopathology of the spleen in non-Hodgkin's lymphoma. (Review.) Histol Histopath 5:113–122, 1990.

Yuen AR, Kamel OW, Halpern J, Horning SJ: Long-term survival after histologic transformation of low-grade follicular lymphoma. J Clin Oncol 13:1726–1733, 1995.

EXTRANODAL MARGINAL ZONE B-CELL LYMPHOMA: LOW GRADE B-CELL LYMPHOMA OF MUCOSA-ASSOCIATED LYMPHOID TISSUE (MALT) TYPE (+/− MONOCYTOID B CELLS)

Synonyms: Rappaport: (not specifically listed) well-differentiated lymphocytic (WDL) or WDL-plasmacytoid, intermediate lymphocytic, poorly differentiated lymphocytic, mixed lymphocytic-histiocytic (nodular or diffuse); Kiel: monocytoid B-cell, immunocytoma (some cases previously classified as centroblastic/centrocytic or centrocytic); Lukes-Collins: small lymphocyte B, lymphocytic-plasmacytic, small lymphocyte B, monocytoid; Working Formulation: (not specifically listed) small lymphocytic (some c/w CLL, some plasmacytoid), small cleaved or mixed small and large cell (follicular or diffuse).

Clinical Features

Extranodal marginal zone B-cell lymphoma (MZL) is the most common low grade lymphoma with which patients present in extranodal sites, comprising the majority of cases previously diagnosed as pseudolymphomas or extranodal small lymphocytic lymphomas. Patients are usually adults, with a slight female predominance overall, although the M:F ratio depends on which anatomic site is affected. Many patients have a history of autoimmune disease, such as Sjögren's syndrome or Hashimoto's thyroiditis, or of *Helicobacter* gastritis. "Acquired MALT" secondary to autoimmune disease or infection in these sites may form the substrate for lymphoma development. Most patients present with localized stage I or II extranodal disease. The stomach is the most common site at presentation; other sites include small and large intestines, lungs, orbits, parotid glands, breasts, thyroid, thymus, liver, gallbladder, skin, and soft tissues. The term "extranodal marginal zone lymphoma" can be used for all extranodal cases, but lymphoma of MALT can be applied properly only to cases involving mucosal sites.

Dissemination occurs in up to 30% of the cases, often in other extranodal sites, with long disease-free intervals. Localized tumors may be cured with local treatment. Studies suggest that proliferation in some early MALT tumors may be antigen-driven and that therapy directed at eradication of the antigen (*Helicobacter pylori* in gastric lymphoma) may result in regression of early lesions. When disseminated, MZL behaves similarly to other disseminated low grade lymphomas. Transformation to large cell lymphoma may occur.

Morphology

MZLs are composed of marginal zone (centrocyte-like) B cells (small, atypical cells with slightly irregular nuclei and relatively abundant, pale cytoplasm, similar to Peyer's patch, mesenteric nodal, or splenic marginal zone cells), with an admixture of variable numbers of monocytoid B cells, small lymphocytes, and plasma cells, and usually, occasional centroblasts or immunoblasts. Reactive follicles are often present, with the neoplastic marginal zone or monocytoid B cells occupying the marginal zone or the interfollicular region. Occasionally, follicles are infiltrated by neoplastic marginal zone or monocytoid cells, producing "follicular colonization." In many extranodal sites, such as the stomach, parotid gland, or thyroid, the marginal zone cells typically infiltrate the epithelium, forming so-called lymphoepithelial lesions. When MZL involves certain other sites, such as lacrimal gland and breast, lymphoepithelial lesions are uncommon.

In lymph nodes MZL may have a perisinusoidal, parafollicular, or marginal zone distribution, reminiscent of the location of marginal zone cells and monocytoid B cells in reactive nodes. Extranodal sites may show alternating bands of light and dark cells (the light cells having more cytoplasm or more developed plasmacytic differentiation). Plasma cells are often distributed in distinct subepithelial or inter-

follicular zones and express monotypic Ig in up to 50% of cases, which is consistent with plasmacytic differentiation of the neoplastic clone. Dutcher bodies are often found in these cases (Figs. 3–25 to 3–30).

Bone marrow involvement in MZL is unusual; however, marrow involvement in the form of small, poorly circumscribed, and occasionally paratrabecular lymphoid aggregates has been described.

High grade transformation has the appearance of diffuse large B-cell lymphoma (Fig. 3–31).

Immunophenotype

Tumor cells are sIg+ (M > G > A), IgD−, cIg+/−, B-cell–associated antigen + (CD19+, CD20+, CD22+, CD79a+), CD5−, CD10−, CD23−, CD43−/+, CD11c+/−. Rare cases of MZL have been CD5+; the significance of this finding is uncertain.

Genetic Features

No rearrangement of bcl-2 or bcl-1 is seen; numerical abnormalities of chromosomes 3, 7, 12, and 18, and t(11;18) have been reported. Ig heavy and light chain genes are rearranged, and the heavy chain variable region shows somatic mutation consistent with a postgerminal center stage of differentiation.

Postulated Normal Counterpart

Peripheral postgerminal center B cell with capacity to differentiate into marginal zone, monocytoid B, and plasma cells.

Text continued on page 99.

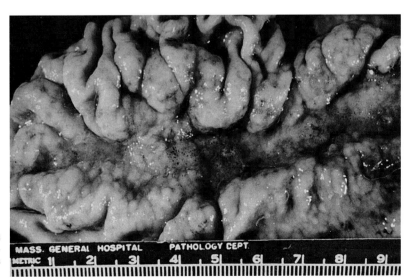

Figure 3–25. Mucosa-associated lymphoid tissue (MALT) lymphoma, stomach. The lymphoma is associated with an ulcer with a nodular base. Gastric folds around the ulcer are thickened by lymphoma.

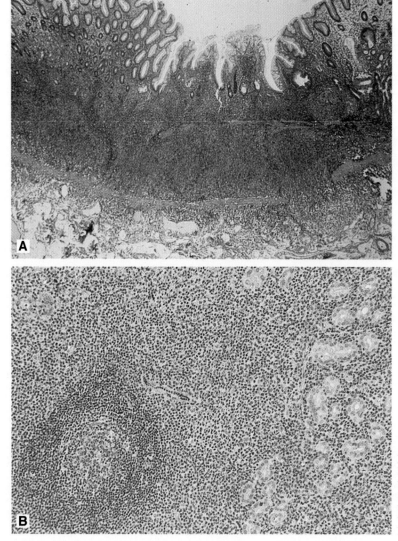

Figure 3–26. Mucosa-associated lymphoid tissue (MALT) lymphoma, stomach. *A,* Lymphoma predominantly involves the lamina propria, which is markedly expanded (Giemsa stain). *B,* A dense infiltrate of marginal zone cells appears in this view, with one reactive lymphoid follicle. The neoplastic cells are pale compared to those in the mantle of the follicle because their cytoplasm is more abundant (H&E stain).

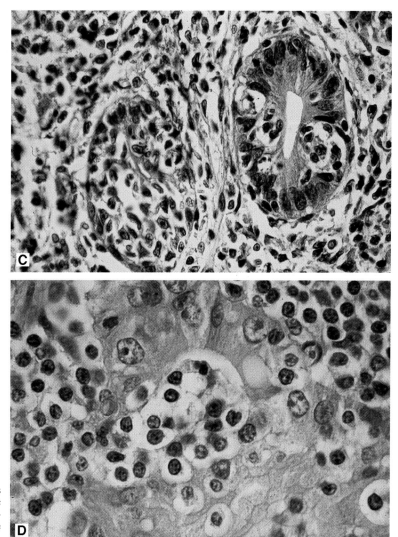

Figure 3–26. *Continued C,* Two lymphoepithelial lesions are visible, one of which has virtually destroyed a gastric gland (H&E stain). *D,* This lymphoepithelial lesion has neoplastic cells with small but slightly irregular nuclei and pale cytoplasm (H&E stain).

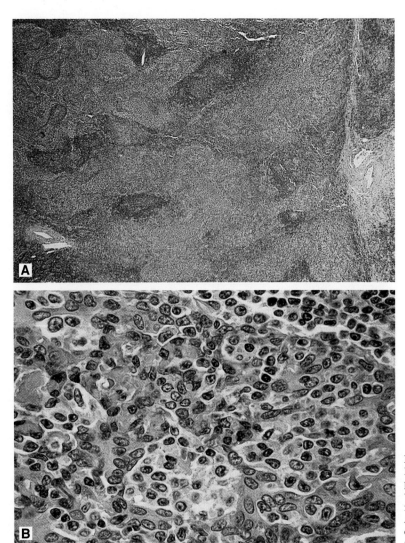

Figure 3–27. Mucosa-associated lymphoid tissue (MALT) lymphoma, parotid gland. *A,* Low power view shows broad, pale bands that correspond to neoplastic lymphoid cells with extensive infiltration of epithelial structures with the formation of multiple epimyoepithelial islands (H&E stain). *B,* Higher power view shows an epimyoepithelial island—a duct with hyperplastic epithelium associated with marginal zone cells/monocytoid B cells (H&E stain).

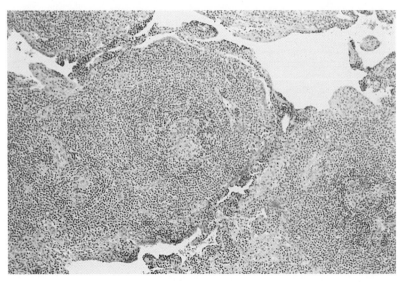

Figure 3–28. Mucosa-associated lymphoid tissue (MALT) lymphoma, lung. An interstitial infiltrate is associated with marked widening of the alveolar septa (H&E stain).

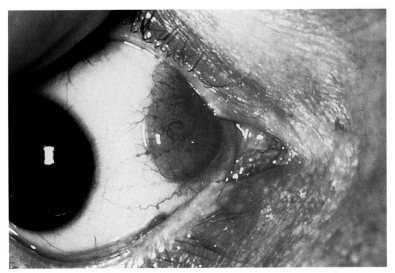

Figure 3–29. Mucosa-associated lymphoid tissue (MALT) lymphoma. A raised red lesion is medial to the pupil on the bulbar conjunctiva.

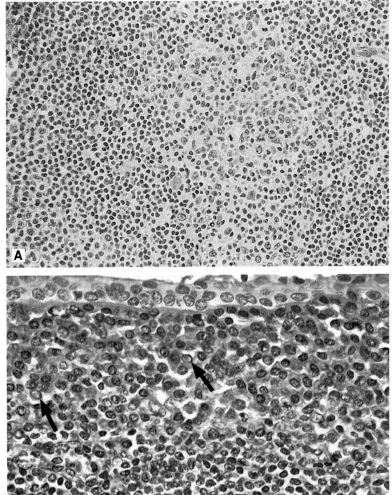

Figure 3–30. Mucosa-associated lymphoid tissue (MALT) lymphoma, ocular adnexa. *A,* This case shows follicular colonization, in which small, pale, uniform marginal zone cells infiltrate a reactive lymphoid follicle (H&E stain). *B,* In this case involving the conjunctiva, a zonation phenomenon occurs, with a deeper layer of small lymphoid cells and a superficial layer with well-developed plasmacytic differentiation. Within the plasma cell layer are occasional Dutcher bodies (*arrows*), which are PAS+ intranuclear protrusions of cytoplasm containing immunoglobulin (PAS stain).

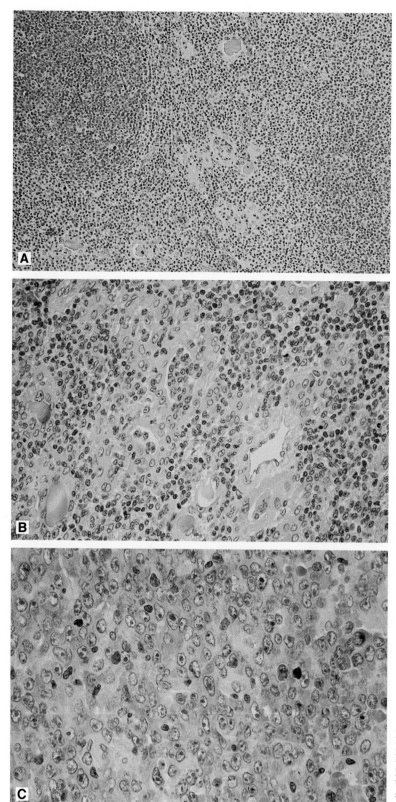

Figure 3–31. Mucosa-associated lymphoid tissue (MALT) lymphoma of the thyroid with large cell transformation. *A,* Much of the thyroid is involved by low grade MALT lymphoma (H&E stain). *B,* Neoplastic lymphoid cells infiltrate thyroid follicles, forming lymphoepithelial lesions (H&E stain). *C,* Aggregates of immunoblasts, consistent with large cell transformation are found in some areas (H&E stain).

Differential Diagnosis

1. B-cell chronic lymphocytic leukemia (B-CLL): The serpiginous, vaguely delineated bands of light and dark cells seen in marginal zone lymphoma may resemble CLL with pseudofollicles. Pseudofollicles are round, rather than band-like, and contain small lymphocytes, prolymphocytes, and paraimmunoblasts, in contrast to the marginal zone cells, plasma cells, and occasional blasts in marginal zone lymphoma. Follicular colonization, lymphoepithelial lesions, and plasmacytic differentiation are frequent in MZL, in contrast to CLL. Peripheral blood and marrow involvement are rare in MZL (except for splenic MZL). Immunophenotyping provides definitive diagnosis (B-CLL: CD5+, CD23+, cIg−; marginal zone lymphoma: CD5−, CD23−, cIg+/−).

2. Other types of low grade B-cell lymphoma, including mantle cell lymphoma, lymphoplasmacytic lymphoma, and follicle center lymphoma: The differential diagnosis of MZL with each of these lymphomas is discussed in the preceding sections corresponding to each of these lymphomas.

References

Bailey EM, Ferry JA, Harris NL, et al: Low-grade B-cell lymphoma of mucosa-associated lymphoid tissue (MALT) type of skin and subcutaneous tissue: a study of 15 patients. Am J Surg Pathol 20:1011–1023, 1996.

Bayerdorffer E, Neubauer A, Rudolph B, et al: Regression of primary gastric lymphoma of mucosa-associated lymphoid tissue type after cure of Helicobacter pylori infection. MALT lymphoma study group. Lancet 345:1591–1594, 1995.

Cogliatti S, Schmid U, Schumacher U, et al: Primary B-cell gastric lymphoma: a clinicopathological study of 145 patients. Gastroenterology 101:1159–1170, 1991.

Ferry JA, Yang WI, Zukerberg LR, et al: CD5+ marginal zone B-cell (MALT) lymphoma. A low grade neoplasm with a propensity for bone marrow involvement and relapse. Am J Clin Pathol 105:31–37, 1996.

Finn T, Isaacson P, Wotherspoon A: Numerical abnormality of chromosomes 3, 7, 12, and 18 in low grade lymphomas of MALT-type and splenic marginal zone lymphomas detected by interphase cytogenetics on paraffin embedded tissue. J Pathol 170:335A, 1993.

Fisher RI, Dahlberg S, Nathwani B, et al: A clinical analysis of two indolent lymphoma entities: mantle cell lymphoma and marginal zone lymphoma (including the mucosa-associated lymphoid tissue and monocytoid B-cell subcategories): a Southwest Oncology Group Study. Blood 85:1075–1082, 1995.

Isaacson PG, Banks PM, Best PV, et al: Primary low-grade hepatic B-cell lymphoma of mucosa-associated lymphoid tissue (MALT)-type. Am J Surg Pathol 19:571–575, 1995.

Li G, Hansmann M, Zwingers T, Lennert K: Primary lymphomas of the lung: morphological, immunohistochemical and clinical features. Histopathology 16:519–531, 1990.

Mattia A, Ferry J, Harris N: Breast lymphoma: a B-cell spectrum including the low grade B-cell lymphoma of mucosa associated lymphoid tissue. Am J Surg Pathol 17:574–587, 1993.

Pelstring R, Essell J, Kurtin P, Banks P: Diversity of organ site involvement among malignant lymphomas of mucosa-associated tissues. Am J Clin Pathol 96:738–745, 1991.

Qin Y, Geriner A, Trunk MJ, et al: Somatic hypermutation in low-grade mucosa-associated lymphoid tissue-type B-cell lymphoma. Blood 86:3528–3534, 1995.

White WL, Ferry JA, Harris NL, Grove AS: Ocular adnexal lymphoma: a clinicopathologic study with identification of lymphomas of mucosa-associated lymphoid tissue (MALT) type. Ophthalmology 102:1994–2006, 1995.

Wotherspoon A, Doglioni C, Diss T, et al: Regression of primary low-grade B-cell gastric lymphoma of mucosa-associated lymphoid tissue type after eradication of Helicobacter pylori. Lancet 342:575–577, 1993.

Zukerberg L, Ferry J, Southern J, Harris N: Lymphoid infiltrates of the stomach: evaluation of histologic criteria for the diagnosis of low-grade gastric lymphoma on endoscopic biopsy specimens. Am J Surg Pathol 14:1087–1099, 1990.

IMMUNOPROLIFERATIVE SMALL INTESTINAL DISEASE (IPSID)

Related terms: Alpha heavy chain disease; Mediterranean lymphoma.

The incidence of intestinal lymphoma in the Middle East is high. A major subtype of these lymphomas is immunoproliferative small intestinal disease (IPSID), a disorder rare outside the Middle East. IPSID is now considered to be a type of MALT lymphoma. It is not included as a separate entity in the R.E.A.L. Classification, but because it has unusual clinical and pathologic features that distinguish it from other marginal zone lymphomas, it is discussed here.

Clinical Features

Patients are young adults who present with malabsorption, diarrhea, and weight loss. There is an association with lower socioeconomic status. In approximately half of cases, the serum contains α heavy chains without associated light chains (α heavy chain disease). Patients have a low grade lymphoma of MALT type involving the small intestine. The disease may be confined to the proximal portion of the small intestine or extend to involve the entire small bowel. Mesenteric lymph nodes are frequently involved. The clinical course is typically prolonged, with lymphoma remaining confined to the abdomen for many years. High grade transformation may occur. In the early stages of the disease, IPSID may respond to broad-spectrum antibiotics, analogous to treatment of gastric MALT lymphomas with eradication of Helicobacter pylori. In later stages (including cases with high grade transformation), the disease is resistant to antibiotics but may respond to chemotherapy.

Morphology

IPSID produces diffuse, uninterrupted thickening of a long segment of the small intestine. The following staging system has been proposed to subclassify the extent of disease in cases of IPSID:

Stage A: Lymphoma is confined to the small intestinal mucosa and mesenteric lymph nodes. The infiltrate consists mainly of plasma cells with relatively small numbers of marginal zone lymphocytes (Fig. 3–32A).

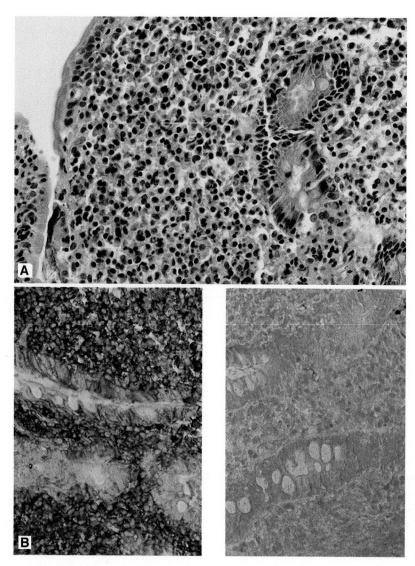

Figure 3–32. Immunoproliferative small intestinal disease (IPSID), stage A. *A,* The lamina propria of the small intestine is filled and expanded by an infiltrate of mature plasma cells (H&E stain). *B,* The plasma cells all show staining for α heavy chain (*left*), but virtually no staining for other heavy chains (μ is shown at *right* for comparison) (immunoperoxidase technique on paraffin section).

Stage B: In addition to the changes found in Stage A, nodular mucosal infiltrates, which may be due to "colonization" of reactive follicles, develop, and the infiltrate invades through the muscularis mucosae. Marginal zone lymphocytes are more prominent and lymphoepithelial lesions may be found.

Stage C: High grade lymphoma develops, producing one or more large masses. The high grade lymphoma is composed of large lymphoid cells, in which immunoblasts sometimes predominate; in other cases, there is a component of large, bizarre cells.

Immunophenotype

The lymphoma usually expresses α heavy chain without a detectable light chain. A minority of cases express monotypic light chain (Fig. 3–32*B*).

Genetic Features

Clonal rearrangement of immunoglobulin heavy and light chain genes has been described, even in early cases responsive to antibiotic therapy, indicating that from the outset IPSID is a lymphoma rather than a florid reactive process.

Differential Diagnosis

See extranodal marginal zone B cell lymphoma.

References

Isaacson PG: Gastrointestinal lymphoma. Hum Pathol 25:1020–1029, 1994.

Isaacson PG, Dogan A, Price SK, Spencer J: Immunoproliferative small intestinal disease: an immunohistochemical study. Am J Surg Pathol 13:1023–1033, 1989.

Malik IA, Shamsi Z, Shafquat A, *et al*: Clinicopathological features and management of immunoproliferative small intestinal lymphoma in Pakistan. Med Pediatr Oncol 25:400–406, 1995.

Martin IG, Aldoori MI: Immunoproliferative small intestinal disease: Mediterranean lymphoma and alpha heavy chain disease. (Review.) Br J Surg 81:20–24, 1994.

Price SK: Immunoproliferative small intestinal disease: a study of 13 cases with alpha heavy chain disease. Histopathology 17:7–17, 1990.

Salem P, el-Hashimi L, Anaissie E, *et al*: Primary small intestinal lymphoma in adults. A comparative study of IPSID versus non-IPSID in the Middle East. Cancer 59:1670–1676, 1987.

Smith WJ, Price SK, Isaacson PG: Immunoglobulin gene rearrangement in immunoproliferative small intestinal disease (IPSID). J Clin Pathol 40:1291–1297, 1987.

Tabbane F, Mourali N, Cammoun M, Najjar T: Results of laparotomy in immunoproliferative small intestinal disease (IPSID). Cancer 61: 1699–1706, 1988.

NODAL MARGINAL ZONE B-CELL LYMPHOMA (+/− MONOCYTOID B CELLS) (PROVISIONAL ENTITY)

Synonym: Miscellaneous: monocytoid B-cell lymphoma.

When MZL involves lymph nodes, the nodes appear identical to those described in cases of nodal monocytoid B-cell lymphoma (Fig. 3–33). When MZL involves the lymph nodes, an extranodal site of involvement can be identified in most cases. Lymph node involvement by this type of lymphoma, however, has occasionally been reported in the

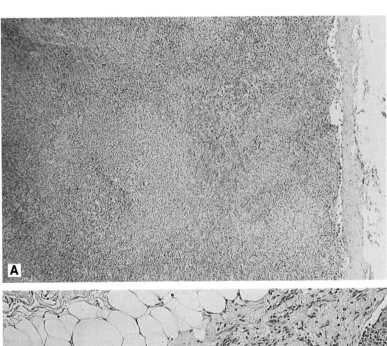

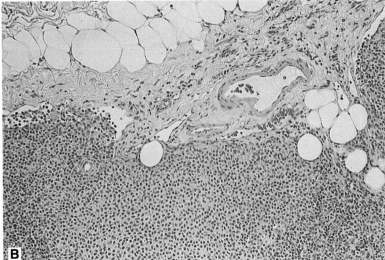

Figure 3–33. Nodal marginal zone B-cell lymphoma. *A,* Low power view shows large pale nodules partially obliterating the architecture of this lymph node (H&E stain). *B,* Neoplastic cells form a broad band just beneath the capsule (H&E stain).

Illustration continued on following page.

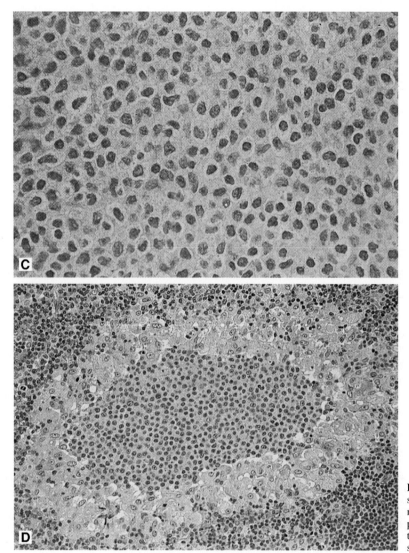

Figure 3–33. *Continued C,* High power examination shows cells with slightly angulated, intermediate-sized nuclei, evenly dispersed chromatin, and abundant pale cytoplasm (H&E stain). *D,* In this case, a ring of epithelioid histiocytes surrounds a cluster of monocytoid B cells (H&E stain).

absence of extranodal disease. These lymphomas may also involve bone marrow and, rarely, peripheral blood; their relationship to extranodal MZL and to other low grade B cell lymphomas remains to be determined.

Differential Diagnosis

1. Other low grade B-cell lymphomas: *See* extranodal marginal zone B-cell lymphoma.
2. Follicle center lymphoma with differentiation to monocytoid B cells: Occasional follicle center lymphomas (FCL) that are otherwise typical have neoplastic follicles with a rim of monocytoid B cells or have subcapsular or parasinusoidal bands of monocytoid B cells. Some investigators consider these lymphomas to be composite lymphomas, and some published series of monocytoid B-cell

lymphoma appear to include cases of this type. Although this entity is controversial, we prefer to designate such cases as follicle center lymphoma and to describe the marginal zone or monocytoid B cell differentiation in a note.

References

Ngan B-Y, Warnke R, Wilson M, *et al*: Monocytoid B-cell lymphoma: a study of 36 cases. Hum Pathol 22:409–421, 1991.

Nizze H, Cogliatti S, von Schilling C, *et al*: Monocytoid B-cell lymphoma: morphological variants and relationship to low-grade B-cell lymphoma of the mucosa-associated lymphoid tissue. Histopathology 18:403–414, 1991.

Sheibani K, Burke J, Swartz W, *et al*: Monocytoid B cell lymphoma. Clinicopathologic study of 21 cases of a unique type of low grade lymphoma. Cancer 62:1531–1538, 1988.

Shin S, Sheibani K, Fishleder A, *et al*: Monocytoid B-cell lymphoma in patients with Sjögren's syndrome: a clinicopathologic study of 13 patients. Hum Pathol 22:422–430, 1991.

SPLENIC MARGINAL ZONE LYMPHOMA, WITH OR WITHOUT VILLOUS LYMPHOCYTES (PROVISIONAL ENTITY)

Synonyms: Rappaport: (not specifically listed) well-differentiated lymphocytic (WDL) or WDL-plasmacytoid; Kiel: not specifically listed; Lukes-Collins: small lymphocyte B, lymphocytic-plasmacytic, small lymphocyte B, monocytoid; Working Formulation: (not specifically listed) SLL (some plasmacytoid).

Clinical Features

This is a recently described disorder whose incidence is unknown; however, it may comprise many cases of chronic B-cell leukemia that lack features of typical B-CLL and most cases of primary splenic low grade B-cell lymphoma. Most patients are older adults (mean age in the seventh decade) who present with marked splenomegaly. Males and females are roughly equally affected. Usually, bone marrow and peripheral blood are involved without peripheral lymphadenopathy, although intra-abdominal lymphadenopathy is common. Circulating villous lymphocytes are identified in some cases. Up to half of patients have a small M-component. The course is reported to be indolent, and splenectomy may result in a prolonged remission. Transformation to large cell lymphoma has been described.

Morphology

Both the mantle and marginal zones of the splenic white pulp are replaced by tumor cells, with a centrally located residual follicle center that may be either atrophic or hyperplastic, or the follicle centers may be obliterated. The neoplastic cells range from small lymphocytes in the mantle zone to larger cells with irregular nuclei and pale cytoplasm in the marginal zone (marginal zone B cells). This zonation phenomenon, with an inner layer of smaller dark cells and an outer layer of slightly larger pale cells, occurs only in the spleen. There may be an admixture of small numbers of large lymphoid cells. In some cases, plasma cells may be identified. Red pulp involvement is common. It may be inconspicuous or prominent, and may take the form of neoplastic cells centered on clusters of epithelioid histiocytes (Fig. 3–34).

Abdominal lymph nodes may be involved in a diffuse, nodular, or marginal zone pattern (Fig. 3–35).

Splenic MZL involving the liver occurs mainly in the portal tracts (Fig. 3–36). Circulating villous lymphocytes are identified in many cases. They are small lymphoid cells with delicate villous projections that tend to be localized toward one end of the cell rather than being circumferential. Cytoplasm is usually slightly more abundant than in normal lymphocytes and is pale to deep blue (Fig. 3–37).

Bone marrow involvement is usually focal, in the form of lymphoid aggregates; in some cases, the aggregates of neoplastic cells contain reactive germinal centers. We have reviewed a case in which SMZL involved the gallbladder (Fig. 3–38).

Immunophenotype

Tumor cells are sIg+, cIg+/− (IgM+, IgD+/−, κ > λ), B antigen+, CD5−, CD10−, CD23−, CD43−, DBA.44−/+, bcl-2 protein+.

Genetic Features

Ig genes are clonally rearranged. Results of cytogenetic analysis have varied in different reports, but trisomy 3 appears to be less frequent than in extranodal MZL. High levels of cyclin D1 mRNA and t(11;14)(q13;q32) have been described in a few cases, but studies suggest that cyclin D1 mRNA+ cases may represent examples of mantle cell lymphoma or B-prolymphocytic leukemia. Bcl-2 is germline. Somatic hypermutation of heavy chain gene variable regions has been described.

Postulated Normal Counterpart

Peripheral B cell with differentiation in part to splenic marginal zone cell.

Differential Diagnosis

1. Hairy cell leukemia: *See* the next discussion.

References

Hammer RD, Glick AD, Greer JP, et al: Splenic marginal zone lymphoma. A distinct B-cell neoplasm. Am J Surg Pathol 20:613–626, 1996.

Isaacson PG, Matutes E, Burke M, Catovsky D: The histopathology of splenic lymphoma with villous lymphocytes. Blood 84:3828–3834, 1994.

Jadayel D, Matutes E, Dyer M, et al: Splenic lymphoma with villous lymphocytes: analysis of bcl-1 rearrangements and expression of the cyclin D1 gene. Blood 83:3664–3671, 1994.

Mollejo M, Menarguez J, Lloret E, et al: Splenic marginal zone lymphoma: a distinctive type of low-grade B-cell lymphoma. A clinicopathologic study of 13 cases. Am J Surg Pathol 19:1146–1157, 1995.

Pawade J, Wilkins BS, Wright DH: Low-grade B-cell lymphomas of the splenic marginal zone: a clinicopathological and immunohistochemical study of 14 cases. Histopathology 27:129–137, 1995.

Pittaluga S, Verhoef G, Criel A, et al: "Small" B-cell non-Hodgkin's lymphomas with splenomegaly at presentation are either mantle cell lymphoma or marginal zone cell lymphoma. A study based on histology, cytology, immunohistochemistry, and cytogenetic analysis. Am J Surg Pathol 20:211–223, 1996.

Schmid C, Kirkham N, Diss T, Isaacson P: Splenic marginal zone cell lymphoma. Am J Surg Pathol 16:455–466, 1992.

Zhu D, Oscier DG, Stevenson FK: Splenic lymphoma with villous lymphocytes involves B cells with extensively mutated Ig heavy chain variable region genes. Blood 85:1603–1607, 1995.

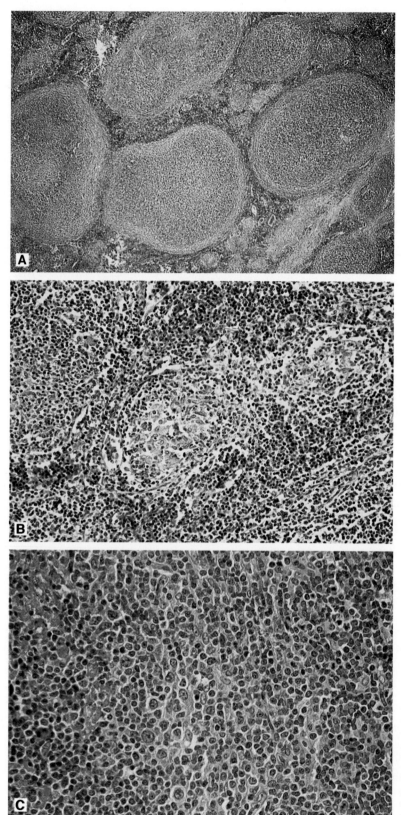

Figure 3–34. Splenic marginal zone lymphoma. *A,* The spleen shows large nodules of lymphoid cells replacing white pulp. The cells at the periphery of the white pulp nodules have slightly more cytoplasm than those in the center, creating a pale rim. Smaller aggregates of neoplastic cells appear in the red pulp (H&E stain). *B,* In the red pulp, aggregates of neoplastic cells are associated with clusters of epithelioid histiocytes (H&E stain). *C,* High power view of the white pulp shows an inner zone of small lymphoid cells with scant cytoplasm (*left*) surrounded by cells with small, slightly irregular nuclei with a moderate amount of pale cytoplasm, and a few large lymphoid cells. Red pulp is at the right (H&E stain).

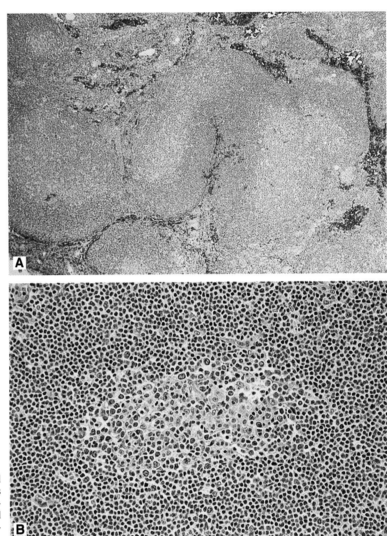

Figure 3–35. Splenic marginal zone lymphoma, periportal lymph node. *A,* Neoplastic cells form broad marginal zones around reactive germinal centers. The paracortex is compressed; some sinuses are patent (H&E stain). *B,* Marginal zone cells encroach on a reactive follicle. The biphasic pattern seen in the splenic white pulp is absent (H&E stain).

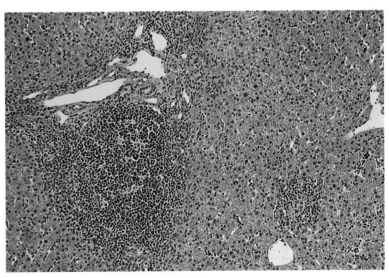

Figure 3–36. Splenic marginal zone lymphoma with hepatic involvement, mainly in the form of periportal aggregates (H&E stain).

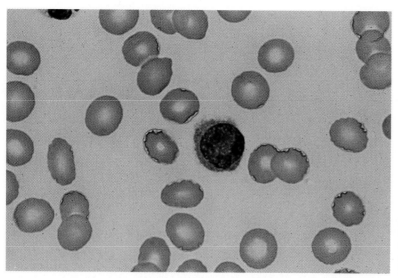

Figure 3–37. Circulating villous lymphocyte. The neoplastic cell is small, with a heterochromatic nucleus and slightly more cytoplasm than a normal lymphocyte. Short villous processes are more prominent at one pole of the cell (Wright-Giemsa stain).

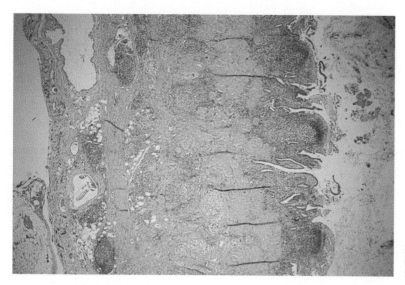

Figure 3–38. Splenic marginal zone lymphoma with involvement of the gallbladder. The wall of the gallbladder is diffusely thickened (H&E stain).

HAIRY CELL LEUKEMIA (HCL)

Clinical Features

Hairy cell leukemia (HCL) is a rare disease that affects middle-aged to older adults (median age 50), although HCL has been reported to affect patients ranging from 24 to 80 years of age. Children are not affected. Men are affected predominantly, with an M:F ratio of 5 to 1. Patients present with abdominal discomfort, which is related to splenomegaly, or with fatigue, easy bruising, or infection, which is related to anemia, thrombocytopenia, neutropenia, and monocytopenia. A wide variety of infectious diseases, in-

cluding infections of bacterial, fungal, parasitic, rickettsial, and atypical mycobacterial origin, have been reported in patients with HCL. Patients appear to have an increased risk for legionnaires' disease. Occasionally, HCL is found incidentally during investigation of an unrelated medical problem. Most patients are pancytopenic at the time of diagnosis. Patients may also have hepatomegaly. Retroperitoneal and mediastinal lymphadenopathy have been reported, but peripheral lymphadenopathy is usually absent. Serum paraprotein is not a feature of HCL. HCL does not respond to conventional lymphoma chemotherapy, but interferon, deoxycoformycin, or 2-chlorodeoxyadenosine can induce long-term remissions.

Morphology

Hairy cells are small to intermediate-sized lymphoid cells that have an oval or bean-shaped nucleus, chromatin slightly more finely dispersed than that of a normal lymphocyte, and abundant, pale cytoplasm with delicate "hairy" projections on smear preparations (Fig. 3–39). Mitotic activity is virtually absent.

The bone marrow is always involved, and the histologic features in this site are sufficiently distinctive to provide a diagnosis in nearly all cases. In the marrow, the infiltrate is interstitial, diffuse, and characterized by small cells that appear widely separated because of their abundant cytoplasm. The appearance has been likened to fried eggs or a honeycomb (Fig. 3–40). The marrow may be normocellular or hypocellular, and the pattern of cellular elements and fat may appear normal on low power examination, although closer inspection reveals the presence of hairy cells. Reticulin is increased, often resulting in a "dry tap." In subtle cases, or in treated cases in which the presence of residual HCL is in question, immunostaining with anti-B-cell antibodies such as L26 or DBA.44 may be useful in detecting neoplastic cells.

In the spleen the tumor involves the red pulp; the white pulp is often atrophic. Dilated red pulp sinuses containing red cells form red cell lakes (Fig. 3–41). Lymph node involvement is uncommon. In lymph nodes, the infiltrate is diffuse and may spare follicles, mimicking marginal zone lymphoma.

Hepatic involvement is frequent in HCL; hairy cells infiltrate both portal tracts and sinusoids. In the sinusoids, hairy cells may replace the normal lining cells and may be associated with an angiomatoid change.

Immunophenotype and Enzyme Histochemistry

The tumor cells are sIg+ (M, M and D, G or A), B antigen+ (CD19+, CD20+, CD22+, CD79a+), CD5−, CD10−, CD23−, CD11c+ (strong), CD25+ (strong), FMC7+, CD103+ (MLA: mucosal lymphocyte antigen, recognized by HML-1, B-ly7, Ber-ACT8, LF61), DBA.44+; tartrate-resistant acid phosphatase (TRAP)+ (*see* Fig. 3–39). A monoclonal antibody, 9C5, has been developed that recognizes TRAP in formalin-fixed, paraffin-embedded tissue; it is reported to be highly sensitive and specific for HCL.

Genetic Features

Ig heavy and light chain genes are rearranged. Ig genes show a moderate degree of somatic mutation. No specific cytogenetic abnormality has been described.

Postulated Normal Counterpart

Peripheral B cell of unknown differentiation (? late) stage.

Differential Diagnosis

1. Low grade B-cell lymphomas: The B-cell lymphomas have nuclear chromatin that is darker and more coarsely clumped than that of HCL. None of them, except for some monocytoid B-cell lymphomas, have such abundant cytoplasm, so that the distinctive fried egg–like appearance of HCL in tissue sections is not observed. A dry tap on attempts to aspirate marrow occurs consistently only in HCL. Strong, diffuse cytoplasmic TRAP

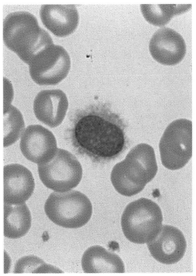 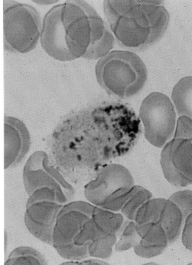

Figure 3–39. Hairy cell leukemia, peripheral blood. The hairy cell has a smooth oval nucleus, and relatively abundant pale blue cytoplasm with numerous, rather long cytoplasmic processes (*left*) (Wright-Giemsa stain) and cytoplasmic reactivity for tartrate-resistant acid phosphatase (TRAP) (*right*).

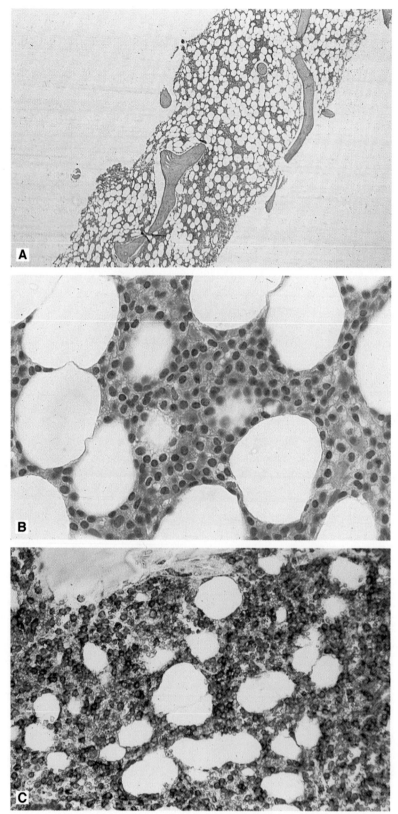

Figure 3–40. Hairy cell leukemia, bone marrow. *A,* On low power examination, the distribution of cellular elements appears normal (H&E stain). *B,* At higher power, however, the majority of cells are hairy cells (H&E stain). *C,* Hairy cells are typically strongly DBA.44+, as seen here (immunoperoxidase technique on paraffin section).

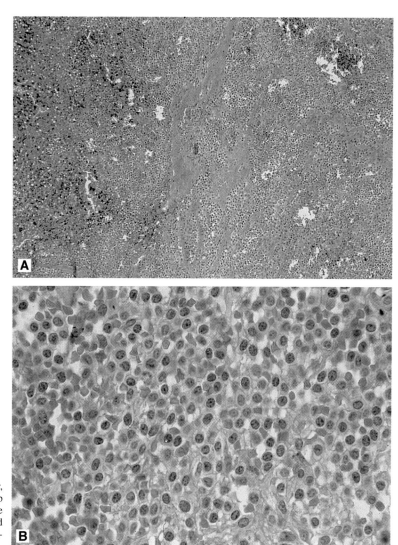

Figure 3–41. Hairy cell leukemia, spleen. *A,* At low power, a diffuse infiltrate of neoplastic cells is visible in the red pulp with red cell lakes (*left*). White pulp is not recognizable (H&E stain). *B,* Higher power examination shows lymphoid cells with round to oval nuclei, fine, pale chromatin, abundant pale cytoplasm, and distinct cell borders (H&E stain).

reactivity is much more common in HCL; however, CD22, CD11c, CD25, FMC7, CD103, and even TRAP may be present in disorders other than HCL.

a. Splenic marginal zone lymphoma with villous lymphocytes (SMZL): Patients with SMZL often have monoclonal gammopathy. In smears, the villous lymphocytes have cytoplasm that is less abundant and more basophilic, with small "villi" that tend to be polar rather than circumferential. White pulp involvement predominates in the spleen. Marrow involvement is usually focal rather than diffuse. DBA.44 is usually negative.

b. Monocytoid B-cell lymphoma/nodal marginal zone cell lymphoma (MZL): Splenomegaly and peripheral blood and marrow involvement are rare, but peripheral lymphadenopathy is common. Few cases of nodal MZL with splenic involvement have been described, but MZL predominantly involves white pulp, not red pulp.

c. B-cell chronic lymphocytic leukemia (B-CLL): Involvement of CLL in the spleen may be nodular or diffuse; diffuse involvement may raise the possibility of HCL. CLL is CD5+, CD23+, and only rarely DBA.44+, in contrast to HCL.

d. Follicle center lymphoma (FCL): FCL tends to involve the marrow focally, often in a paratrabecular location, and involves the white pulp of the spleen. The nuclei of FCL cells are more irregular than those of hairy cells.

e. Mantle cell lymphoma (MCL): Nuclei may be more irregular than those of hairy cells, cytoplasm is scant, and mitoses may be frequent. MCL involves splenic white pulp, expresses CD5, and lacks CD11c.

2. Monocytic leukemias: The morphology of monocytic leukemia cells may overlap that of HCL, but neoplastic monocytes express lysozyme and other monocyte-associated antigens. Usually mitoses are found easily.

3. Mast cell disease: Usually, discrete aggregates of mast cells are mixed in the marrow with eosinophils, lymphocytes, and plasma cells. Although some oval mast cells may resemble hairy cells, others often have the shape of fibroblasts. With Giemsa stain or chloroacetate esterase stain, mast cells show a granular cytoplasm. *See also* Mast Cell Disease, in Chapter 7.

References

Chang KL, Stroup R, Weiss LM: Hairy cell leukemia: current status. (Review.) Am J Clin Pathol 97:719–738, 1992.

Falini B, Pileri S, Flenghi L, *et al*: Selection of a panel of monoclonal antibodies for monitoring residual disease in peripheral blood and bone marrow of interferon-treated hairy cell leukemia patients. Br J Haematol 76:460–468, 1990.

Hounieu H, Chittall SM, Al Saati T, *et al*: Hairy cell leukemia: diagnosis of bone marrow involvement in paraffin-embedded sections with monoclonal antibody DBA.44. Am J Clin Pathol 28:26–33, 1992.

Janckila AJ, Cardwell EM, Yam LT, Li C-Y: Hairy cell identification by immunohistochemistry of tartrate-resistent acid phosphatase. Blood 85:2839–2844, 1995.

Korsmeyer S, Greene W, Cossman J: Rearrangement and expression of immunoglobulin genes and expression of Tac antigen in hairy cell leukemia. Proc Natl Acad Sci USA 80:4522–4528, 1983.

Kraut EH, Grever MR, Bouroncle BA: Long term follow-up of patients with hairy cell leukemia after treatment with 2′-deoxycoformycin. Blood 84:4061–4063, 1994.

Mason D, Cordell J, Tse A, *et al*: The IgM-associated protein mb-1 as a marker of normal and neoplastic B-cells. J Immunol 147(8):2474–2482, 1991.

Piro L, Carrera C, Carson D, Beutler E: Lasting remissions in hairy cell leukemia induced by a single infusion of 2′-chlorodeoxyadenosine. Cancer 332:1117–1121, 1990.

PLASMACYTOMA/PLASMA CELL MYELOMA

Clinical Features

Plasma cell neoplasms are most often disseminated bone marrow tumors of older adults (multiple myeloma). Some patients present with solitary bone or extramedullary tumors (plasmacytoma). Lymph node involvement is rare. Most cases of solitary bone plasmacytomas show progression to multiple myeloma, while only 10% to 20% of solitary extramedullary plasmacytomas show such progression.

Infrequently, patients have one or more sclerotic plasmacytomas (osteosclerotic myeloma). Such cases may be associated with POEMS syndrome (polyneuropathy, organomegaly, endocrinopathy, monoclonal gammopathy, and skin changes). In POEMS syndrome, the neuropathy is a progressive demyelinating sensorimotor polyneuropathy. The organomegaly consists of hepatomegaly, splenomegaly, or lymphadenopathy. The most common manifestations of the endocrinopathy are hypogonadism and hypothyroidism. The monoclonal gammopathy is almost always IgAλ or IgGλ. Skin changes include hyperpigmentation, hypertrichosis, skin thickening, Raynaud's phenomenon, and clubbing of the fingers. The survival rate of patients with osteosclerotic myeloma is significantly longer than that of patients with myeloma of the usual type; this may correlate with the lack of extensive marrow involvement distant from the osteosclerotic lesions that occurs in most cases.

Morphology

Plasmacytoma/myeloma is composed of cells that resemble mature or immature plasma cells (plasmablasts). In some cases, cells may have cleaved or lobated nuclei or cells that resemble immunoblasts. The presence of neoplastic cells that are immature or that have marked cytologic atypia, frequent mitoses, and masses of plasma cells (packed marrow) are adverse prognostic indicators. When the plasma cells form a discrete extramedullary or osseous mass, a diagnosis of plasmacytoma is appropriate. A diagnosis of plasma cell myeloma should be made when collections of plasma cells large enough to fill the space between fat cells and displace normal elements are discovered on a random biopsy specimen of iliac crest bone marrow. If an aspirate smear contains more than 30% plasma cells (greater than 10% in the presence of biopsy-proven plasmacytoma or a large serum M-component (IgG >3.5 g/dL, IgA > 2g/dL), or Bence-Jones proteinuria), a diagnosis of myeloma can be made. Among patients with the full-blown clinical syndrome of multiple myeloma (multiple lytic bone lesions due to osseous plasmacytomas, large M-component, hypercalcemia, and renal failure), demonstration of bone marrow plasmacytosis is not required to establish a diagnosis (Figs. 3–42 and 3–43).

In cases of osteosclerotic myeloma, marrow distant from the bone lesions may not have significantly increased numbers of plasma cells (usually less than 5%). Among patients with POEMS syndrome with lymphadenopathy, the lymph nodes may show changes of the plasma cell type of Castleman's disease (*see* Castleman's Disease, Chapter 2).

Rarely, neoplastic cells are found in the peripheral blood (plasma cell leukemia) (Fig. 3–44).

Immunophenotype

Neoplastic cells are sIg−, cIg+ (G > A > light chain only; rarely D or E), most B-cell-associated antigen negative (CD19, CD20, CD22), but CD79a+/−; CD45−/+, CD45-RO−/+, HLA-DR−/+, CD38+, EMA−/+, CD43+/−, CD56+/−. The light chain ratio (number of plasma cells expressing the light chain of the myeloma compared with the number of plasma cells expressing the opposite light chain) is almost always 16 or greater. CD30 may be detected in paraffin sections using the BerH2 antibody. The immunoglobulin expressed in cases associated with POEMS syndrome is almost always IgGλ or IgAλ.

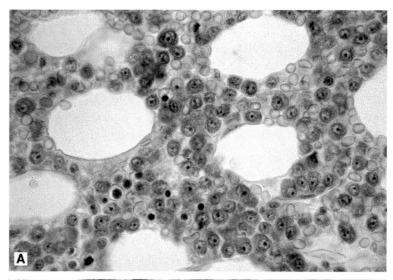

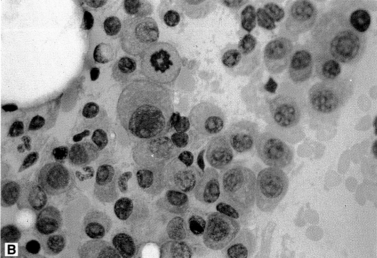

Figure 3–42. Plasma cell myeloma, bone marrow. *A,* This bone marrow biopsy specimen shows extensive interstitial infiltrate of immature plasma cells with eccentrically placed, vesicular nuclei, prominent central nucleoli, and amphophilic cytoplasm. Only a few normal hematopoietic elements remain (Giemsa stain). *B,* A specimen from bone marrow aspirate in another case shows slightly immature plasma cells, although abnormally large plasma cells are present occasionally (Wright-Giemsa stain).

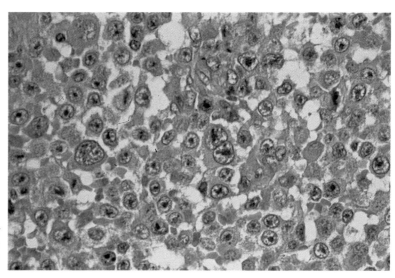

Figure 3–43. Anaplastic plasmacytoma, composed of sheets of highly atypical plasma cells that have vesicular nuclei and prominent nucleoli; occasional bizarre binucleated cells also appear (H&E stain).

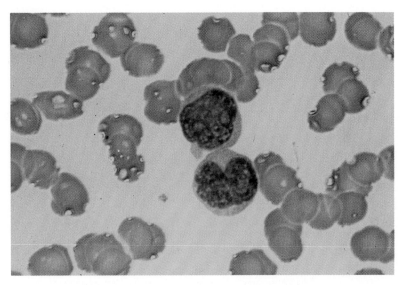

Figure 3–44. Plasma cell leukemia. The leukemic cells in this case have lobated, heterochromatic nuclei with small nucleoli and a moderate amount of blue cytoplasm (Wright-Giemsa stain).

Genetics

Ig heavy and light genes are rearranged or deleted. Cytogenetic abnormalities are frequent. Rarely, t(11;14) and cyclin D1 overexpression are found.

Postulated Normal Counterpart

Plasma cell.

Differential Diagnosis

1. Diffuse large B-cell lymphoma, composed of immunoblasts with plasmacytic features: Presentation with lymphadenopathy favors lymphoma. Presentation with lytic bone lesions or diffuse marrow disease with an M-component favors plasmacytoma/myeloma. Lymphomas are more often sIg+, cIg−/+ (IgM is most frequent), B-antigen+, CD45+. Plasmacytomas are more often sIg−, cIg+ (especially IgG or IgA), B-antigen−, CD45−.
2. Carcinoma: Usually, carcinoma and plasma cell neoplasms can be distinguished on routinely stained sections. Occasionally, however, plasma cell neoplasms contain large bizarre cells, and this differential diagnostic possibility may arise. In addition, some plasma cell neoplasms are CD45−, EMA+, an immunophenotype that raises the question of carcinoma. Immunostains for cytokeratin and Ig should establish the diagnosis.
3. Acute myelogenous leukemia (AML): Some cases of myeloma show cleaved or multilobated nuclei (*see* Fig. 3–44), and in the presence of diffuse marrow involvement, they can resemble AML, especially myelomonocytic (M4) or monocytic (M5). Neoplastic plasma cells have more heterochromatic nuclei and lack cytoplasmic granularity, myeloperoxidase, and lysozyme.
4. Reactive plasmacytosis: Increased numbers of plasma cells may be found in the bone marrow in association with a variety of conditions, including infections, autoimmune diseases, and acquired immunodeficiency syndrome. Relative to other marrow elements, plasma cells may be abundant following chemotherapy for leukemia. Reactive plasma cells tend to be sprinkled evenly throughout the marrow, with some predilection for a perivascular localization, and tend not to displace hematopoietic precursors. Their appearance is almost always that of mature plasma cells. In difficult cases, immunohistochemical staining can be employed; reactive plasma cells express polyclonal immunoglobulin (normal light chain ratio is 4 or less).
5. Monoclonal gammopathy of uncertain significance (MGUS): Patients are older adults with an M-component, but without plasma cell myeloma, malignant lymphoma, or amyloidosis. Paraprotein in the serum is almost always less than 3g/dL; a monoclonal protein is found in the urine in only a minority of cases, and when present, it is a small amount. There are no bone lesions, renal disease, or cytopenias unless due to unrelated causes. In the marrow, plasma cells comprise 1% to 10% of the cellular population; they occur singly or in small clusters and appear mature or slightly immature. In one study, immunohistochemical staining showed that the light chain ratio was less than 16 in 96% of cases. Many patients have a stable course over a long period of time or die of unrelated causes, but a few develop a neoplasm so patients with MGUS should have regular clinical follow-up with serial quantitation of their paraprotein. In one large series, the actuarial risk for development of myeloma (or, less often, lymphoma or a related disorder) was 17% at 10 years and 33% at 20 years.

Patients with MGUS may have a variety of medical problems, with no single type predominating. MGUS does occur frequently in patients with Gaucher's disease. In a study of a large series of such patients treated at the Massachusetts General Hospital, nearly all were found to have a serum M-component, and the bone marrow biopsy specimens often showed increased numbers of plasma cells (Fig. 3–45). Despite long follow-up, the development of plasma cell myeloma in these patients was encountered only rarely (D. Kuter, personal communication).

References

Grogan TM, Spier CM: The B cell immunoproliferative disorders, including multiple myeloma and amyloidosis. *In:* Knowles DM, ed. Neoplastic hematopathology. Baltimore: Williams & Wilkins, 1992; 1235–1265.

Harris N, Bhan A: B-cell neoplasms of the lymphocytic, lymphoplasmacytoid, and plasma cell types: immunohistologic analysis and clinical correlation. Hum Pathol 16:829–837, 1985.

Kyle RA: "Benign" monoclonal gammopathy—after 20 to 35 years of follow-up. Mayo Clin Proc 68:26–36, 1993.

Lai JL, Zandecki M, Mary JY, *et al*: Improved cytogenetics in multiple myeloma: a study of 151 patients including 117 patients at diagnosis. (Review.) Blood 85:2490–2497, 1995.

Miralles GD, O'Fallon JR, Talley NJ: Plasma-cell dyscrasia with polyneuropathy: the spectrum of POEMS syndrome. N Engl J Med 327: 1919–1923, 1992.

Peterson LC, Brown BA, Crosson JT, Mladenovic J: Application of immunoperoxidase technic to bone marrow trephine biopsies in the classification of patients with monoclonal gammopathies. Am J Clin Pathol 85:688–693, 1986.

Sailer M, Vykoupil KF, Peest D, *et al*: Prognostic relevance of a histologic classification system applied in bone marrow biopsies from patients with multiple myeloma: a histopathological evaluation of biopsies from 153 untreated patients. Eur J Haematol 54:137–146, 1995.

Sukpanichant S, Cousar JB, Leelasiri A, *et al*: Diagnostic criteria and histologic grading in multiple myeloma: histologic and immunohistologic analysis of 176 cases with clinical correlation. Hum Pathol 25:308–318, 1994.

Tsuchiya J, Murakami H, Kanoh T, *et al*: Ten-year survival and prognostic factors in multiple myeloma. Br J Haematol 87:832–834, 1994.

Zukerberg L, Ferry J, Conlon M, Harris N: Plasma cell myeloma with cleaved, multilobated, and monocytoid nuclei. Am J Clin Pathol 93: 657–661, 1990.

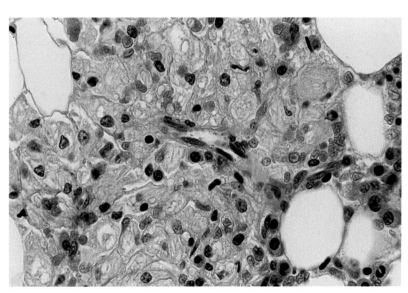

Figure 3–45. Gaucher's disease. The marrow contains numerous histiocytes with abundant, filamentous-appearing cytoplasm. The number of mature plasma cells is slightly increased (H&E stain).

DIFFUSE LARGE B-CELL LYMPHOMA (DLBCL)

Synonyms: Rappaport: diffuse histiocytic, occasional diffuse mixed lymphocytic-histiocytic; Kiel: centroblastic, B-immunoblastic, large cell anaplastic (B cell); Lukes-Collins: large cleaved or large noncleaved follicular center cell, B-immunoblastic; Working Formulation: large cell cleaved, noncleaved, or immunoblastic; occasionally diffuse mixed small and large cell.

Clinical Features

Large B-cell lymphomas affect patients over a broad age range from childhood to old age; the median age is in the sixth decade. They account for 30% to 40% of non-Hodgkin's lymphomas in adults. DLBCL is also one of the major types of lymphoma to affect children and adolescents. Patients typically present with a rapidly enlarging mass at a single nodal or extranodal site; DLBCL is extranodal in up to 40% of cases. A wide variety of extranodal sites may be affected, including gastrointestinal tract, bone, Waldeyer's ring, male and female genital tracts, central nervous system, spleen, and other sites (Figs. 3–46 and 3–47). In many cases, patients present with localized disease, but disseminated disease also occurs and is associated with a worse outcome. Large B-cell lymphomas are aggressive but potentially curable with aggressive therapy. Cases of multilobated B-cell type are often primary in bone.

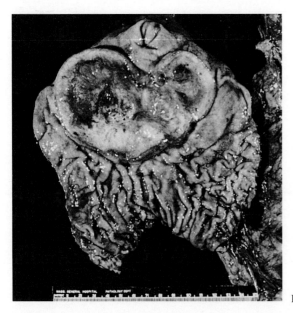

Figure 3–46. Diffuse large B-cell lymphoma associated with a huge gastric ulcer.

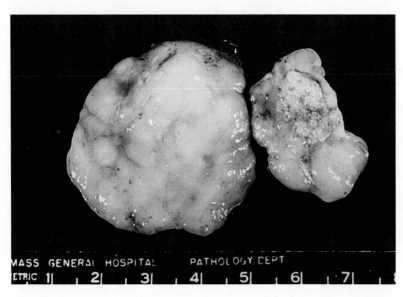

Figure 3–47. Diffuse large B-cell lymphoma. Pale, lobulated tissue has nearly entirely replaced both ovaries.

Morphology

Most diffuse large B-cell lymphomas are composed of large blastic cells with vesicular chromatin, prominent nucleoli, and basophilic cytoplasm with a Giemsa stain. Cells in most cases resemble centroblasts (large noncleaved cells) or immunoblasts, but some may be composed of large centrocytes (which typically have scant, pale, rather than basophilic, cytoplasm), multilobated cells, or a mixture of these (Figs. 3–48 to 3–51). Occasional cases are composed of anaplastic large cells identical to those of T- or null-cell anaplastic large cell lymphoma. Some cases of large B-cell lymphoma may be rich in small T lymphocytes or histiocytes, creating a resemblance to either T-cell lymphoma or Hodgkin's disease of the lymphocyte predominance type (T-cell-rich large B-cell lymphoma). (T-cell-rich large B-cell lymphoma is discussed in a separate section.)

The histologic features of bone marrow involvement in patients presenting with DLBCL in an extramedullary site vary. In many cases, marrow involvement takes the form of paratrabecular and nonparatrabecular aggregates of small irregular lymphoid cells with a few admixed large cells ("discordant marrow"). The prognosis for patients with discordant marrow involvement is similar to that for patients with staging bone marrow biopsy specimens free of lymphoma. In a minority of cases, the staging bone marrow biopsy reveals DLBCL; this is associated with a poor prognosis (Figs. 3–52 and 3–53).

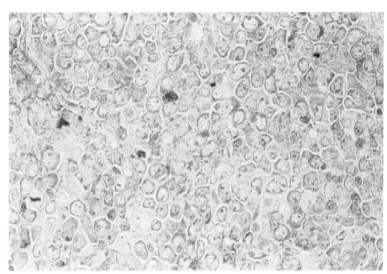

Figure 3–48. Diffuse large B-cell lymphoma composed of centroblasts. Nuclei are oval and vesicular, having one to several peripherally placed nucleoli and a narrow but distinct rim of basophilic cytoplasm (Giemsa stain).

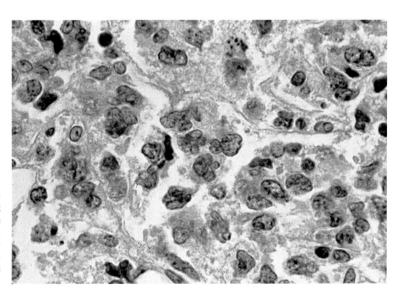

Figure 3–49. Diffuse large B-cell lymphoma with a predominance of multilobated cells. Nuclei show prominent nuclear lobation, the chromatin is fine, the nucleoli are inconspicuous, and the cytoplasm is scant (H&E stain). (From Harris NL, Jaffe ES, Stein H, *et al*: A revised European-American classification of lymphoid neoplasms: A proposal from the International Lymphoma Study Group. Blood 84:1361–1392, 1994.)

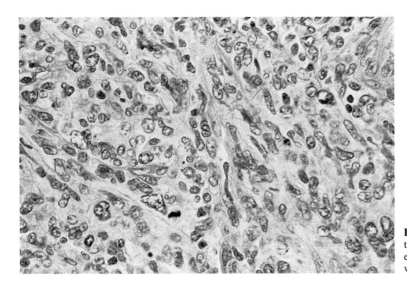

Figure 3–50. Diffuse large B-cell lymphoma with large centrocytes (large cleaved cells). Many of the neoplastic cells are elongated with a spindle shape. The lymphoma is associated with sclerosis (H&E stain).

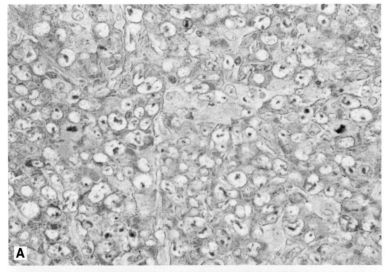

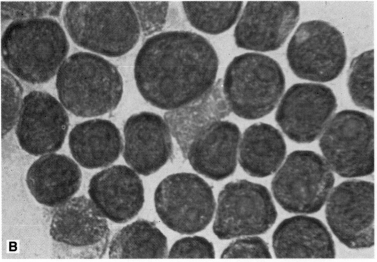

Figure 3–51. Diffuse large B-cell lymphoma composed of immunoblasts. *A,* In this testicular lymphoma, the neoplastic cells have oval vesicular nuclei, prominent central nucleoli, and basophilic cytoplasm that is slightly more abundant than in centroblasts (Giemsa stain). *B,* In this touch preparation from an ovarian lymphoma, the neoplastic cells have round nuclei, prominent nucleoli, and intensely basophilic cytoplasm (Wright-Giemsa stain).

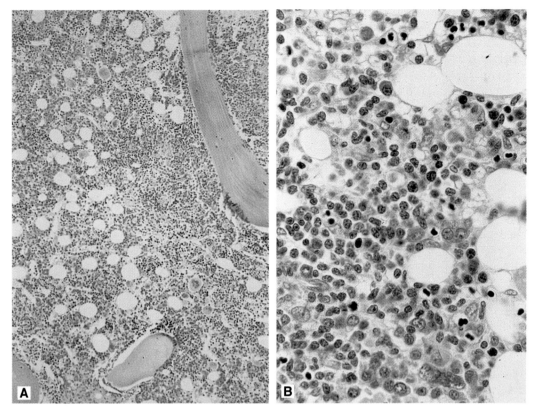

Figure 3–52. Bone marrow involvement by low grade lymphoma in a patient with an extramedullary diffuse large B-cell lymphoma (DLBCL). *A,* Low power view shows a poorly circumscribed, paratrabecular lymphoid aggregate in the upper right of the illustration (Giemsa stain). *B,* Higher power examination shows that the aggregate is composed mainly of small lymphocytes and small irregular lymphoid cells (Giemsa stain).

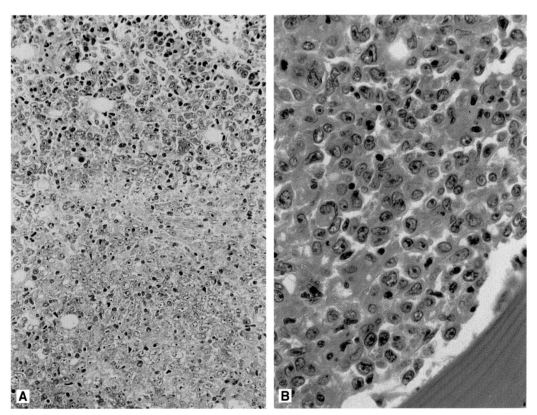

Figure 3–53. Bone marrow involvement by diffuse large B-cell lymphoma (DLBCL). *A,* Low power view shows a large irregular area of lymphoma that is paler and more homogeneously stained than the surrounding hematopoietic marrow (Giemsa stain). *B,* High power examination shows a monomorphous population of large lymphoid cells; many have the appearance of immunoblasts (H&E stain).

When a patient with DLBCL presents with splenic involvement, the disease usually is in the form of one or more large, destructive nodules, with frequent transgression of the splenic capsule and invasion of adjacent structures (Fig. 3–54).

Immunophenotype

Tumor cells are sIg+/−, cIg−/+, B-cell-associated antigens+ (CD19+, CD20+, CD22+, CD79a+), CD45+/−, CD5−/+, CD10−/+. Only a minority of cases with anaplastic morphology are DLBCL (most are T-lineage; *see* Chapter 4, Anaplastic Large Cell Lymphoma).

Genetic Features

Ig heavy and light chain genes are rearranged. The bcl-2 gene is rearranged in about 30%; in some cases c-myc is rearranged. A novel proto-oncogene, bcl-6, which codes for a zinc finger transcription factor, may be involved in the pathogenesis in up to one third of cases. Bcl-6 rearrangement has been associated with extranodal presentation and longer freedom from progression; bcl-2 rearrangement has been associated with a worse outcome.

Postulated Normal Counterpart

Proliferating peripheral B cell. (Rearrangement of the bcl-2 gene has been interpreted as evidence for a follicle center origin of some cases.)

Differential Diagnosis

Nonlymphoid neoplasms, including undifferentiated carcinoma, thymoma, granulocytic sarcoma, melanoma, and seminoma/dysgerminoma, are the most important entities in the differential diagnosis of DLBCL. In general, cohesive growth favors carcinoma (or thymoma), whereas lymphoid cells are discohesive. Cytologic features in favor of lymphoma are the presence of nuclei corresponding to centroblasts, immunoblasts, large centrocytes, or multilobated lymphoid cells with cytoplasm that usually appears deep blue on Giemsa stain. Immunoperoxidase stains are helpful in equivocal cases, but because both lymphoid and nonlymphoid tumors may lack some normal antigens, a broad panel of antibodies may be required.

1. Carcinoma: Cytokeratin+, CD45−.
2. Granulocytic sarcoma: Myeloperoxidase+, lysozyme+ (*see also* Granulocytic Sarcoma, Chapter 7).
3. Melanoma: S-100+, HMB-45+, CD45−.
4. Seminoma/dysgerminoma: This type of neoplasm has a distinctive pattern of growth, with nests or bands of tumor cells separated by fibrous septa containing small lymphocytes. The abundant pale cytoplasm is glycogen-rich. Seminoma/dysgerminoma is placental alkaline phosphatase (PLAP)+, CD45−.
5. Spindle cell sarcoma: Occasionally, especially in extranodal sites, DLBCL is composed of elongated cells resembling fibroblasts and is associated with sclerosis, which may be marked. In some cases, the neoplastic lym-

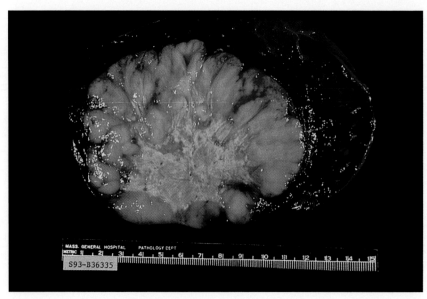

Figure 3–54. Spleen with diffuse large B-cell lymphoma (DLBCL). The tumor mass is large, tan, and centrally necrotic.

phoid cells acquire a storiform pattern of growth, and the appearance closely mimics that of fibrosarcoma or malignant fibrous histiocytoma. Careful attention to the

nuclear features of the neoplastic cells can help to establish the correct diagnosis, but frequently immunohistochemistry is required (Fig. 3–55).

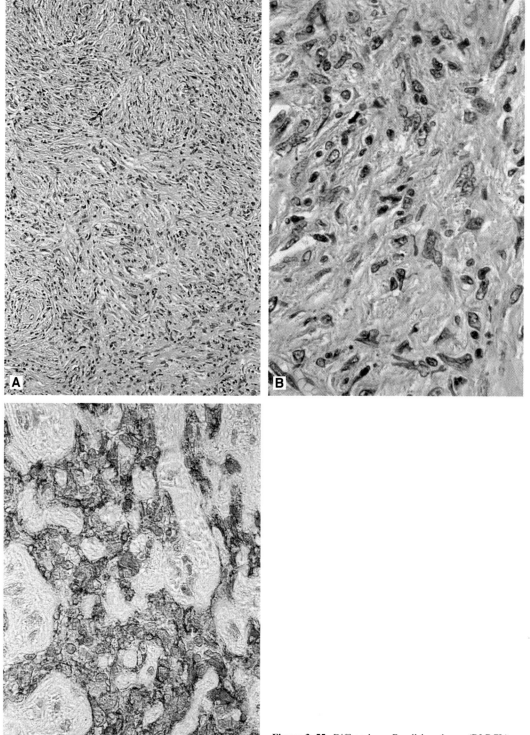

Figure 3–55. Diffuse large B-cell lymphoma (DLBCL) presenting in the vagina, mimicking spindle cell sarcoma. *A,* The tumor shows marked sclerosis and a vague storiform pattern (H&E stain). *B,* Most neoplastic cells have a spindle shape (H&E stain). *C,* Immunohistochemical staining confirmed the diagnosis of lymphoma (L26 shown here; immunoperoxidase technique on paraffin section).

References

Ferry JA, Harris NL, Picker LJ, *et al*: Intravascular lymphomatosis (malignant angioendotheliomatosis). A B-cell neoplasm expressing surface homing receptors. Mod Pathol 1:444–452, 1988.

Fisher DE, Jacobson JO, Ault KA, Harris NL. Diffuse large cell lymphoma with discordant bone marrow histology. Clinical features and biological implications. Cancer 64:1879–1887, 1989.

Harris NL, Aisenberg AC, Meyer JE, *et al*. Diffuse large cell (histiocytic) lymphoma of the spleen. Clinical and pathological characteristics of ten cases. Cancer 54:2460–2467, 1984.

Lennert K, Feller A: Histopathology of non-Hodgkin's lymphomas. New York: Springer-Verlag, 1992.

McBride JA, Rodriguez J, Luthra R, *et al*: T-cell-rich B large-cell lymphoma simulating lymphocyte-rich Hodgkin's disease. Am J Surg Pathol 20:193–201, 1996.

Non-Hodgkin's Lymphoma Pathologic Classification Project: National Cancer Institute sponsored study of classifications of non-Hodgkin's lymphomas: summary and description of a Working Formulation for clinical usage. Cancer 49:2112–2135, 1982.

Offit K, Lo Coco F, Louie DC, *et al*: Rearrangement of the bcl-6 gene as a prognostic marker in diffuse large-cell lymphoma. (See comments.) N Engl J Med 331:74–80, 1994.

Pettit C, Zukerberg L, Gray M, *et al*: Primary lymphoma of bone: a B cell tumor with a high frequency of multilobated cells. Am J Surg Pathol 14:329–334, 1990.

van Krieken JHJM: Histopathology of the spleen in non-Hodgkin's lymphoma. (Review.) Histol Histopath 5:113–122, 1990.

Ye BH, Lista F, Lo Coco F, *et al*: Alteration of a zinc-finger encoding gene, bcl-6, in diffuse large cell lymphoma. Science 262:747–750, 1993.

Yunis J, Mayer M, Arnesen M: Bcl-2 and other genomic alterations in the prognosis of large-cell lymphoma. N Engl J Med 320:1047–1054, 1989.

PRIMARY MEDIASTINAL (THYMIC) LARGE B-CELL LYMPHOMA

Clinical Features

Mediastinal B-cell lymphoma tends to affect young adults with a male:female ratio of about 1:2. Patients present with symptoms related to a locally invasive mass originating in the thymus, often with airway obstruction, superior vena cava syndrome, and pulmonary infiltration. The tumor is usually localized (Stage I or II) at presentation. Relapses are often extranodal, affecting the central nervous system, liver, gastrointestinal tract, kidneys, and ovaries (Figs. 3–56 and 3–57). The tumor is aggressive, but intensive treatment regimens yield cure rates similar to those of other forms of diffuse large B-cell lymphoma (DLBCL).

Morphology

The tumor is composed of large cells with nuclei that may be either round, angulated, or multilobated. The cytoplasm is often pale or clear. Less frequently, the tumor cells resemble immunoblasts. Reed-Sternberg-like cells may be present. Many cases have fine, compartmentalizing sclerosis (Figs. 3–58 and 3–59).

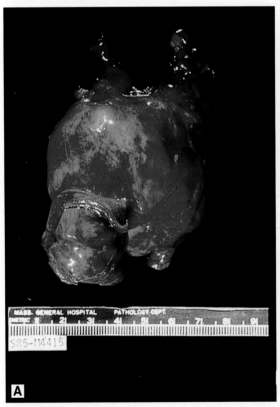
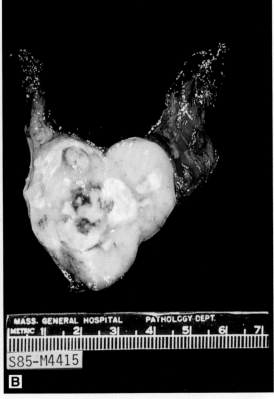

Figure 3–56. Mediastinal large B-cell lymphoma, gross appearance of a thymectomy specimen. *A,* External examination reveals a large, bulging tumor that replaces much of the thymus. *B,* Cross section of the specimen shows a pale yellow, lobulated tumor with a central chalky yellow area of necrosis.

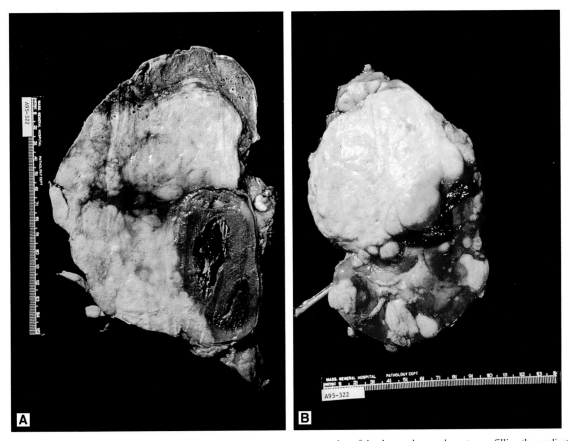

Figure 3–57. Mediastinal large B-cell lymphoma, fatal case. *A,* At autopsy, a cross section of the thorax shows a huge tumor filling the mediastinum, partially encasing the heart (*lower right*) and markedly compressing one lung (*top*). *B,* This patient had multiple extranodal sites of involvement, including the kidney, in which the parenchyma was nearly totally replaced by lymphoma.

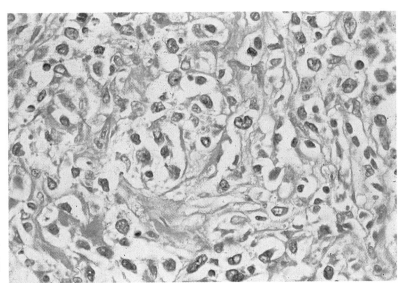

Figure 3–58. Mediastinal large B-cell lymphoma, composed of lymphoid cells with abundant clear cytoplasm, in a background of compartmentalizing sclerosis (H&E stain).

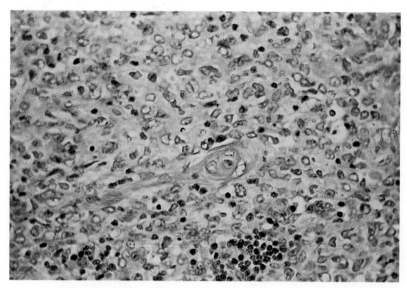

Figure 3–59. Mediastinal large B-cell lymphoma. The neoplastic cells surround a Hassall's corpuscle (*center*) (H&E stain).

Immunophenotype

Tumor cells are Ig−/+, B-cell-associated antigens+ (CD19+, CD20+, CD22+, CD79a+), CD45+/−, CD30−/+, CD15−.

Genetic Features

Ig heavy and light chain genes are rearranged.

Postulated Normal Counterpart

Putative thymic (medullary) B cell.

Differential Diagnosis

The differential diagnosis is the same as that for diffuse large B-cell lymphoma (DLBCL) in the preceding section.

References

Cazals-Hatem D, Lepage E, Brice P, *et al*: Primary mediastinal large B-cell lymphoma: a clinical and pathological study of 141 cases compared with nonmediastinal large B-cell lymphomas, a GELA ("groupe d'etude des lymphomes de l'adulte") study. Am J Surg Pathol 20:877–888, 1996.

Falini B, Venturi S, Martelli M, *et al*: Mediastinal large B-cell lymphoma: clinical and immunohistological findings in 18 patients treated with different third-generation regimens. Br J Haematol 89:780–789, 1995.

Jacobson J, Aisenberg A, Lamarre L, *et al*: Mediastinal large cell lymphoma: an uncommon subset of adult lymphoma curable with combined modality therapy. Cancer 62:1893–1898, 1988.

Lamarre L, Jacobson J, Aisenberg A, Harris N: Primary large cell lymphoma of the mediastinum. Am J Surg Pathol 13:730–739, 1989.

Rodriguez J, Pugh WC, Romaguera JE, Cabanillas F: Primary mediastinal large cell lymphoma. (Review.) Hematol Oncol 12:175–184, 1994.

T-CELL-RICH LARGE B-CELL LYMPHOMA (TCR-BCL); T-CELL/HISTIOCYTE-RICH LARGE B-CELL LYMPHOMA (T/HR-BCL)

Synonyms and Related Terms: T-cell-rich B-cell lymphoma; histiocyte-rich B-cell lymphoma; pseudo-T-cell lymphoma; Hodgkin's-like B-cell lymphoma; Working Formulation: diffuse mixed small and large cell, some cases; Rappaport: diffuse mixed lymphocytic and histiocytic, some cases.

The term "T-cell-rich B-cell lymphoma" was introduced in 1988 by Ramsay and co-workers to describe cases of large B-cell lymphoma with a striking infiltrate of T cells (90% or more), which obscured the neoplastic population and gave rise to a differential diagnosis of peripheral T-cell lymphoma. Since that time, many publications have been devoted to this topic, although criteria for the definition of T-cell-rich B-cell lymphoma have varied from study to study, with the proportion of T cells described as ranging from 90% or more to simply a "majority" of T cells. Although the lymphomas in most cases were entirely diffuse, some series included cases with a nodular component. Moreover, the neoplastic B cells were exclusively large cells in most cases described in these studies, but a few cases included in this category had an admixture or even a predominance of small B cells. Most cases occurred de novo, but some had a previous or subsequent history of follicle center lymphoma. A few cases were considered to be related to immunocytoma or chronic lymphocytic leukemia. Rarely, patients had lymphocyte predominance Hodgkin's disease concurrent with T-cell-rich B-cell lymphoma.

This heterogeneous group of cases can be sorted roughly into three categories: (1) diffuse large B-cell lymphoma with an unusually prominent infiltrate of reactive T cells; (2) low grade B-cell lymphomas (usually follicle center cell or lymphoplasmacytic) with many T cells; and (3) a rare disorder resembling or equivalent to diffuse lymphocyte predominance Hodgkin's disease. The last group might represent an important clinicopathologic entity, whereas the other categories are probably morphologic variants of familiar B-cell lymphomas.

We therefore recommend that the term T-cell-rich large B-cell lymphoma (TCR-BCL) be confined to cases in which the lymphoma has a predominantly diffuse architecture and the B cells are all large, transformed cells present singly in a background of non-neoplastic T cells. In some cases, histiocytes as well as T cells form a prominent component of the reactive infiltrate, so that an equally appropriate designation is T-cell/histiocyte-rich large B-cell lymphoma (T/HR-BCL). The information that follows is based on cases that fit this description.

Clinical Features

TCR-BCL (or T/HR-BCL) is estimated to constitute 1% of non-Hodgkin's lymphomas. Most patients are middle-aged to elderly adults (median age usually in the sixth decade) with a male preponderance. Occasionally, young adults are affected. Most patients present with lymphadenopathy, although extranodal presentations also occur. B symptoms (fever, night sweats, weight loss) are common. Patients usually have widespread disease (stage III or IV) at presentation; hepatosplenomegaly is common.

The course of the lymphoma is moderately aggressive, with most patients dying of disease despite intensive therapy. Some patients have responded to combination chemotherapy of the type used for diffuse large cell lymphoma, such as CHOP.

Morphology

The lymphoma has a diffuse pattern, typically obliterating the normal architecture of the lymph node or extranodal structure. Vague nodularity is sometimes seen. The T cells are small lymphocytes or sometimes slightly enlarged lymphoid cells with irregular nuclei. The B cells usually have the appearance of centroblasts or immunoblasts; some of them may resemble L and H ("popcorn") cells. Reed-Sternberg-like or bizarre cells, or large cells with irregular nuclei may be found, but diagnostic Reed-Sternberg cells are infrequent. Histiocytes, which may be epithelioid, are sometimes abundant, and some cases show plasma cells and eosinophils. Vascularity may be prominent. Necrosis has been described in a few cases. Fine, fibrillar sclerosis may be seen (Fig. 3–60). In a 1995 report by Schmidt and associates, two cases of TCR-BCL had foci resembling lymphocyte predominance Hodgkin's disease.

Immunophenotype

B cells may be difficult to appreciate on frozen sections; they are more readily visualized on paraffin sections. The B cells express pan B-cell antigens (L26, CD79a) and, often, EMA. CD15 is negative and CD30 is almost always negative. In some cases, monotypic Ig expression can be demonstrated, but in others, the B cells appear Ig-negative (Fig. 3–60C).

Most cells are T cells (CD3+, CD45RO+, CD43+), usually with a predominance of CD4+ over CD8+ cells (Fig. 3–60D). Expression of CD25 and HLA-DR, consistent with an activated state, has been described. Whether the numerous T cells represent an exuberant host response to the B-cell lymphoma or whether they are attracted to the lymphoma by cytokine release is a topic of debate. Against the former hypothesis is the relatively poor prognosis of TCR-BCL patients; in favor of the latter, one group using paraffin section immunohistochemistry has found interleukin 4 (IL-4) in tumor cells and histiocytes in nearly all cases of TCR-BCL but infrequently in control cases. These workers postulated that IL-4 secretion was responsible for the T-cell infiltrate. Since IL-4 also reportedly has an antiproliferative effect on activated neoplastic B cells, the same workers also suggested that IL-4 may play a role in the small number of B cells present.

Genotype

Clonal Ig heavy chain gene rearrangement has been demonstrated in some cases but not in others, most likely because of the small number of B cells. Clonal rearrangements of TCR genes are almost always absent (clonal rearrangement of TCR genes is found infrequently in cases of B-cell lymphoma).

Bcl-2 rearrangement usually is not found. Occasional cases contain EBV genetic material.

Differential Diagnosis

1. B-cell lymphomas with abundant T cells, other than TCR-BCL: Some non-Hodgkin's lymphomas contain a large component of non-neoplastic T cells but do not fulfill the criteria for TCR-BCL and should not be designated as such. Follicle center lymphomas, for example, frequently have numerous T cells, which may even compose greater than 50% of the cellular population. The appropriate diagnosis in such cases, however, is follicle center lymphoma. Occasionally, diffuse large B-cell lymphomas have typical areas as well as areas that contain numerous T cells resembling TCR-BCL. These cases should be designated diffuse large B-cell lymphoma with T-cell-rich areas.
2. Peripheral T-cell lymphoma (PTCL): The mixture of cells that may be seen in TCR-BCL and the occasionally prominent vascularity raise the possibility of angioim-

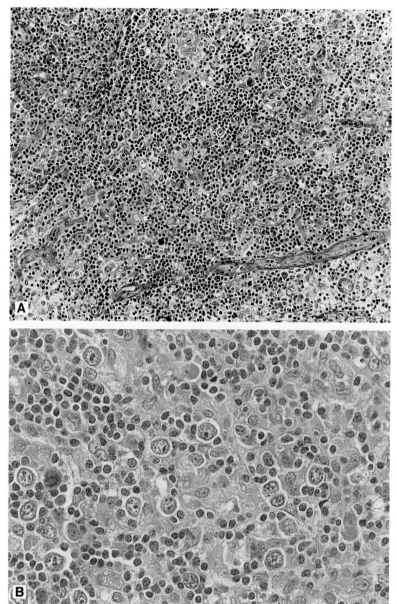

Figure 3–60. T-cell-rich large B-cell lymphoma. *A,* At low power, numerous small lymphocytes are visible as well as small clusters of histiocytes and increased high endothelial venules. Only a few large cells are present (H&E stain). *B,* The neoplastic cells are centroblasts and immunoblasts, scattered singly among reactive cells (H&E stain).

munoblastic T-cell lymphoma (AIL-TCL) (*see* Chapter 4). The presence of numerous histiocytes in some cases may suggest Lennert's lymphoma (*see* Peripheral T-cell Lymphoma, Unspecified, Chapter 4) or lymphohistiocytic T-cell lymphoma (histiocyte-rich variant of anaplastic large cell lymphoma) (*see* Anaplastic Large Cell (CD30+) Lymphoma, Chapter 4). The main problem in distinguishing TCR-BCL from PTCL, however, is that the few B cells may be overlooked, especially if the diagnosis is based on immunophenotyping performed on frozen sections alone. Paraffin section immunohistochemistry readily reveals that the atypical cells are B

cells. Some T cells may be slightly enlarged and have irregular nuclei, which is consistent with an activated state, but they do not show significant atypicality compared with the large B cells. The clear cells characteristic of AIL-TCL are not found.

3. Hodgkin's disease (HD), classic types (especially mixed cellularity and lymphocyte-rich classic HD): Diagnostic Reed-Sternberg cells are infrequent in TCR-BCL, and the large cells are B cells that are virtually always negative for CD15 and CD30 and positive for EMA, in contrast to Reed-Sternberg cells. The background population is more consistently polymorphous in HD, mixed cellu-

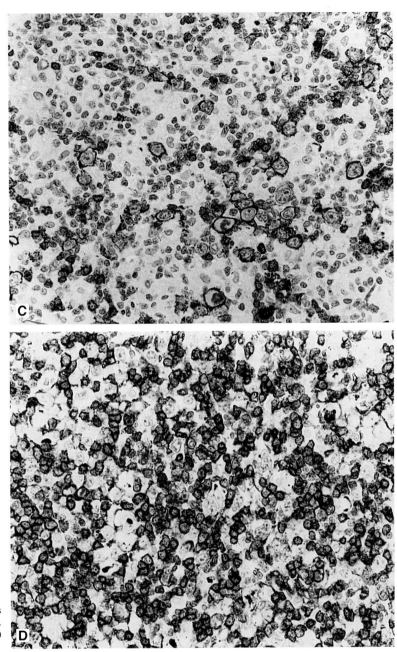

Figure 3–60. *Continued C,* The large cells are B cells (L26+) (immunoperoxidase technique on paraffin section). *D,* The reactive lymphocytes are T cells (CD45RO+) (immunoperoxidase technique on paraffin section).

larity, than in TCR-BCL, in which eosinophils and plasma cells may be infrequent.

Patients with TCR-BCL usually present with widespread disease, which may involve extranodal sites typically spared by HD. The distinction is important, because TCR-BCL is unlikely to respond to therapy directed against HD (*see also* Chapter 5).

4. HD, lymphocyte predominance (LPHD): In virtually all cases of LPHD, the lymphoma is partially or entirely nodular. L and H cells are usually uncommon in TCR-BCL. TCR-BCL may contain eosinophils and plasma cells, which are absent in LPHD. LPHD reportedly has

significantly larger numbers of small lymphoid cells expressing CD57, which sometimes form collarettes around L and H cells. Small numbers of CD57+ cells are found in TCR-BCL, and they do not surround the large B cells. Many of the small lymphocytes in LPHD are B cells, in contrast to TCR-BCL. LPHD contains meshworks of follicular dendritic cells that can be highlighted with antibodies to CD21; such meshworks are absent in TCR-BCL. (*See also* Lymphocyte Predominance HD, Chapter 5.)

5. Histiocyte-rich B-cell lymphoma (HR-BCL): In 1992, Delabie and co-workers described six cases they desig-

nated as HR-BCL and suggested that HR-BCL is a distinct entity that may be derived from the subset of B cells that gives rise to LPHD. HR-BCL appears to be equivalent to TCR-BCL (or T/HR-BCL), as described previously.

6. Reactive paracortical hyperplasia: Lymphoid hyperplasia in reaction to viruses or vaccinations may produce paracortical expansion, distorting the normal architecture with immunoblasts in a background of smaller lymphoid cells, raising the possibility of TCR-BCL. In lymphoid hyperplasias, however, the sinuses typically remain patent and often contain immunoblasts and the paracortex contains cells of a spectrum of sizes between small lymphocytes and immunoblasts.

References

Baddoura FK, Chan WC, Masih AS, *et al*: T-cell-rich B-cell lymphoma. A clinicopathologic study of eight cases. Am J Clin Pathol 103:65–75, 1995.

Chittal SM, Brousset P, Voigt J-J, Delsol G: Large B-cell lymphoma rich in T-cells and simulating Hodgkin's disease. Histopathology 19:211–220, 1991.

Delabie J, Vandenberghe E, Kennes C, *et al*: Histiocyte-rich B-cell lymphoma. A distinct clinicopathologic entity possibly related to lymphocyte predominant Hodgkin's disease, paragranuloma subtype. Am J Surg Pathol 16(1):37–48, 1992.

Jaffe ES, Longo DL, Cossman J, *et al*: Diffuse large B-cell lymphomas with T-cell predominance in patients with follicular lymphoma or "pseudo T-cell lymphoma." Lab Invest 50:27A–28A, 1984.

Kamel OW, Gelb AB, Shibuya RB, Warnke RA: Leu 7 (CD57) reactivity distinguishes nodular lymphocyte predominance Hodgkin's disease from nodular sclerosing Hodgkin's disease, T-cell-rich B-cell lymphoma and follicular lymphoma. Am J Pathol 142:541–546, 1993.

Macon WR, Cousar JB, Waldron JA, Jr., Hsu S-M: Interleukin-4 may contribute to the abundant T-cell reaction and paucity of neoplastic B cells in T-cell-rich B-cell lymphomas. Am J Pathol 141(5):1031–1036, 1992.

Macon WR, Williams ME, Greer JP, et al: T-cell-rich B-cell lymphomas. A clinicopathologic study of 19 cases. Am J Surg Pathol 16(4):351–363, 1992.

Mirchandani I, Palutke M, Tabaczka P, *et al*: B-cell lymphomas morphologically resembling T-cell lymphomas. Cancer 56:1578–1583, 1985.

Ng CS, Chan JKC, Hui PK: Large B-cell lymphomas with a high content of reactive T cells. Hum Pathol 20:1145–1154, 1989.

Ramsay AD, Smith WJ, Isaacson PG: T-cell-rich B-cell lymphoma. Am J Surg Pathol 12(6):433–443, 1988.

Schmidt U, Metz KA, Leder L-D: T-cell-rich B-cell lymphoma and lymphocyte-predominant Hodgkin's disease: two closely related entities? Br J Haematol 90:398–403, 1995.

INTRAVASCULAR LARGE B-CELL LYMPHOMA

Synonyms and Related Terms: Intravascular lymphomatosis; angiotropic lymphoma; malignant angioendotheliomatosis; neoplastic angioendotheliosis; systemic angioendotheliomatosis.

Intravascular lymphoma is a rare type of large B-cell lymphoma in which the neoplastic cells are exclusively or predominantly confined to the lumens of blood vessels. The lymphoma is usually widespread, affecting multiple extranodal sites, and symptoms relate to the resulting ischemia. For many years this disorder was thought to be a proliferation of endothelial cells. Another theory concerning the ori-

gin of the tumor was that it was a carcinoma from an occult primary site with extensive vascular invasion. Immunohistochemistry has established the lymphoid nature of this tumor. Why the neoplastic cells tend to remain within blood vessels is uncertain, but a defect in homing receptors has been suggested.

Clinical Features

Patients are middle-aged to older adults who present with symptoms related to extranodal disease, most often of the central nervous system, with the brain involved more often than the spinal cord. Patients may also have weight loss, fever, renal failure, pulmonary insufficiency, hypoadrenalism, and gastrointestinal hemorrhage.

Intravascular lymphoma does not respond well to therapy; the course usually progresses rapidly, with death most often due to neurologic deterioration. Among patients treated with combination chemotherapy appropriate for high grade lymphomas, however, a sustained complete remission may sometimes be attained. A less aggressive cutaneous form of this disease also exists.

Morphology

The sites most commonly involved are the brain, spinal cord, meninges, kidneys, lungs, adrenals, gastrointestinal tract, and soft tissue. Involvement of lymph nodes, peripheral blood, spleen, or bone marrow is uncommon. Large lymphoid cells with the appearance of centroblasts or immunoblasts fill the blood vessels, which are often dilated. Most vessels show no thrombosis. Although hemorrhage and necrosis of the surrounding tissue may occur, in most cases the tissue is viable and lacks obvious ischemic damage. In some cases, a small extravascular tumor may be identified, but in others, the tumor appears confined completely to vascular spaces (Figs. 3–61 and 3–62).

Immunophenotype

Nearly all cases have been B-cell lymphomas, although a few T-lineage cases have been described.

Differential Diagnosis

1. Nasal/nasal type T/NK cell lymphoma: Nasal-type lymphoma is associated with invasion and destruction of the walls of blood vessels and with extensive necrosis of the surrounding tissue. The usual lineage is natural killer (NK) cell or possibly NK-like T cell, not B cell.

2. Lymphomatoid granulomatosis: Lymphomatoid granulomatosis, like nasal-type lymphoma, is associated with angioinvasion and angiodestruction, not with plugging of vascular lumens by neoplastic cells. As in intravascular lymphoma, however, the neoplastic cells in lymphomatoid granulomatosis may be B cells.

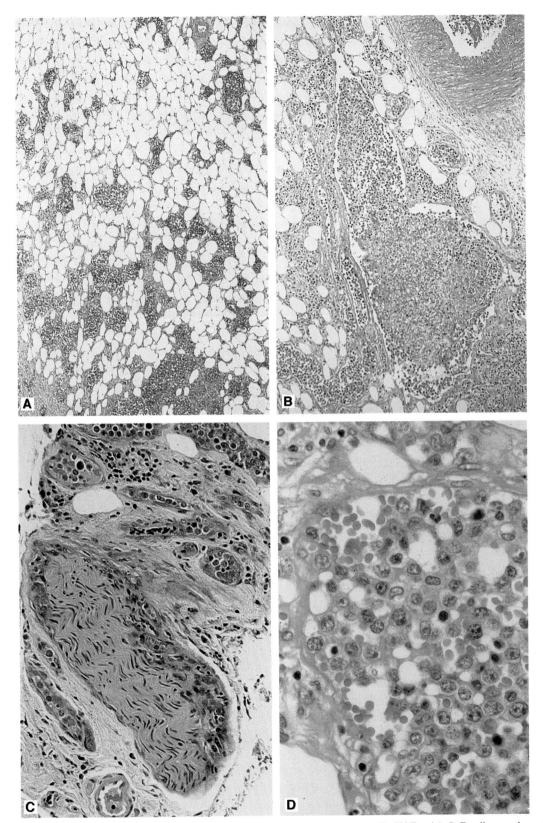

Figure 3–61. Intravascular lymphoma, soft tissue. *A,* Multiple blood vessels are filled with tumor cells (H&E stain). *B,* Focally, vessels containing tumor cells are thrombosed (H&E stain). *C,* Tumor cells are found in blood vessels within and surrounding small nerves (H&E stain). *D,* High power view shows a population of centroblasts and immunoblasts (H&E stain).

Illustration continued on following page.

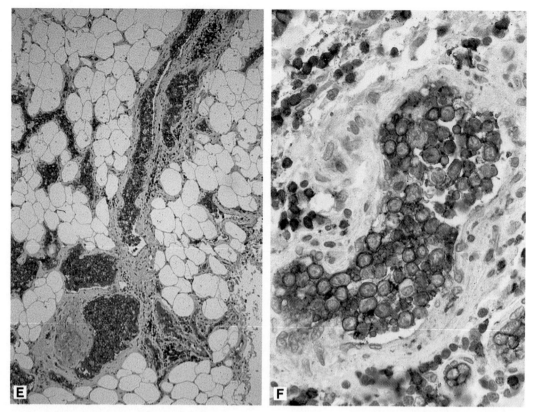

Figure 3–61. *Continued E,* Intravascular tumor cells throughout the soft tissue are positive for L26 (immunoperoxidase technique on paraffin section). *F,* Higher power view of the L26-stained section shows that the neoplastic cells are much larger than the non-neoplastic small lymphocytes located outside the blood vessel (immunoperoxidase technique on paraffin section).

References

Bhawan J, Wolff SM, Ucci AA, Bhan AK: Malignant lymphoma and malignant angioendotheliomatosis: one disease. Cancer 55:570–576, 1985.

Case Records of the Massachusetts General Hospital. Case 39–1986. N Engl J Med 315:874–885, 1986.

DiGiuseppe JA, Nelson WG, Seifter EJ, *et al*: Intravascular lymphomatosis: A clinicopathologic study of 10 cases and assessment of response to chemotherapy. J Clin Oncol 12:2573–2579, 1994.

Ferry JA, Harris NL, Picker LJ, *et al*: Intravascular lymphomatosis (malignant angioendotheliomatosis). A B-cell neoplasm expressing surface homing receptors. Mod Pathol 1:444–452, 1988.

Tateyama H, Eimoto T, Tada T, *et al*: Congenital angiotropic lymphoma (intravascular lymphomatosis) of the T-cell type. Cancer 67:2131–2136, 1991.

Wick MR, Mills SE, Scheithauer BW, *et al*: Reassessment of malignant "angioendotheliomatosis." Evidence in favor of its reclassification as "intravascular lymphomatosis." Am J Surg Pathol 10:112–123, 1986.

Sheibani K, Battifora H, Winberg CD, *et al*: Further evidence that "malignant angioendotheliomatosis" is an angiotropic large-cell lymphoma. N Engl J Med 314:943–948, 1986.

Wrotnowski U, Mills SE, Cooper PH: Malignant angioendotheliomatosis. An angiotropic lymphoma? Am J Clin Pathol 83:244–248, 1985.

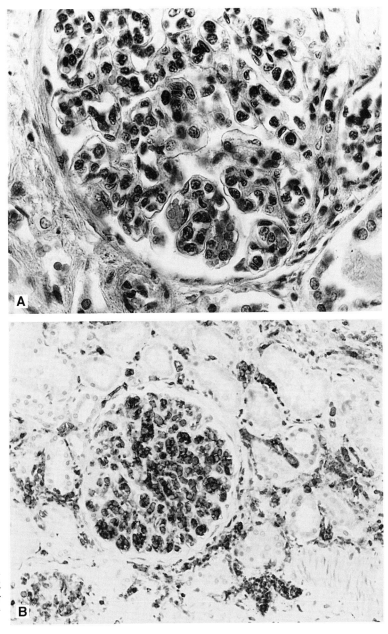

Figure 3–62. Intravascular lymphoma, kidney. *A,* Large lymphoid cells fill and distend the glomerular capillaries (H&E stain). *B,* Numerous large cells in glomerular and peritubular capillaries are stained by an anti-CD20 antibody (immunoperoxidase technique on frozen section).

PRIMARY EFFUSION LYMPHOMA

Synonyms and Related Terms: Body cavity-based lymphoma; primary serosal lymphoma; primary lymphomatous effusion.

Kaposi's sarcoma–associated herpes virus (human herpes virus type 8 [HHV-8]) has been associated with three diseases—Kaposi's sarcoma, multicentric Castleman's disease, and primary effusion lymphoma, all of which can be found in patients infected with human immunodeficiency virus (HIV). HHV-8 is a recently recognized virus that has partial homology with two other herpes viruses, Epstein-Barr virus (EBV) and herpes virus saimiri, a squirrel monkey virus.

The discovery of HHV-8 represents a critical step forward in the understanding of the pathogenesis of these diseases, suggesting that the development of Kaposi's sarcoma, multicentric Castleman's disease, and primary effusion lymphoma may be linked to a transmissible agent. This hypothesis would explain, for example, the puzzling question of why Kaposi's sarcoma is so much more common among HIV-positive homosexual and bisexual males compared with patients in other HIV risk groups.

Clinical Features

Patients with primary effusion lymphoma are nearly all HIV-positive young and middle-aged men. In most cases, patients have been homosexuals; intravenous drug abusers have also been affected. Most have a diagnosis of AIDS before the development of lymphoma. Overall, approximately half have had Kaposi's sarcoma, often accompanied by one or more opportunistic infections prior to presentation with lymphoma. Rarely, patients are HIV-negative and have no history of any other specific immunodeficiency.

Patients present with pleural effusion, pericardial effusion, ascites, or a combination of these, usually without a discrete mass that can be attributed to lymphoma. Follow-up information is not available in many cases, but the outcome has been virtually universally poor, with a median survival of only a few months. Death is due to lymphoma or, in these profoundly immunosuppressed patients, to Kaposi's sarcoma or opportunistic infection.

Morphology

The lymphoma is composed of large cells, usually described as resembling immunoblasts or having an anaplastic appearance. Tumor cells may be relatively uniform or pleomorphic, having binucleated, multinucleated, or Reed-Sternberg-like cells.

The neoplastic cells are usually best visualized in cytologic preparations of the effusions. A few scattered neoplastic cells may be seen in the pleura, but they do not form a substantial mass (Figs. 3–63 to 3–65).

Immunophenotype

In most cases, the neoplastic cells have a null immunophenotype, expressing CD45 and often CD30 and HLA-DR, but not B- or T-cell specific antigens. In a few cases, tumor cells express B-cell-associated antigens (Fig. 3–65B). In one case reported by Green and associates, the lymphoma was of T-lineage (CD3+, CD4+, CD5+), but the HHV-8 status of the patient was not known.

Genetic Features

Nearly all cases (including cases with a null immunophenotype) demonstrate Ig heavy and light chain gene rearrangement, confirming B-lineage. In addition, the neoplastic cells contain clonal EBV and HHV-8 genetic sequences. C-myc rearrangement is not found. EBV and HHV-8 may function together in the pathogenesis of this unusual lymphoma.

Differential Diagnosis

1. Pyothorax-associated lymphoma: Patients who have had longstanding pyothorax or marked chronic inflammation of the pleura, typically due to tuberculosis, may develop pleural lymphomas. These patients often have a history of pleural or pulmonary tuberculosis treated with pneumothorax. The lymphomas usually develop three or more decades after the onset of pleuritis. The lymphomas are large cell lymphomas of B-lineage and characteristically contain EBV. Unlike primary effusion lymphoma, however, pyothorax-associated lymphoma more often affects elderly men with no HIV risk factors; the lymphoma forms a solid pleural mass; the neoplastic cells more often have a B-cell, rather than null, immunophenotype; and HHV-8 is absent. Most reported pyothorax-associated lymphoma cases are from Japan; only a few such cases have been observed in any Western populations.

2. Secondary lymphomatous effusions: Any of a variety of high and low grade lymphomas in immunodeficient and immunocompetent patients can secondarily involve mesothelial-covered surfaces and be associated with effusions. In the absence of the large cell morphology and immunophenotype described previously, primary effusion lymphoma is unlikely. The presence of a contiguous tumor mass at the time of presentation excludes primary effusion lymphoma. If the patient has, or has had, a discrete lymphomatous mass in another site, the diagnosis of primary effusion lymphoma should be made with caution, although Cesarman and colleagues, in their 1995 report, include one case in which the patient had a submandibular lymphoma 5 months prior to presentation with a primary effusion lymphoma containing HHV-8.

3. Burkitt's and Burkitt-like lymphoma presenting as lymphomatous effusions: AIDS patients infrequently present with a lymphomatous effusion in which the morphology

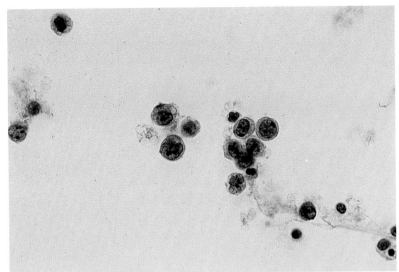

Figure 3–63. Primary effusion lymphoma in a young man with AIDS. The patient died 3 months after the diagnosis of lymphoma. Pleural fluid contains multiple large atypical lymphoid cells (Papanicolaou stain).

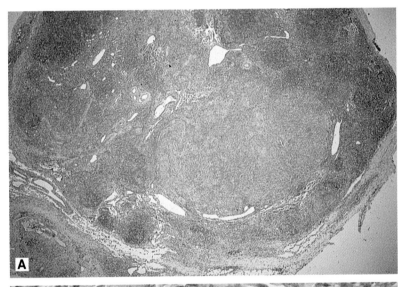

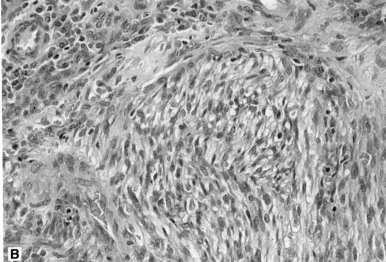

Figure 3–64. Same case as Figure 3–63. The patient also had Kaposi's sarcoma and multiple opportunistic infections. *A,* On low power examination, a nodule of Kaposi's sarcoma occupies a portion of a lymph node (H&E stain). *B,* On higher power examination, the Kaposi's sarcoma is composed of short fascicles of spindle cells with a few extravasated red blood cells (H&E stain).

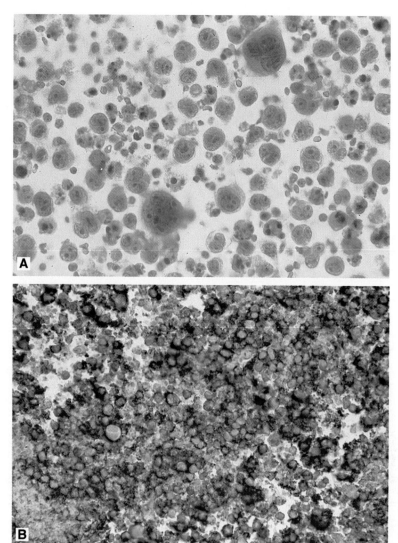

Figure 3–65. Primary effusion lymphoma in an elderly man of Italian descent with no HIV risk factors. *A,* The pleural fluid shows numerous large, atypical, sometimes multinucleated, lymphoid cells (Papanicolaou stain). *B,* An unusual feature of this case is the expression of the B-cell antigen, CD20 (immunoperoxidase technique on paraffin section).

of the neoplastic cells resembles Burkitt's or Burkitt-like lymphoma cells. In contrast to the primary effusion lymphomas described here, these lymphomas have c-myc rearrangement and lack HHV-8.

References

Ansari MQ, Dawson DB, Nador R, *et al*: Primary body cavity-based AIDS-related lymphomas. Am J Clin Pathol 105:221–229, 1996.

Cesarman E, Chang Y, Moore PS, *et al*: Kaposi's sarcoma-associated herpesvirus-like DNA sequences in AIDS-related body-cavity-based lymphomas. N Engl J Med 332:1186–1191, 1995.

Cesarman E, Nador RG, Aozasa K, *et al*: Kaposi's sarcoma-associated herpes virus in non-AIDS-related lymphomas occurring in body cavities. Am J Pathol 149:53–57, 1996.

Green I, Espiritu M, Ladanyi M, *et al*: Primary lymphomatous effusions in AIDS: a morphological, immunophenotypic and molecular study. Mod Pathol 8:39–45, 1995.

Jaffe ES: Primary body cavity-based AIDS-related lymphomas. Evolution of a new disease entity. (Editorial.) Am J Clin Pathol 105:141–143, 1996.

Martin A, Capron F, Liguory-Brunaud M-D, *et al*: Epstein-Barr virus-associated primary malignant lymphomas of the pleural cavity occurring in longstanding pleural chronic inflammation. Hum Pathol 25:1314–1318, 1994.

Ohsawa M, Tomita Y, Kanno H, *et al*: Role of Epstein-Barr virus in pleural lymphomagenesis. Mod Pathol 8:848–853, 1995.

BURKITT'S LYMPHOMA (BL)

Synonyms: Rappaport: undifferentiated lymphoma, Burkitt's type; Kiel: Burkitt's lymphoma; Lukes-Collins: small noncleaved follicular center cell; Working Formulation: small noncleaved cell, Burkitt's type; FAB: ALL, L3.

Clinical Features

Burkitt's lymphoma (BL) occurs in two settings: as an endemic disease in equatorial Africa and as a sporadic disease outside Africa. Sporadic BL may occur in normal or immunocompromised hosts. In both groups, most cases are found in the first two decades of life, although BL can affect patients of any age. Males are affected two to three times more often than females. Patients with either endemic or sporadic cases frequently present with high stage disease involving lymph nodes and extranodal sites; in endemic BL, the jaw, the kidneys, and the ovaries are involved most frequently, whereas in sporadic BL, the gastrointestinal tract is involved most often (Fig. 3–66). The tumor is highly aggressive but potentially curable. Rarely, a patient with the features of BL presents with involvement of bone marrow and peripheral blood. Such cases are designated acute lymphoblastic leukemia (ALL), L3. ALL, L3 has a poor prognosis.

Morphology

BL has a diffuse growth pattern; occasional cases show a focal follicular pattern. This tumor has an extremely high mitotic rate as well as a high rate of spontaneous cell death.

A starry-sky pattern is usually present, imparted by numerous tingible body macrophages that have ingested apoptotic debris. The tumor cells are monomorphic, medium-sized cells, with round nuclei, multiple nucleoli, and relatively abundant basophilic cytoplasm with lipid-containing vacuoles that can be seen on specimens from smears or touch preparations (Fig. 3–67).

In patients presenting with ALL, L3, bone marrow involvement is diffuse and extensive (Fig. 3–68).

Immunophenotype

Tumor cells are sIgM+, B antigen+ (CD19+, CD20+, CD22+, CD79a+), CD10+, CD5−, CD23−.

Genetic Features

Ig heavy and light chain genes are rearranged. Most cases have a translocation of c-*myc* from chromosome 8 to the Ig heavy chain region on chromosome 14 [t(8;14)], or less commonly, to light chain loci on chromosome 2 [t(2;8)] or 22 [t(8;22)]. In endemic cases, the breakpoint on chromosome 14 involves the heavy chain joining region, suggesting that the translocation occurs in an early B cell, before complete Ig gene rearrangement. In sporadic cases, the translocation involves the Ig heavy chain switch region, consistent with a translocation occurring at a later stage of B-cell development. Epstein-Barr virus (EBV) genomes can be demonstrated in the tumor cells in most endemic cases, but they are found infrequently in sporadic cases in immunocompetent patients.

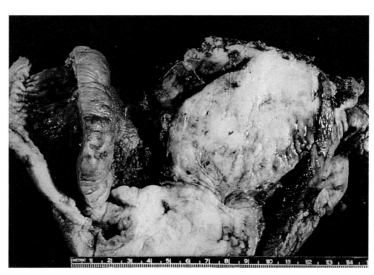

Figure 3–66. Burkitt's lymphoma, with a large mass involving the terminal ileum.

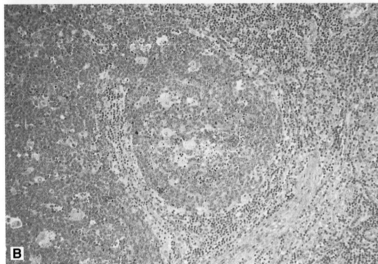

Figure 3–67. Burkitt's lymphoma. *A,* Low power view shows a diffuse infiltrate of tumor cells with a prominent starry-sky pattern (Giemsa stain). *B,* In this case from a 4-year-old child with congenital HIV infection, the lymphoma focally has a follicular pattern (H&E stain).

Both sporadic and endemic forms have had heavy chain genes with mutated variable regions, with a mutation frequency lower than that of follicle center lymphomas.

Postulated Normal Counterpart

B cell of unknown differentiation stage; possibly B-cell blast of early germinal center reaction.

Differential Diagnosis

1. High grade B-cell lymphoma, Burkitt-like: Distinction from BL on routine sections can be subjective; however, a uniform population of medium-sized neoplastic cells favors BL, while variation in nuclear size with an admixture of cells approaching the size of large lymphoid cells favors Burkitt-like lymphoma. In children, BL is more likely, whereas in adults, the Burkitt-like type is more common. Burkitt-like lymphoma is discussed in greater detail in the section that follows.

2. Lymphoblastic lymphoma (LBL), T- or B-cell type: In LBL, chromatin is dispersed more finely, nucleoli are less conspicuous, and cytoplasm is less abundant and less intensely basophilic than in BL. BL cells are positive for B-cell-associated antigens (CD19+, CD20+, CD22+, CD79a+), sIg+, TdT−, whereas B-LBL is typically sIg−, TdT+, and CD19+, although other B-cell antigens may be absent. T-LBL is sIg−, TdT+, T antigen+ and does not express B-cell-associated antigens.

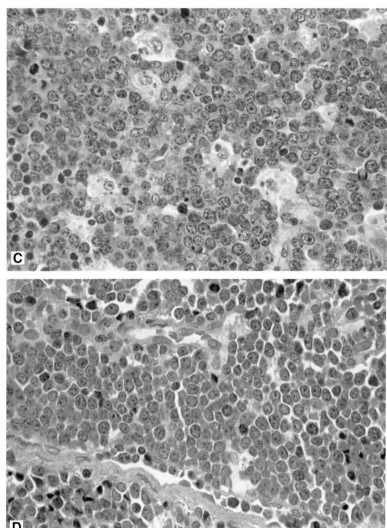

Figure 3–67. *Continued C,* Neoplastic cells are intermediate in size and have round nuclei, granular chromatin, and small nucleoli. The size of the tumor cell nuclei is similar to that of the interspersed tingible body macrophages. The mitotic rate is high (H&E stain). *D,* In this specimen, some areas form a mosaic pattern, with the cytoplasm of neighboring cells "squared off" (H&E stain).

References

Dayton VD, Arthur DC, Gajl-Peczalska KJ, Brunning R: L3 acute lymphoblastic leukemia. Comparison with small noncleaved cell lymphoma involving the bone marrow. Am J Clin Pathol 101:130–139, 1994.

Garcia C, Weiss L, Warnke R: Small noncleaved cell lymphoma: an immunophenotypic study of 18 cases and comparison with large cell lymphoma. Hum Pathol 17:454–461, 1986.

Magrath I, Shiramizu B: Biology and treatment of small non-cleaved cell lymphoma. Oncology 3:41–53, 1989.

Neri A, Barriga F, Knowles D, *et al*: Different regions of the immunoglobulin heavy-chain locus are involved in chromosomal translocations in distinct pathogenetic forms of Burkitt lymphoma. Proc Natl Acad Sci USA 85:2748–2752, 1988.

Tamaru J, Hummel M, Marafioti T, *et al*: Burkitt's lymphomas express VH genes with a moderate number of antigen-selected somatic mutations. Am J Pathol 147:1398–1407, 1995.

Wright D: Gross distribution and hematology. *In* Burkitt D, Wright D, eds. Burkitt's Lymphoma. London: E & S Livingstone, 1970; 64–81.

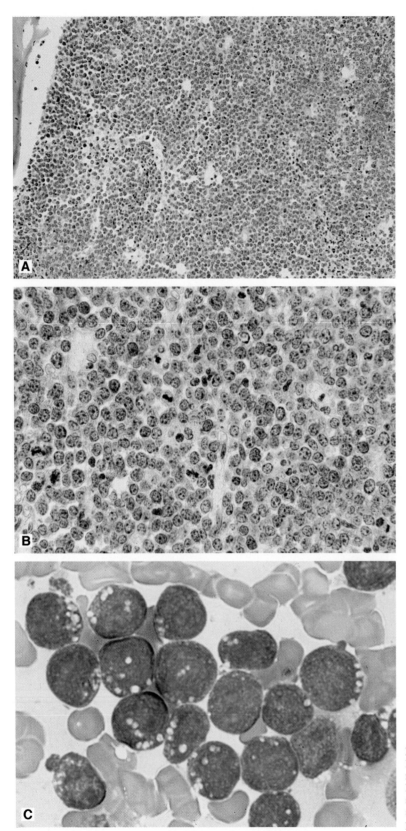

Figure 3–68. Burkitt's lymphoma, bone marrow (acute lymphoblastic leukemia L3). *A,* The normal marrow elements are virtually replaced by lymphoma (Giemsa stain). *B,* High power view shows a population of uniform, medium-sized cells with a high mitotic rate (Giemsa stain). *C,* The smear from aspirate contains blasts with basophilic cytoplasm and cytoplasmic vacuoles (Wright-Giemsa stain).

HIGH GRADE B-CELL LYMPHOMA, BURKITT-LIKE (PROVISIONAL CATEGORY)

Synonyms: Rappaport: undifferentiated, non-Burkitt; Kiel: Burkitt's lymphoma with cytoplasmic Ig (?); Lukes Collins: small noncleaved follicular center cell; Working Formulation: small noncleaved cell, non-Burkitt.

Clinical Features

Compared with Burkitt's lymphoma, patients with Burkitt-like lymphoma are more likely to be adults and to present with nodal disease. In children, these lymphomas behave similarly to classic Burkitt's tumor, but in adults, they are highly aggressive and often fatal, although encouraging results have been reported with the use of aggressive combination chemotherapy.

Morphology

Cases included in this group are diffuse, high grade lymphomas with a high mitotic rate and, often, a starry-sky pattern. Cytologic features are intermediate between those of large cell lymphoma composed of centroblasts or immunoblasts and classic Burkitt's lymphoma. Nuclei may be more pleomorphic than those of Burkitt's lymphoma, and nucleoli may be more prominent (Fig. 3–69).

Immunophenotype

Tumor cells are sIg+/− (may have cIg), B-cell-associated antigens+, CD5−, and usually CD10−.

Genetic Features

Rearrangement of c-*myc* is uncommon; the bcl-2 gene is rearranged in 30%, suggesting that these tumors are probably related more closely to large B-cell lymphoma than to true Burkitt's lymphoma.

Postulated Normal Counterpart

Proliferating peripheral B cell.

Differential Diagnosis

1. Burkitt's lymphoma (*see* preceding section).
2. Diffuse large B-cell lymphoma (DLBCL): The differentiation of DLBCL from Burkitt-like lymphoma may be difficult, and in fact this category is reserved, in effect, for borderline cases between BL and DLBCL. A diagnosis of DLBCL is made when large cells having nuclei larger than the nuclei of reactive histiocytes predominate. A diagnosis of Burkitt-like lymphoma is made when the neoplastic cells, on average, have nuclei smaller than, or the same size as, those of histiocytes, with an unusually high mitotic rate.

References

Hutchison R, Murphy S, Fairclough D, *et al*: Diffuse small noncleaved cell lymphoma in children, Burkitt's versus non-Burkitt's types. Cancer 64:23–38, 1989.

Longo DL, Duffey PL, Jaffe ES, *et al*: Diffuse small noncleaved cell, non-Burkitt's lymphoma in adults: a high grade lymphoma responsive to Pro-MACE-based combination chemotherapy. J Clin Oncol 12:2153–2159, 1994.

Yano T, van Krieken J, Magrath I, *et al*: Histogenetic correlations between subcategories of small noncleaved cell lymphomas. Blood 79:1282–1290, 1992.

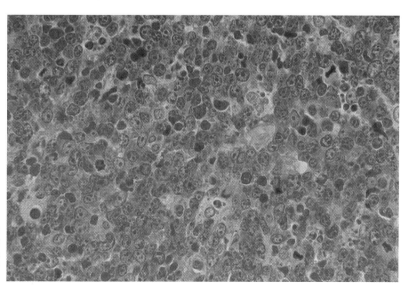

Figure 3–69. Burkitt-like lymphoma. The neoplastic cells show slightly more variation in size, more vesicular nuclei and more prominent nucleoli than occur in Burkitt's lymphoma. Numerous mitoses and tingible body macrophages are present (H&E stain).

CHAPTER 4

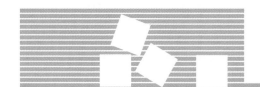

Non-Hodgkin's Lymphomas: T-Cell and Putative Natural Killer-Cell (NK) Neoplasms

In this chapter, as in Chapter 3, lymphomas are classified according to the R.E.A.L. (Revised European-American Lymphoma) Classification. R.E.A.L. diagnostic categories for T-cell neoplasms are shown with the corresponding diagnoses in the Kiel Classification and the Working Formula-tion in Table 4–1. A summary of clinical and pathologic features of T-cell neoplasms is given in Table 4–2. As with B-cell lymphomas, the different types of T-cell lymphomas are thought to represent malignant transformation of T cells at various stages of differentiation (Fig. 4–1).

Table 4–1

COMPARISON OF T-CELL NEOPLASMS IN THE REVISED EUROPEAN-AMERICAN LYMPHOMA CLASSIFICATION
WITH THE KIEL CLASSIFICATION AND THE WORKING FORMULATION

Kiel Classification	Revised European-American Lymphoma Classification	Working Formulation
T-lymphoblastic	Precursor T-lymphoblastic lymphoma/leukemia	Lymphoblastic
T-lymphocytic, CLL type T-lymphocytic, prolymphocytic leukemia	T-cell chronic lymphocytic leukemia/ prolymphocytic leukemia	*Small lymphocytic* Diffuse small cleaved cell

T-lymphocytic, CLL type	Large granular lymphocyte leukemia
	  T-cell type
	  NK-cell type
		Small lymphocytic
		Diffuse, small cleaved cell

Small cell cerebriform (mycosis fungoides, Sézary syndrome)	Mycosis fungoides/Sézary syndrome	Mycosis fungoides
T-zone Lymphoepithelioid Pleomorphic, small T cell *Pleomorphic, medium-sized and large T cell* T-immunoblastic	Peripheral T-cell lymphomas, unspecified (including provisional subtype: subcutaneous panniculitic T-cell lymphoma) Hepatosplenic γδ T-cell lymphoma (provisional entity)	Diffuse, small cleaved cell *Diffuse, mixed small and large cell* Diffuse, large cell *Large cell immunoblastic*
Angioimmunoblastic (angioimmunoblastic lymphadenopathy, lymphogranu-lomatosis X)	Angioimmunoblastic T-cell lymphoma	*Diffuse, mixed small and large cell* Diffuse, large cell *Large cell immunoblastic*
*	Nasal/nasal type T/NK-cell lymphoma	Diffuse, small cleaved cell *Diffuse, mixed small and large cell* Diffuse, large cell *Large cell immunoblastic*
*	Intestinal T-cell lymphoma	Diffuse, small cleaved cell Diffuse, mixed small and large cell Diffuse, large cell *Large cell immunoblastic*
Pleomorphic small T cell, HTLV-1+ *Pleomorphic medium-sized and large T cell, HTLV-1+*	Adult T-cell lymphoma/leukemia	Diffuse, small cleaved cell *Diffuse, mixed small and large cell* Diffuse, large cell *Large cell immunoblastic*
Large T-cell anaplastic (Ki-1)+	Anaplastic large cell lymphoma, T- and null-cell types	Large cell immunoblastic

When more than one Kiel or Working Formulation category is listed, those in *italic* type constitute the majority of the cases.

*Not listed in classification, but discussed as rare or ambiguous type.

Modified from Table 2 in Harris NL, Jaffe ES, Stein H, *et al*: A revised European-American Classification of lymphoid neoplasms: A proposal from the International Lymphoma Study Group. Blood 84:1361–1392, 1994.

Table 4-2
T-CELL AND NATURAL KILLER (NK)-CELL NEOPLASMS

Category	Neoplastic Cells	Usual Immuno-phenotype	Genetic Features	Patients Affected	Sites Affected	Usual Behavior
1. Precursor T-lymphoblastic lymphoma/leukemia	T lymphoblasts	TdT+, CD1a+, CD3+, CD7+, CD4+, CD8+	TCR-R (most) or G; IgH-R or G (most)	Adolescent and young adults>older adults, M>F	Mediastinum, lymph nodes, marrow, blood	Highly aggressive, but potentially curable
2. T-cell chronic lymphocytic leukemia/T-cell prolymphocytic leukemia	Prolymphocytes or small lymphocytes	CD3+, CD5+/−, CD7+, most CD4+	TCR-R; inv 14(q11;q32) is common	Adults	Marrow, spleen, liver, blood, lymph nodes, mucosal sites, skin	More aggressive than B-CLL, not curable
3. T-cell large granular lymphocyte leukemia	Large granular lymphocytes	CD3+, CD5+/−, CD7−, TCRαβ+, CD4−, CD8+, CD16+, CD56−, CD57+/−	TCR-R	Adults>children	Blood, spleen (red pulp)	Indolent
4. NK-cell large granular lymphocyte leukemia	Large granular lymphocytes	CD2+, CD3−, TCRαβ−, CD4−, CD8+/−, CD16+, CD56+/−, CD57+/−	TCR-G, some EBV+	Young adults>children, more common in Asians	Blood; may spread to liver and spleen	May be indolent but EBV+ cases are aggressive
5. Mycosis fungoides/Sézary syndrome	Small +/− large cerebriform cells	CD3+, CD5+, CD7−/+, CD4+, CD8−	TCR-R	Adults	Skin with/without blood, lymph nodes, and other sites late in course	Indolent
6. Peripheral T-cell lymphoma, unspecified	Small, medium, or large atypical cells	CD3, CD2, CD5, CD7, CD45RO variably +, CD4>CD8	TCR-R	Adults	Lymph nodes and extranodal sites	Variable, usually aggressive
7. Hepatosplenic γδ T-cell lymphoma	Medium-sized cells with pale cytoplasm	TCRγδ+, CD2+, CD3+, CD5−/+, CD7−/+, CD4−, CD8−/+	TCR-R, iso 7q	Young men	Liver (sinuses), spleen (red pulp), marrow (sinusoids)	Aggressive
8. Subcutaneous panniculitic T-cell lymphoma	Small, medium or large cells with karyorrhexis	As for peripheral T-cell lymphoma, unspecified; TCRαβ+, EBV−	TCR-R	Adults	Subcutaneous tissue	May be indolent, but if associated with hemophagocytosis, prognosis is poor
9. Angioimmunoblastic T-cell lymphoma	Medium-sized clear cells, some blasts	CD3+, CD4+, prominent CD21+ FDC network	TCR-R; IgH-R rarely; EBV often present	Adults	Lymph nodes (generalized); marrow and extranodal sites may be involved	Moderately aggressive
10. Nasal-type T/NK-cell (angiocentric) lymphoma	Small, medium, or large cells	CD2+, sCD3− but cCD3+, CD56+	TCR-G, IgH-G, EBV+	Adults, rarely children; Asians>Caucasians	Nose, palate, skin, other extranodal sites	Often aggressive, occasionally indolent; potentially curable
11. Intestinal T-cell lymphoma	Small, medium, or large cells; sometimes anaplastic cells	CD3+, CD8+/−, CD4−, CD103+	TCR-R	Adults, often with history of celiac sprue	Proximal small intestine, other extranodal sites	Aggressive
12. Adult T-cell lymphoma/leukemia	Small, medium, or large cells, "flower" cells	CD3+, CD4+, CD25+, CD7−/+	TCR-R, HTLV-1+	Adults, especially from Japan and Caribbean	Blood, lymph nodes, often disseminated	Highly aggressive
13. Anaplastic large cell lymphoma	Large, pleomorphic or monomorphic cells, sometimes RS-like	T-cell antigen+, or null; CD30+, EMA+	TCR-R, IgH-G; occasionally TCR and IgH-G; t(2;5) common	Adults and children	Lymph nodes, skin and other extranodal sites	Aggressive, but potentially curable

Abbreviations: TCR, T-cell receptor genes; IgH, Ig heavy chain genes; R, clonally rearranged; G, germline; M, male; F, female; c, cytoplasmic; s, surface; TCRαβ, T-cell receptor αβ heterodimer; TCRγδ, T-cell receptor γδ heterodimer; EBV, Epstein-Barr virus; FDC, follicular dendritic cell; RS, Reed-Sternberg cell.

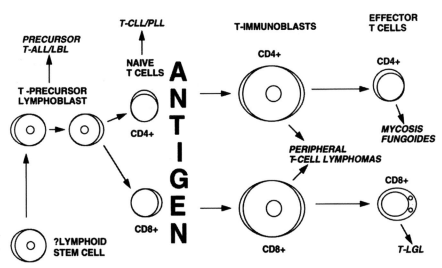

Figure 4–1. T-cell differentiation with postulated neoplastic counterparts (noted in italics). Compare with Figure 1–2.

Precursor T-Cell Neoplasm

PRECURSOR T LYMPHOBLASTIC LYMPHOMA/LEUKEMIA (T-LBL)

Synonyms: Rappaport: poorly differentiated lymphocytic, diffuse (modified to lymphoblastic); Kiel: T lymphoblastic; Lukes-Collins: convoluted T lymphocytic; Working Formulation: lymphoblastic, convoluted or NOS; FAB: ALL, L1 and L2.

Clinical Features

Precursor T lymphoblastic lymphoma/leukemia (T-LBL) constitutes 40% of childhood lymphomas and 15% of acute lymphoblastic leukemia (ALL). Most patients are adolescent and young adult males, but older adults may be affected. As for B-precursor LBL, in cases in which patients have discrete tumors but more than 25% bone marrow lymphoblasts, a diagnosis of ALL is made. Patients present with rapidly enlarging, mediastinal (thymic) masses and/or peripheral lymphadenopathy or with acute leukemia. If untreated, most cases of lymphoma progress to acute leukemia; CNS involvement is common. The tumor is rapidly fatal if untreated but potentially curable with chemotherapy.

Morphology

T-LBL has a diffuse pattern of growth. The tumor cells have round or convoluted nuclei, finely dispersed chromatin, inconspicuous nucleoli, scant cytoplasm, and high mitotic rate (Fig. 4–2). They are morphologically indistinguishable from precursor B lymphoblasts.

Among patients presenting with ALL, marrow involvement is usually extensive, and only small numbers of normal hematopoietic precursors may be recognizable.

Immunophenotype

Most cases are CD7+, CD3+ (cytoplasmic CD3+, surface CD3+/−) TdT+, CD1a+/−, CD2+/−, CD5+/−, CD10−/+, Ig−, B-cell antigens−, CD4+, CD8+ (double positive), or CD4−, CD8− (double negative) (Fig. 4–2, C and D). They may express either αβ or γδ T-cell receptor molecules, or express neither. Expression of NK antigens (CD16, CD57) has been reported and may be associated with a worse prognosis. Leukemic cases tend to have a more immature phenotype than lymphoma cases. Many cases of T-ALL express the SCL/TAL-1 (stem cell leukemia/T-cell acute leukemia) protein, which, among leukemias and lymphomas, is highly specific for T-ALL.

Genetic Features

Rearrangement of TCR genes is usually found; Ig heavy chain gene rearrangement is seen in a minority of cases. Some cases are diploid, but recurring abnormalities include those involving 14q11 (TCR αδ), 7q32-q36 (TCR β), 11p15 (tcl-2 oncogene), and 1p32 (tal-1 gene), and abnormalities of 9p.

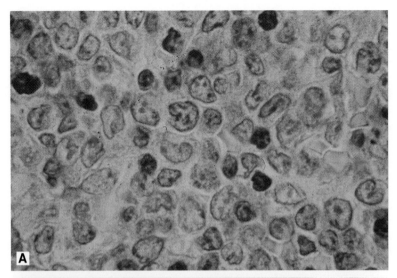

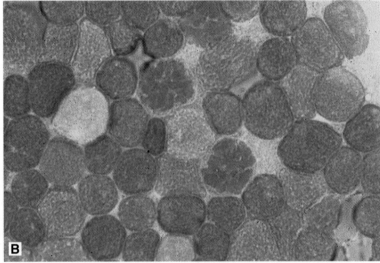

Figure 4–2. T-precursor lymphoblastic lymphoma (LBL). *A,* In a tissue section, the tumor cells are small, with pale, often angulated, and deeply indented nuclei and scant cytoplasm. Nucleoli are relatively small (Giemsa stain). *B,* In a touch preparation of a specimen from another case, nuclei are round to occasionally deeply indented, with finely dispersed chromatin. Cytoplasm is scant and the mitotic rate is high (Wright-Giemsa stain).

Postulated Normal Counterparts

Precursor T cells (antigen-independent stage), including prothymocyte, early thymocyte, and common thymocyte.

Differential Diagnosis

1. Precursor B lymphoblastic lymphoma: See Chapter 3, Precursor B Lymphoblastic Leukemia/Lymphoma.
2. Mantle cell lymphoma (MCL): MCL of blastoid type can be difficult to distinguish from LBL of either B or T pre-

cursor type on routine light microscopy. T-LBL tends to affect younger patients and to appear in different anatomic sites (mediastinum, marrow, peripheral blood) at presentation than MCL (lymph nodes, gastrointestinal tract). Immunohistochemistry readily distinguishes T-LBL from MCL: T-LBL is usually CD1a+, CD3+, CD7+, CD4+, CD8+, TdT+; MCL is Ig+, B antigen+, CD5+.
3. Granulocytic sarcoma: Granulocytic sarcomas composed of blasts, without recognizable myeloid maturation, may be difficult to distinguish from LBL. Granulocytic sarco-

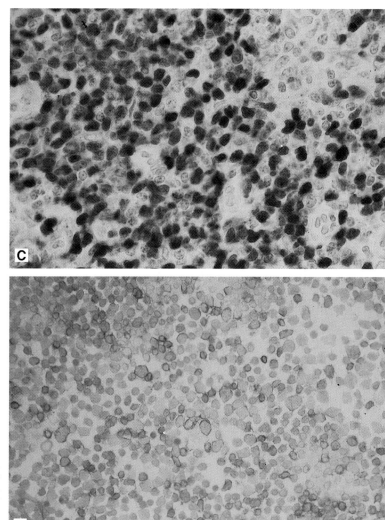

Figure 4–2. *C,* Strong staining for TdT occurs in the nuclei of neoplastic cells; adjacent normal lymphocytes are negative (immunoperoxidase technique on paraffin sections). *D,* A pleural effusion from a patient with a mediastinal T-precursor LBL shows distinct staining of many cells with an antibody to CD1a, confirming the presence of neoplastic cells (immunoperoxidase technique on cytospin preparations).

mas, unlike T-LBL, are CAE+, myeloperoxidase+, lysozyme+.

References

Chetty R, Pulford K, Jones M, *et al*: SCL-Tal-1 expression in T-acute lymphoblastic leukemia: an immunohistochemical and genotypic study. Hum Pathol 26:994–998, 1995.

Falini B, Flenghi L, Fagioli M, *et al*: T-lymphoblastic lymphomas expressing the non-disulfide-linked form of the T-cell receptor. Blood 74(7):2501–2507, 1989.

Gouttefangeas C, Bensussan A, Boumsell L: Study of the CD3-associated T-cell receptors reveals further differences between T-cell acute lymphoblastic lymphoma and leukemia. Blood 74:931–934, 1990.

Nathwani B, Diamond L, Winberg C, *et al*: Lymphoblastic lymphoma: a clinicopathologic study of 95 patients. Cancer 48:2347–2357, 1981.

Pulford K, Lecointe N, Leroy-Viard K, *et al*: Expression of TAL-1 proteins in human tissues. Blood 85:675–684, 1995.

Sheibani K, Nathwani B, Winberg C: Antigenically defined subgroups of lymphoblastic lymphoma: relationship to clinical presentation and biological behavior. Cancer 60:183–190, 1987.

Sixth International Workshop on Chromosomes in Leukemia: London, England, May 11–18, 1987: Selected papers. Cancer Genet Cytogenet 40:171–216, 1989.

Swerdlow S, Habeshaw J, Richards M, *et al*: T lymphoblastic lymphoma with Leu-7 positive phenotype and unusual clinical course: a multiparameter study. Leuk Res 9:167–173, 1985.

Peripheral T-Cell Neoplasms

T-CELL CHRONIC LYMPHOCYTIC LEUKEMIA (T-CLL)/T-PROLYMPHOCYTIC LEUKEMIA (T-PLL)

Synonyms: Rappaport: Well-differentiated lymphocytic, poorly differentiated lymphocytic; Kiel: T-cell CLL/PLL; Lukes-Collins: small lymphocyte, T, prolymphocytic; Working Formulation: small lymphocytic, c/w CLL; diffuse small cleaved cell; FAB: T-PLL.

Clinical Features

Only 1% of cases of CLL, but up to 20% of PLL, are of T lineage. Patients have a very high peripheral white blood count (often > 100,000) and, frequently, cutaneous or mucosal infiltrates. Bone marrow, spleen, liver, and lymph nodes may be involved. T-CLL/T-PLL is more aggressive than B-CLL and not usually curable with available therapy.

Morphology

A minority of cases are morphologically similar to typical B-CLL and are classified as T-CLL (Fig. 4–3). Most cases have irregular nuclei, prominent nucleoli, and relatively abundant cytoplasm; these are classified as T-PLL. The cells are usually nongranular, but show focal granular paranuclear positivity with acid phosphatase and nonspecific esterase stains. Lymph node involvement is diffuse and often prefer-entially paracortical, sparing the follicles. Unlike B-CLL, there are no pseudofollicles. High endothelial venules may be numerous and often contain atypical lymphoid cells (Fig. 4–4). Splenic red pulp and hepatic sinusoids may be infiltrated. Bone marrow involvement is usually diffuse and may be accompanied by increased reticulin.

Immunophenotype

Neoplastic cells are T-cell-associated antigen+ (CD2+, CD3+, CD5+, CD7+), CD25−, CD4+ CD8− > CD4+ CD8+ > CD4− CD8+.

Genetic Features

Clonal rearrangement of TCR genes is present; inv14(q11;q32) is found in 75% of cases, and trisomy 8q is common.

Postulated Normal Counterpart

Circulating peripheral T cell.

Differential Diagnosis

1. B-cell chronic lymphocytic leukemia (B-CLL): Immunophenotyping is required for definitive diagnosis of T-CLL/PLL. The presence of pseudofollicles in tissue sections supports B-CLL and excludes T-CLL.

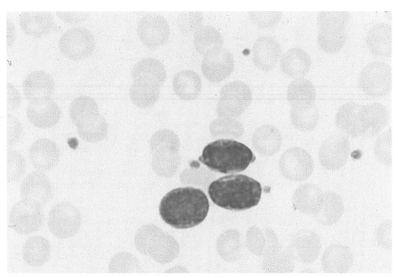

Figure 4–3. T-cell chronic lymphocytic leukemia/prolymphocytic leukemia, peripheral blood. The neoplastic cells are small lymphocytes with heterochromatic nuclei and scant cytoplasm (Wright-Giemsa stain).

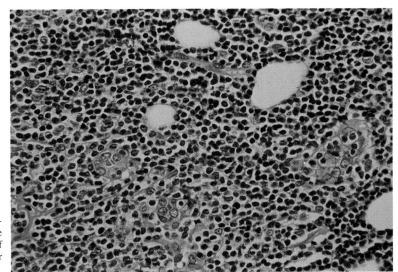

Figure 4–4. T-cell chronic lymphocytic leukemia/prolymphocytic leukemia, axillary lymph node. There is a diffuse infiltrate of small lymphocytes with increased numbers of high endothelial venules (H&E stain). (Courtesy of Dr. Peter Banks, Carolinas Medical Center, Charlotte, NC.)

2. Mycosis fungoides/Sézary syndrome (MF/SS): Patients with MF/SS usually present with skin involvement; after a chronic course, the disease may spread to extracutaneous sites. The white count is usually elevated only moderately. Patients with T-CLL/PLL usually present with marked peripheral lymphocytosis, often accompanied by widespread disease. In the skin, T-CLL/PLL lacks the distinctive histologic features of MF. In peripheral blood, nuclear convolutions are more prominent in SS than in T-CLL/PLL. Compared with T-PLL, Sézary cells have less conspicuous nucleoli and less cytoplasm. The cells of MF/SS are typically negative for CD7.

3. Adult T-cell lymphoma/leukemia (ATLL): ATLL mainly affects patients from Japan and the Caribbean; it is associated with a positive serologic test for HTLV-1. In the peripheral blood, ATLL cells have distinctive multilobated nuclei ("flower cells"). CD7 is typically absent.

4. Large granular lymphocyte leukemia (LGL): In the peripheral blood, the leukemic cells have cytoplasmic azurophilic granules. They have the immunophenotype of natural killer cells or T cytotoxic-suppressor cells. CD4 expression is not seen.

References

Bennett J, Catovsky D, Daniel M-T, *et al*: Proposals for the classification of chronic (mature) B and T lymphoid leukemias. J Clin Pathol 42:567–584, 1989.

Matutes E, Brito-Babapulle V, Swansbury J, *et al*: Clinical and laboratory features of 78 cases of T-prolymphocytic leukemia. Blood 78:3269–3274, 1991.

Suchi T, Lennert K, Tu L-Y: Histopathology and immunohistochemistry of peripheral T-cell lymphomas: a proposal for their classification. J Clin Pathol 40:995–1015, 1987.

LARGE GRANULAR LYMPHOCYTE LEUKEMIA (LGL), T-CELL AND NK-CELL TYPES

Synonyms: Rappaport: chronic lymphocytic leukemia; Kiel: T-CLL; Lukes-Collins: small lymphocyte, T; Working Formulation: small lymphocytic, c/w CLL; FAB: T-CLL, T-LGL; Other: Large granular lymphocytosis, T8 lymphocytosis with neutropenia, CD8 or Tγ lymphoproliferative disease.

Clinical Features

Large granular lymphocyte leukemia (LGL) occurs in two forms: T-cell LGL (T-LGL) and natural killer-cell LGL (NK-LGL). T-LGL affects patients from childhood to old age, with a median of 55 years and a roughly equal male to female ratio. Patients usually have modest, stable, peripheral lymphocytosis, mild to moderate splenomegaly, neutropenia (which may be severe), and less often, anemia and thrombocytopenia. These patients also have defects in cellular immunity and NK activity; these combined with neutropenia, result in the infections that are the most common presenting complaint in this group. More than one-quarter of patients also have rheumatoid arthritis. The course is usually indolent. In patients in whom cytopenias have been severe, successful treatment has been reported with single-agent chemotherapy.

Most patients with increased numbers of CD3-negative NK antigen+ large granular lymphocytes (NK-LGL) have an indolent clinical course. Preliminary investigations, however, suggest that these cases may be reactive, rather than neoplastic, disorders. An aggressive clonal form of NK-

LGL that tends to occur among Asians has been described: affected patients are slightly younger than those with T-LGL; anemia and thrombocytopenia are more common, and severe neutropenia is less common than in T-LGL. Patients present with rapidly progressive disease, high fever, hepatosplenomegaly, jaundice, and ascites. The course is rapidly progressive and usually fatal.

Morphology

Peripheral blood cells have slightly eccentric, round, or oval nuclei slightly larger than those of normal lymphocytes, as well as slightly paler chromatin, rare nucleoli, and abundant pale blue cytoplasm with azurophilic granules (Fig. 4–5). The cells are acid phosphatase positive with a granular pattern and are nonspecific esterase negative or weakly positive. Bone marrow infiltration is typically subtle, with mild lymphocytosis or a few small lymphoid aggregates that may be poorly circumscribed. There may be myeloid maturation arrest or erythroid hypoplasia. Neoplastic cells may infiltrate splenic red pulp (Fig. 4–6) and hepatic sinuses.

Immunophenotype

T cell: CD2+, CD3+, CD5+/−, CD7−, TCRαβ+, CD4−, CD8+, CD16+, CD56−, CD57+/−, CD25− (Fig. 4–5B).

NK cell: CD2+, CD3−, TCRαβ−, CD4−, CD8+/−, CD16+, CD56+/−, CD57+/−.

Genetic Features

T-LGL: TCR genes are rearranged.

NK-LGL: TCR genes are germline. Cytogenetic abnormalities and clonal integration of EBV are reported in aggressive cases of NK-LGL in Asian patients.

Postulated Normal Counterpart

T-cell type: peripheral CD8+ T lymphocyte with suppressor, but no NK function.

NK-cell type: NK cell.

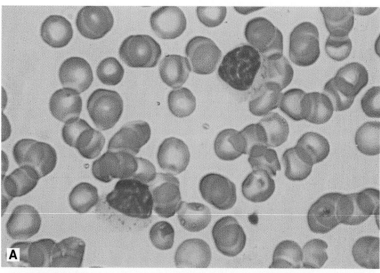

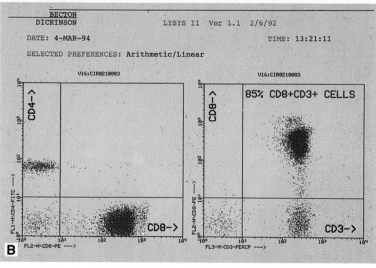

Figure 4–5. T-large granular lymphocyte leukemia, peripheral blood. *A,* A smear shows increased numbers of lymphoid cells that are larger than normal lymphocytes and have dark nuclei and abundant, pale blue, nonvacuolated cytoplasm containing azurophilic granules (Wright-Giemsa stain). *B,* In the same case, flow cytometric analysis shows a predominant population of CD3+ CD8+ lymphoid cells. The CD8 expression of this population is slightly less intense than that of the small population of normal T-suppressor cells. (Flow cytometric data courtesy of Dr. F. Preffer.)

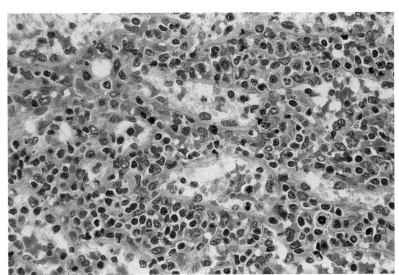

Figure 4–6. T-large granular lymphocyte leukemia, spleen. The red pulp cords are expanded by a population of small- to intermediate-sized atypical lymphoid cells. The white pulp was normal (H&E stain).

Differential Diagnosis

1. T-CLL/PLL: See preceding section.
2. B-CLL: In B-CLL, the cytoplasm is less abundant and lacks granules and the nuclei have more condensed chromatin. If prolymphocytes are present, they have more prominent nucleoli than large granular lymphocytes. When cytopenia is present, it is usually caused by extensive marrow involvement. There is no association with rheumatoid arthritis. The immunophenotype is completely different.
3. Adult T-cell lymphoma/leukemia (ATLL): All cases are associated with HTLV-1; no cases are associated with EBV. ATLL is usually an acute illness with hypercalcemia and extensive lymphadenopathy; the lymphocytosis is often much higher than seen in LGL. The leukemic cells are "flower cells" with agranular cytoplasm. ATLL is typically CD4+, lacking CD8 and NK-cell markers.
4. Non-neoplastic large granular lymphocytosis: Atypical lymphocytosis with increased numbers of large granular lymphocytes may occur in reactive conditions, e.g., viral infections. In addition to clinical features, assessment of TCR genes may be helpful in establishing a diagnosis in CD3+ cases. In CD3− cases, finding clonal EBV supports a neoplastic process. Preliminary studies suggest that assessment of the pattern of X-chromosome inactivation may be helpful in establishing a diagnosis in female patients.

References

Agnarsson B, Loughran T, Starkebaum G, Kadin M: The pathology of large granular lymphocyte leukemia. Hum Pathol 20:643–651, 1989.

Bennett J, Catovsky D, Daniel M-T, et al: Proposals for the classification of chronic (mature) B and T lymphoid leukemias. J Clin Pathol 42:567–584, 1989.

Kelly A, Richards SJ, Sivakumaran M, et al: Clonality of CD3 negative large granular lymphocyte proliferations determined by PCR based X-inactivation studies. J Clin Pathol 45:399–404, 1994.

Loughran T: Clonal diseases of large granular lymphocytes. Blood 82:1–14, 1993.

MYCOSIS FUNGOIDES/SÉZARY SYNDROME (MF/SS)

Synonyms: Rappaport: mycosis fungoides/Sézary syndrome; Kiel: small cell, cerebriform; Lukes-Collins: cerebriform T; Working Formulation: mycosis fungoides.

Clinical Features

Mycosis fungoides/Sézary syndrome (MF/SS) is the most common form of primary cutaneous lymphoma. Most patients are adults who present with multiple cutaneous plaques or nodules or with generalized erythroderma. Disease may appear to be confined to the skin for years; lymphadenopathy is usually a late occurrence. Peripheral blood involvement may be subtle in mycosis fungoides or prominent in Sézary syndrome. Large cell transformation may occur; it is associated with a poor prognosis. An association with Hodgkin's disease and lymphomatoid papulosis has also been reported.

Morphology

In the skin, MF typically produces a superficial dermal, lichenoid infiltrate of small lymphoid cells that have dark,

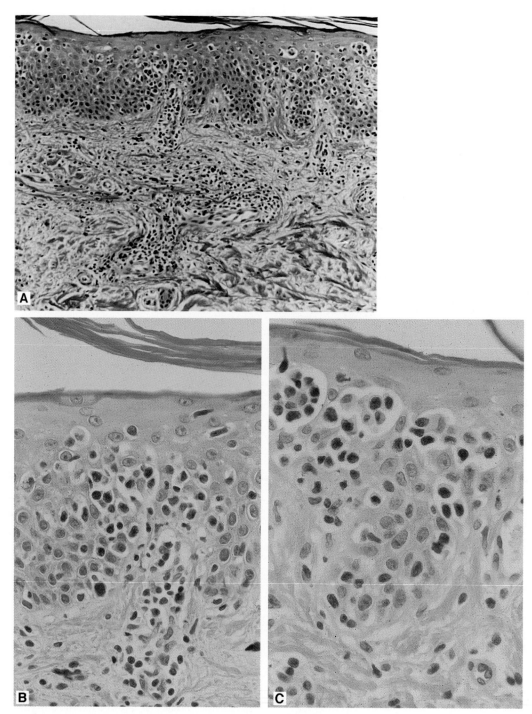

Figure 4–7. Mycosis fungoides, skin. *A,* Low power examination shows a superficial perivascular lymphoid infiltrate and numerous lymphoid cells infiltrating the epidermis, without prominent spongiosis (H&E stain). *B,* "Haloed" lymphoid cells with dark, irregular nuclei infiltrate the epidermis singly and in small clusters; they are significantly larger than the lymphocytes in the dermis (H&E stain). *C,* In some areas, Pautrier's collections are prominent (H&E stain).

irregular nuclei and scant cytoplasm. Cells that are similar or slightly larger infiltrate the epidermis in variable numbers; clusters of them are called Pautrier's collections. Intraepidermal lymphoid cells are often surrounded by a clear space ("haloed lymphocytes") (Fig. 4–7). The epidermis frequently shows parakeratosis but only minimal spongiosis. One-micron sections or electron microscopy shows that the cells have deeply indented and convoluted ("cerebriform") nuclei. Similar cells may be found in the paracortex of lymph nodes or in the peripheral blood (Sézary cells) (Fig. 4–8). The bone marrow usually is not involved. Early lymph node involvement by MF may be indistinguishable from dermatopathic lymphadenopathy by light microscopic and immunohistochemical studies (see Dermatopathic Lymphadenopathy, Chapter 2). With disease progression, nodal involvement may become obvious, with distortion of the normal architecture by cerebriform cells. In cases of large cell transformation, the neoplastic cells resemble immunoblasts or anaplastic large cells. The morphology and immunophenotype may be identical to anaplastic large cell lymphoma (Fig. 4–9).

Immunophenotype

Neoplastic cells are positive for T-cell-associated antigens (CD2+, CD3+, CD5+), CD4+ CD8− (rarely CD4− CD8+), CD25− (rarely CD25+); one-third of cases are CD7+. Admixed S-100+, CD1a+ interdigitating dendritic, and Langerhans' cells are present.

Genetic Features

TCR genes are clonally rearranged.

Postulated Normal Counterpart

Peripheral epidermotropic CD4+ T cell.

Differential Diagnosis

1. T-CLL/PLL: See previous discussion.
2. Adult T-cell lymphoma/leukemia (ATLL): ATLL is typically associated with a rapid clinical course and widespread disease at presentation. Skin involvement may be present. ATLL mainly affects patients from Japan and the Caribbean and is associated with HTLV-1. Although the morphology may overlap with MF/SS, neoplastic cells in ATLL are usually larger and have either lobated or rounded nuclei. ATLL is usually CD25+; otherwise, the immunophenotype is similar to MF/SS.
3. Inflammatory dermatoses: The distinction between dermatitis and MF may be difficult. Features that are significantly more frequent in MF include Pautrier's collections, haloed lymphocytes, disproportionate epidermitropism of lymphoid cells compared with the extent of the dermal infiltrate, single lymphoid cells in the basal layer, and hyperconvoluted lymphoid cells. Immunophenotyping is not definitive in many cases because of the overlap in results between MF and some dermatoses.

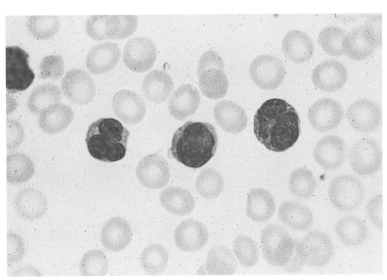

Figure 4–8. Mycosis fungoides/Sézary syndrome. Atypical lymphoid cells with convoluted nuclei are found in the peripheral blood (Wright-Giemsa stain).

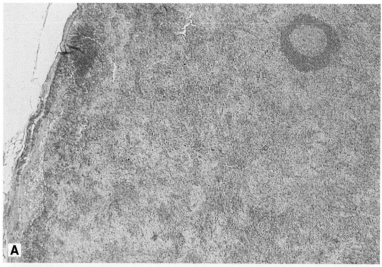

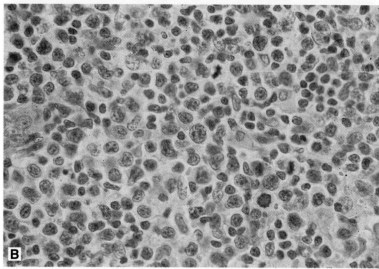

Figure 4–9. Mycosis fungoides, lymph node. *A,* The para-cortex is markedly expanded; rare residual lymphoid follicles are seen (H&E stain). *B,* High power view shows intermediate- and large-sized atypical lymphoid cells and frequent mitoses (H&E stain).

Genotyping may be helpful, but a relatively sparse infiltrate may not yield sufficient cells for analysis. Examination of 1-μm sections to assess the degree of nuclear convolution can be helpful.

References

Burke J, Khalil S, Rappaport H: Dermatopathic lymphadenopathy. An immunophenotypic comparison of cases asssociated and unassociated with mycosis fungoides. Am J Pathol 123:256–263, 1986.

Davis T, Morton C, Miller-Cassman R, *et al*: Hodgkin's disease, lymphomatoid papulosis, and cutaneous T-cell lymphoma derived from a common T-cell clone. N Engl J Med 326:1115–1122, 1992.

Ralfkiaer E, Wantzin G, Mason D, *et al*: Phenotypic characterization of lymphocyte subsets in mycosis fungoides. Am J Clin Pathol 84:610–619, 1985.

Scheffer E, Meijer CJLM, Van Vloten WA: Dermatopathic lymphadenopathy and lymph node involvement in mycosis fungoides. Cancer 45:137–148, 1980.

Smoller BR, Bishop K, Glusac E, *et al*: Reassessment of histologic parameters in the diagnosis of mycosis fungoides. Am J Surg Pathol 19:1423–1430, 1995.

Weiss L, Hu E, Wood G, Moulds C, *et al*: Clonal rearrangements of T cell receptor genes in mycosis fungoides and dermatopathic lymphadenopathy. N Engl J Med 313:539–544, 1985.

PERIPHERAL T-CELL LYMPHOMAS, UNSPECIFIED (PTCL) (PROVISIONAL CYTOLOGIC CATEGORIES: MEDIUM-SIZED CELL, MIXED MEDIUM AND LARGE CELL, LARGE CELL)

Synonyms: Rappaport: diffuse poorly differentiated lymphocytic, diffuse mixed lymphocytic-histiocytic, histiocytic; Kiel: T-zone lymphoma, lymphoepithelioid cell lymphoma, pleomorphic small, medium, and large cell, T-immunoblastic; Lukes-Collins: T-immunoblastic lymphoma; Working Formulation: diffuse small cleaved cell, diffuse mixed small and large cell, large cell immunoblastic (polymorphous or clear cell).

The term "peripheral T-cell lymphoma of unspecified type" is used to describe a nonlymphoblastic T-cell lymphoma that does not fall into one of the distinctive categories of T-cell lymphoma described previously or in the following sections.

Clinical Features

These tumors comprise less than 10% of lymphoma cases in most European and United States studies, but are more common in other parts of the world. Most patients are adults who present with generalized disease. Lymph nodes, skin or subcutis, liver, spleen, and other viscera may be involved. Occasional patients have eosinophilia, pruritus, or hemophagocytic syndrome. The clinical course is usually aggressive, although PTCL is potentially curable. Patients with B-cell lymphomas tend to have fewer relapses than patients with T-cell lymphomas of similar histologic grade.

Morphologic Features

Specimens of PTCL typically show a diffuse or an occasionally interfollicular proliferation of atypical small, medium-sized, or large cells or a mixture of these; most contain a mixed population of small and large atypical cells; and even those with a predominance of medium-sized or large cells often contain a broad spectrum of cell sizes (Fig. 4–10). Admixed eosinophils or epithelioid histiocytes may be numerous. Cases in which the neoplastic cells are predominantly small and medium-sized and have numerous clusters of epithelioid histiocytes have been called lymphoepithelioid cell (Lennert's) lymphoma (Fig. 4–11). The neoplastic cells vary in size and shape and have irregular nuclei. Large, hyperchromatic cells that resemble Reed-Sternberg (RS) cells may be present, but true RS cells are rare or absent. Although this category is clearly heterogeneous and probably consists of multiple different diseases, reproducible morphologic criteria for subclassification do not exist at this time. It is recommended that these cases be distinguished by the size of the predominant neoplastic cells, as medium, mixed medium and large, and large cell types.

Immunophenotype

Neoplastic cells are positive for T-cell-associated antigens (CD3+, CD2+, CD5+, CD45RO+, CD7+) although in any case, one or more, or even all, T-cell antigens may be lost; CD4+ > CD8+ > CD4− CD8−; CD1−; negative for B-cell antigens. Exceptions include CD45RA expression in some cases (CD45RA is present on virgin T cells as well as B cells) and rare cases of CD20+ T-cell lymphoma, which may be derived from a small normal population of dim CD20+ T cells.

Genetic Features

TCR genes are usually clonally rearranged. Ig heavy and Ig light chain genes are germline.

Postulated Normal Counterpart

Peripheral T cells in various stages of transformation.

Differential Diagnosis

1. Reactive hyperplasia: Greater extent of architectural distortion and more severe cytologic atypia favor lymphoma. Loss of one or more pan-T-cell antigens (CD2+, CD3+, CD5+) strongly favors lymphoma, as does lack of both CD4 and CD8. CD7 is not a pan-T-cell antigen, and its absence is unusual, but not diagnostic of lymphoma. In difficult cases, molecular genetic analysis for TCR gene rearrangement is often necessary.
2. Diffuse B-cell lymphomas: PTCL and diffuse B-cell lymphomas, including lymphoplasmacytic, follicle center, and diffuse large B-cell types, are frequently indistinguishable on routine sections; immunophenotyping is recommended to separate B- from T-cell lymphomas.
3. Hodgkin's disease (HD): When the small lymphoid population lacks cytologic atypia and a morphologic hiatus exists between small cells and large cells (Reed-Sternberg cells), a diagnosis of HD is favored. When a morphologic continuum occurs from small to medium to large cells and the large cells do not closely resemble classic Reed-Sternberg cells, a non-Hodgkin's lymphoma is favored. Expression of T-cell antigens on large cells favors PTCL. Loss of one or more pan-T antigens by small- or medium-sized T cells surrounding Reed-Sternberg-like cells confirms T-cell lymphoma. Clonal TCR gene rearrangement strongly favors T-cell lymphoma.
4. True histiocytic lymphoma (THL)/malignant histiocytosis (MH): THL and MH are neoplasms derived from histiocytes; THL is used for patients who present primarily with lymphadenopathy and more localized disease. MH is used for neoplasms that diffusely and extensively involve the reticuloendothelial system. Acceptable examples in either category are rare. Malignant histiocytes are said to have the capacity for erythrophagocytosis, and THL and MH may enter the differential diagnosis of PTCL associated with a hemophagocytic syndrome. The phagocytic histiocytes in cases of PTCL may appear activated, having slightly enlarged nuclei and small nucleoli, but they are cytologically benign. They are often admixed with cytologically malignant T cells, and careful examination of immunostained sections is necessary to identify the immunophenotype of the malignant population. Occasionally, hemophagocytosis occurs in

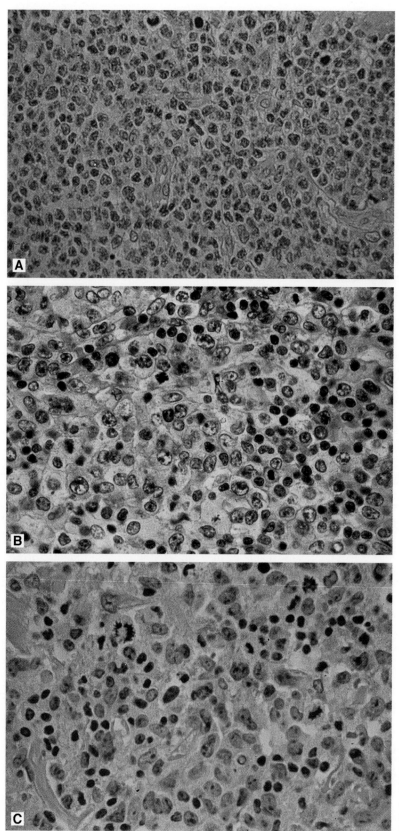

Figure 4–10. Peripheral T-cell lymphoma (PTCL), unspecified. *A,* PTCL, medium-sized cell type. Tumor cells have irregular nuclei and distinct rims of clear cytoplasm. They are intermediate in size between normal lymphocytes and large lymphoid cells (H&E stain). *B,* PTCL, mixed medium- and large-cell type (H&E stain). *C,* PTCL, large-cell type (H&E stain).

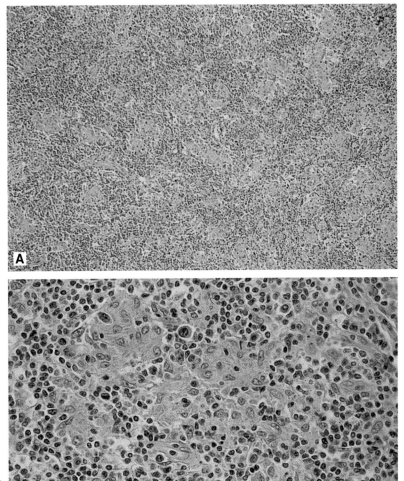

Figure 4–11. Lymphoepithelioid cell (Lennert's) lymphoma. *A,* Low power examination shows obliteration of the nodal architecture by an infiltrate of lymphocytes and histiocytes (H&E stain). *B,* Higher power examination shows clusters of epithelioid histiocytes surrounded by small- to medium-sized lymphoid cells, some with slightly irregular nuclei (H&E stain).

anatomic sites distant from sites involved by PTCL, and a specific diagnosis cannot be made unless additional tissue is obtained.

References

Armitage J, Greer J, Levine A, *et al*: Peripheral T-cell lymphoma. Cancer 63:158–163, 1989.

Cabacadas J, Isaacson P: Phenotyping of T-cell lymphomas in paraffin sections—which antibodies? Histopathology 19:419–424, 1991.

Chott A, Dragosics B, Radaszkiewicz T: Peripheral T-cell lymphomas of the intestine. Am J Pathol 141:1361–1371, 1992.

Coiffier B, Brousse N, Peuchmaur M, *et al*: Peripheral T-cell lymphomas have a worse prognosis than B-cell lymphomas: a prospective study of 361 immunophenotyped patients treated with the LNH-84 regimen. Ann Oncol 1:45–50, 1990.

Falini B, Pileri S, De Solas I, *et al*: Peripheral T-cell lymphoma associated with hemophagocytic syndrome. Blood 75:434–444, 1990.

Hastrup N, Ralfkiaer E, Pallesen G: Aberrant phenotypes in peripheral T cell lymphomas. J Clin Pathol 42:398–402, 1989.

Patsouris E, Noel H, Lennert K: Histological and immunohistological findings in lymphoepithelioid cell lymphoma (Lennert's lymphoma). Am J Surg Pathol 12:341–350, 1988.

Said J, Shintaku P, Parekh K, Pinkus G: Specific phenotyping of T-cell proliferations in formalin-fixed paraffin-embedded tissues. Use of antibodies to the T-cell receptor βF1. Am J Clin Pathol 93:382–386, 1990.

Suchi T, Lennert K, Tu L-Y: Histopathology and immunohistochemistry of peripheral T-cell lymphomas: a proposal for their classification. J Clin Pathol 40:995–1015, 1987.

Weiss L, Picker L, Grogan T, *et al*: Absence of clonal beta and gamma T-cell receptor gene rearrangements in a subset of peripheral T-cell lymphomas. Am J Pathol 130:436–443, 1988.

HEPATOSPLENIC γδ T-CELL LYMPHOMA (PROVISIONAL SUBTYPE)

Clinical Features

This rare lymphoma mainly affects adolescent and young adult males, who present with hepatosplenomegaly with inconspicuous peripheral lymphadenopathy. Peripheral blood involvement and cytopenias have been described. Combination chemotherapy can cause complete remissions, although most patients subsequently experience relapse. The mortality rate is high.

Morphology

The neoplastic cells are medium-sized or occasionally large, having oval nuclei with moderately dispersed chromatin and abundant pale cytoplasm. In the liver, the infiltrate is sinusoidal; in the spleen, it involves the red pulp (Fig. 4–12). Marrow involvement may be subtle; it may be predominantly sinusoidal.

Immunophenotype

By definition, neoplastic cells express the γδ T-cell-receptor (TCR) heterodimer and lack the αβ TCR. Typically, tumor cells are also CD2+, CD3+, CD5−/+, CD7−/+, CD16+/−, CD56+/−, CD57−, CD4−, CD8−/+.

Genotype

Rearrangement of TCRδ and TCRγ chain genes usually can be detected; clonal rearrangement of β chain gene of TCR (TCRβ) is often present. Isochromosome 7q has been found frequently.

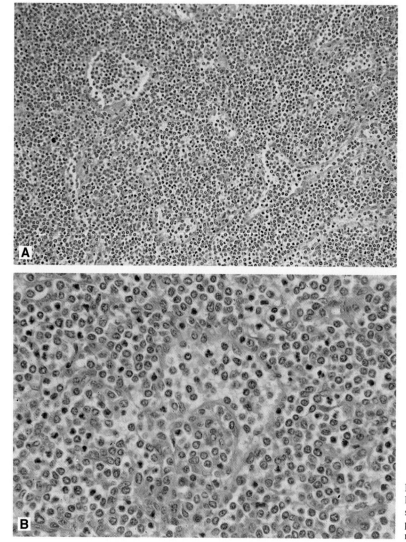

Figure 4–12. Hepatosplenic γδ T-cell lymphoma. *A,* The lymphoma diffusely infiltrates the splenic red pulp; dilated sinuses contain neoplastic cells (H&E stain). *B,* The lymphoma is composed of relatively bland cells with oval nuclei and pale cytoplasm (H&E stain).

Postulated Normal Counterpart

Post-thymic γδ T cell, possibly NK-like γδ T cell (most circulating T cells are αβ type; <5% are γδ T cells, although γδ cells are more numerous in mucosal sites and spleen).

Differential Diagnosis

Hairy cell leukemia (HCL): The distribution of disease is similar to that of HCL. HCL, however, usually affects older patients and behaves in a more indolent fashion. Hepatosplenic lymphoma cells may be more irregular and lack villous processes. Immunophenotyping provides a definitive diagnosis.

References

Farcet J, Gaulard P, Marolleau J, *et al*: Hepatosplenic T-cell lymphoma: sinusal/sinusoidal localization af malignant cells expressing the T-cell receptor γδ. Blood 75:2213–2219, 1990.

Jaffe ES: Classification of natural killer (NK) cell and NK-like T-cell malignancies. Blood 87:1207–1210, 1996.

Wang CC, Tien HF, Lin MT, *et al*: Consistent presence of isochromosome 7q in hepatosplenic T gamma/delta lymphoma: a new cytogenetic-clinicopathologic entity. Genes Chrom Cancer 12:161–164, 1995.

Wong KF, Chan JKC, Matutes E, *et al*: Hepatosplenic γδ T cell lymphoma. A distinctive aggressive lymphoma type. Am J Surg Pathol 19:718–726, 1995.

SUBCUTANEOUS PANNICULITIC T-CELL LYMPHOMA WITH HEMOPHAGOCYTOSIS (PROVISIONAL SUBTYPE)

Synonyms and Related Terms: Cytophagic histiocytic panniculitis (?).

Clinical Features

This rare lymphoma affects young to middle-aged adults, both males and females. Patients present with subcutaneous nodules, 1 to 12 cm in greatest dimension, often involving the extremities; even with disease progression, tumor remains confined to the subcutis. The course is frequently complicated by a hemophagocytic syndrome, which may exist at presentation or may develop years after the onset of the lymphoma; it is often fatal. In one case, high serum levels of γ interferon were attributed to the lymphoma, which may have played a role in the pathogenesis of the patient's fever and leukopenia.

The disorder called "cytophagic histiocytic panniculitis," which was considered an inflammatory disorder primarily of histiocytes, may actually represent subcutaneous panniculitic T-cell lymphoma.

Morphology

Subcutaneous tissue contains atypical small and large lymphoid cells in solid aggregates or infiltrating between adipocytes. In addition, fat necrosis and karyorrhectic debris are seen, sometimes with granuloma formation (Fig. 4–13). Neoplastic cells often infiltrate small blood vessels, although prominent angiocentric growth and angiodestruction are not seen. Hemophagocytosis may occur in the bone marrow, liver, spleen, lymph nodes, or skin.

Immunophenotype

Neoplastic cells are CD2+, CD3+, CD5+, CD7+, CD45RO+, CD43+, CD4+/−, CD8−/+, CD30−, often with loss of one or more of the preceding pan-T antigens. In one case thought to be of γδ origin, the neoplastic cells were CD1+, CD3+, CD4−, CD5−, CD8−, CD30+, CD25+, CD56+, TCRδ chain+. B-cell antigens are absent.

Genotype

Relatively few cases have been tested, but T-cell-receptor (TCR) genes have been clonally rearranged. In the case of γδ origin, clonal TCR δ chain rearrangement was shown.

Postulated Normal Counterpart

Peripheral T cell of unknown stage.

Differential Diagnosis

1. Panniculitis: Low power microscopic examination and admixture of histiocytes with fat necrosis suggest an inflammatory process, but higher power examination reveals lymphoid cells with cytologic atypia in excess of that expected for a reactive infiltrate. In the absence of sufficient cytologic atypia, demonstration of pan-T antigen loss or clonal TCR gene rearrangement confirms T-cell lymphoma.

2. Nasal-type lymphoma (angiocentric lymphoma): Nasal-type lymphoma may involve the subcutaneous tissue and enter the differential diagnosis of subcutaneous panniculitic T-cell lymphoma. Nasal-type lymphoma, however, often involves the dermis as well as the subcutis when it affects the skin and frequently involves anatomic sites distant from the skin. Both lymphomas may show angioinvasion, but subcutaneous panniculitic T-cell lymphoma is less likely to be angiodestructive.

   Nasal-type lymphoma is composed of cells expressing the NK-associated antigen CD56 and a limited number of T-cell-associated antigens; it shows no clonal rearrangement of T-cell-receptor genes. Subcutaneous panniculitic T-cell lymphoma, however, has a T-cell immunophenotype and shows clonal rearrangement of TCR genes. Nasal-type lymphoma contains clonal EBV, unlike subcutaneous T-cell lymphoma.

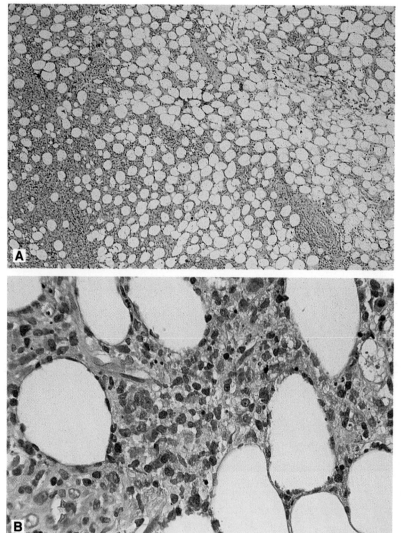

Figure 4–13. Subcutaneous panniculitic T-cell lymphoma. *A,* At low power examination, a subcutaneous lymphohistiocytic infiltrate ranges from relatively sparse to dense (H&E stain). *B,* At high power, the infiltrate consists of histiocytes, cellular debris, and atypical lymphoid cells (H&E stain).

References

Burg G, Dummer R, Wilhelm M, *et al*: A subcutaneous delta-positive T-cell lymphoma that produces interferon gamma. N Engl J Med 325: 1078–1081, 1991.

Crotty CP, Winkelmann RK: Cytophagic histiocytic panniculitis with fever, cytopenia, liver failure and terminal hemorrhagic diathesis. J Am Acad Dermatol 4:181–194, 1981.

Gonzalez C, Medeiros L, Braziel R, Jaffe E: T-cell lymphoma involving subcutaneous tissue: a clinicopathologic entity commonly associated with hemophagocytic syndrome. Am J Surg Pathol 15:17–27, 1991.

Medeiros LJ, Greiner TG, Gonzalez CL, *et al*: T-cell lymphoma involving subcutaneous tissue: an update. Mod Pathol 7:116A, 1994.

ANGIOIMMUNOBLASTIC T-CELL LYMPHOMA

Synonyms and Related Disorders: Rappaport: not listed (diffuse mixed lymphocytic-histiocytic, histiocytic); Kiel: T-cell, angioimmunoblastic; lymphogranulomatosis X (LgX); Lukes-Collins: immunoblastic lymphadenopathy (IBL)-like T-cell lymphoma; Working Formulation: not listed (diffuse mixed small and large cell, diffuse large cell, large cell immunoblastic); other: immunoblastic lymphadenopathy; angioimmunoblastic lymphadenopathy with dysproteinemia (AILD).

Clinical Features

Initially, this disorder was considered an abnormal immune reaction (angioimmunoblastic lymphadenopathy with dysproteinemia [AILD], or immunoblastic lymphadenopathy [IBL]), but it is now generally accepted that most cases represent T-cell lymphoma. Patients are usually middle-aged to older adults (median age in the sixth or seventh decade), although younger adults are affected occasionally. There is a slight male preponderance. Patients typically have generalized lymphadenopathy, fever, weight loss, skin rash, polyclonal hypergammaglobulinemia, hemolytic anemia, and infectious complications. The course is moderately aggressive, but some patients respond to chemotherapy or steroid therapy. In a study performed by Siegert and co-workers, 64% of angioimmunoblastic T-cell lymphoma (AIL-TCL) patients attained a complete response with combination chemotherapy, whereas a much smaller proportion attained a response to prednisone alone. The median survival time was 15 months; most patients died of infectious complications rather than lymphoma. Spontaneous remissions have been reported. Progression to high grade lymphoma with a predominance of large T or occasionally B cells occurs in some instances.

Morphology

The nodal architecture is largely effaced, although "burnt-out" germinal centers, predominantly containing follicular dendritic cells (FDCs) are sometimes found at the periphery of the node. Although the infiltrate often extends into perinodal soft tissue, the subcapsular sinus is typically patent. The node has a pale, depleted appearance on low power examination. Numerous small, arborizing, high endothelial venules (HEV), many of which show thickened or hyalinized PAS+ walls, are present. Occasional large, irregular aggregates of FDCs may be scattered among the atypical lymphoid cells and may surround the proliferating blood vessels. The lymphoid infiltrate usually appears relatively sparse, compared with other lymphomas, probably because of the large number of FDCs. The lymphoid population is composed of small lymphocytes, immunoblasts, and clusters of characteristic atypical "clear" cells having round to slightly indented nuclei and abundant, pale, or clear cytoplasm. Epithelioid histiocytes, plasma cells, and eosinophils may be admixed (Fig. 4–14).

When this type of lymphoma affects the bone marrow, involvement is in the form of focal or occasionally diffuse infiltrates having a cellular composition similar to that found in lymph nodes. The surrounding marrow may show erythroid hyperplasia (particularly in patients with hemolytic anemia) or myeloid hyperplasia.

Some cases of AIL-TCL may be preceded by atypical lymphoid hyperplasia not readily recognizable as AIL-TCL. We reviewed the case of an elderly man whose presenting complaints were related to atherosclerotic cardiovascular disease. Work-up revealed leukocytosis, predominantly consisting of increased neutrophils, although a few plasma cells, some of them atypical, were found on the peripheral smear. A bone marrow biopsy sample showed myeloid hyperplasia with an increase in mature plasma cells. The patient had multiple, slightly enlarged lymph nodes with a marked increase in plasma cells, including some that were immature (plasmablasts) and some that were binucleate, filling the medullary cords, extending into the paracortex, and occasionally entering sinuses. A few primary follicles were pres-

ent, and T cells were compressed into a few perivascular aggregates. Despite the atypia and extent of the plasma cells, they expressed polytypic immunoglobulin. A definite diagnosis was not made (Fig. 4–15). One month later, the patient returned with markedly enlarged lymph nodes that showed the typical picture of AIL-TCL.

In retrospect, T cells in the first lymph node biopsy specimen did have slightly irregular nuclei, and the subcapsular sinus was widely patent, with some of the infiltrate extending beyond the nodal capsule. These features, though not specific, suggest that the first lymph node probably contained an abnormal T-cell population and represented very early involvement by AIL-TCL (Fig. 4–16).

Immunophenotype

Tumor cells are positive for T-cell antigens, often with loss of one or more pan-T antigens and are usually CD4+. Immunoblasts may be positive for Epstein-Barr virus latent membrane protein (EBV-LMP); FDCs are CD21+ and CD23+ (*see* Figs. 4–14 and 4–16).

Genetic Features

TCR genes are rearranged in 75% of cases; Ig heavy chain genes, in 10%. EBV genomes are frequently detected. In two cases of EBV+ AILD that progressed to immunoblastic lymphoma of B-cell type, sequence analysis of the LMP1 gene showed deletions and point mutations of the type found in nasopharyngeal carcinoma and aggressive Hodgkin's disease. These investigators suggested that the LMP1 deletion mutant may have been involved in the transformation to immunoblastic lymphoma, analogous to the proposed role of the LMP1 deletion mutant in the behavior of nasopharyngeal carcinoma and Hodgkin's disease.

Postulated Normal Counterpart

Peripheral T cell of unknown subset in various stages of transformation.

Differential Diagnosis

This includes reactive hyperplasia, B-cell lymphoma, and Hodgkin's disease, as described for the differential diagnosis of peripheral T-cell lymphoma, unspecified (see previous discussion).

Occasionally, architectural changes similar to those described previously occur without sufficient cytologic atypia to permit a confident diagnosis of malignant lymphoma. In these cases, genetic studies should be done to evaluate T-cell clonality. If such studies have negative results, these cases should be designated atypical lymphoid hyperplasia with features of AILD; they may regress or progress to angioimmunoblastic T-cell lymphoma.

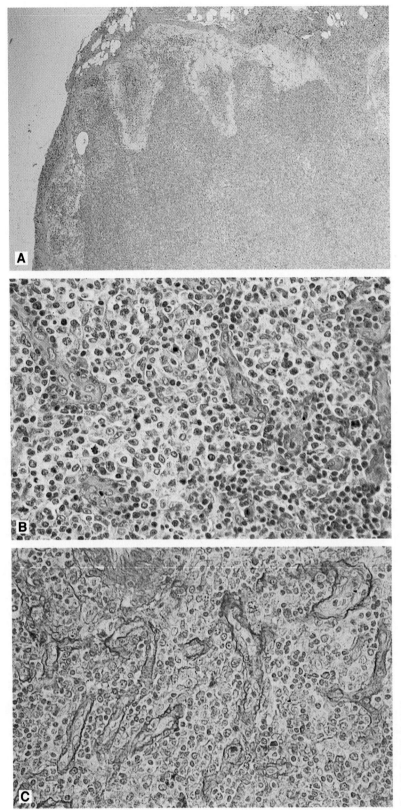

Figure 4–14. Angioimmunoblastic T-cell lymphoma. *A,* Low power view shows diffuse infiltration of the lymph node, with extension of the atypical lymphoid infiltrate into surrounding soft tissue, although the subcapsular sinus is widely patent (H&E stain). *B,* Higher power examination shows atypical lymphoid cells with clear cytoplasm and increased numbers of small blood vessels (H&E stain). *C,* With a PAS stain, large numbers of blood vessels are demarcated.

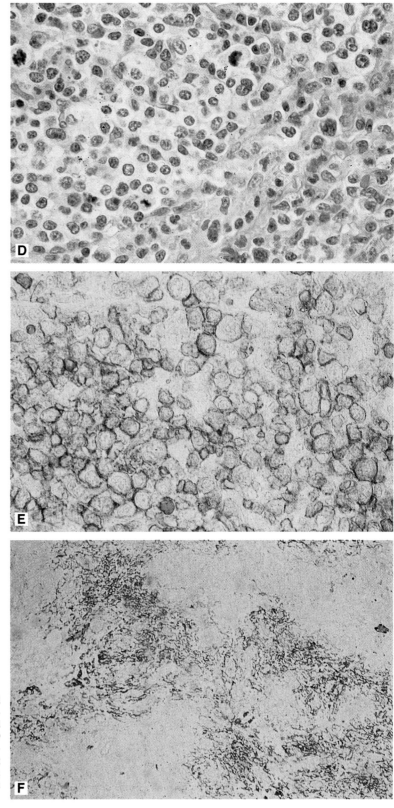

Figure 4–14. *D,* The "clear cells" are intermediate-sized lymphoid cells with nuclei that are usually smoothly contoured. Also present are occasional large lymphoid cells and a few eosinophils (H&E stain). *E,* An antibody to CD45RO (T cells) highlights the intermediate and large cells (immunoperoxidase technique on paraffin sections). *F,* Staining with an antibody to CD21 (FDCs) shows large, irregular, dendritic aggregates (immunoperoxidase technique on frozen sections).

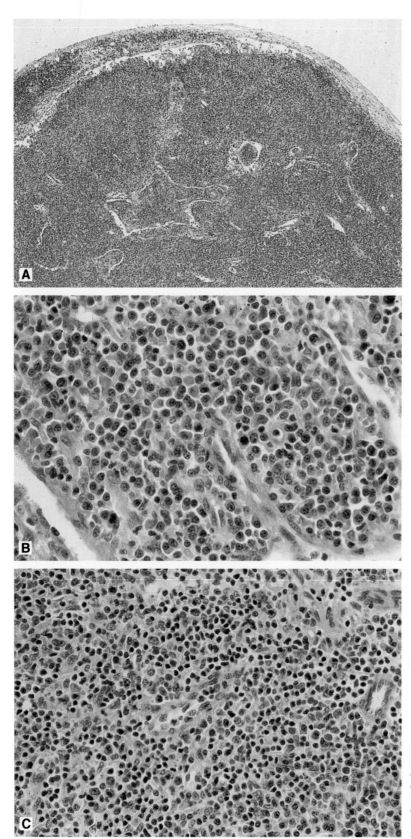

Figure 4–15. Atypical lymphoid infiltrate, probably representing early nodal involvement by angioimmunoblastic T-cell lymphoma. *A,* On low power examination, the paracortex and medullary cords are expanded, follicles are inconspicuous, and sinuses are patent (H&E stain). *B,* Most of the cells are plasma cells (H&E stain). *C,* In some areas, mainly around blood vessels, lymphoid cells predominate rather than plasma cells (H&E stain).

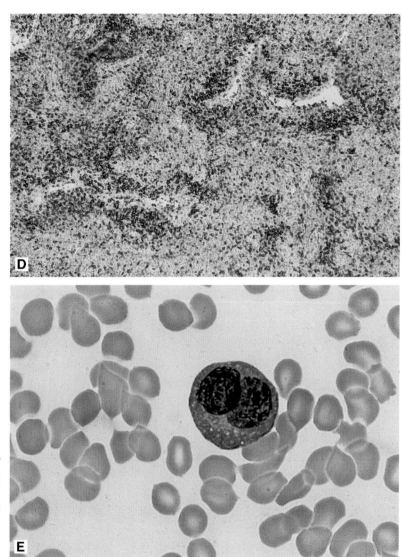

Figure 4–15. *D,* Staining with an antibody to CD45RO demonstrates that most of the lymphoid cells are T cells, although they are not abundant (immunoperoxidase technique on paraffin sections). *E,* The peripheral blood contains small numbers of plasma cells, some of which are atypical. A binucleate plasma cell is illustrated here. Despite findings suggesting plasma cell dyscrasia, immunoperoxidase stains showed that the plasma cells expressed polytypic immunoglobulin (Wright-Giemsa stain).

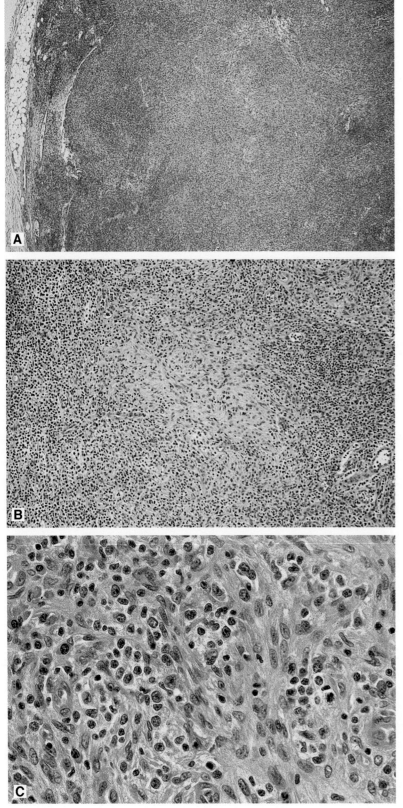

Figure 4–16. Angioimmunoblastic T-cell lymphoma (AIL-TCL). Six weeks after the biopsy illustrated in Figure 4–15, the patient's lymphadenopathy dramatically increased. *A,* The nodal architecture is effaced, although the subcapsular sinus is patent (H&E stain). *B,* A pale, irregular aggregate of follicular dendritic cells, resembling a burnt-out germinal center, is surrounded by atypical lymphoid cells (H&E stain). *C,* Higher power examination shows spindle-shaped follicular dendritic cells intimately admixed with clusters of atypical lymphoid cells that have pale cytoplasm ("clear cells") (H&E stain).

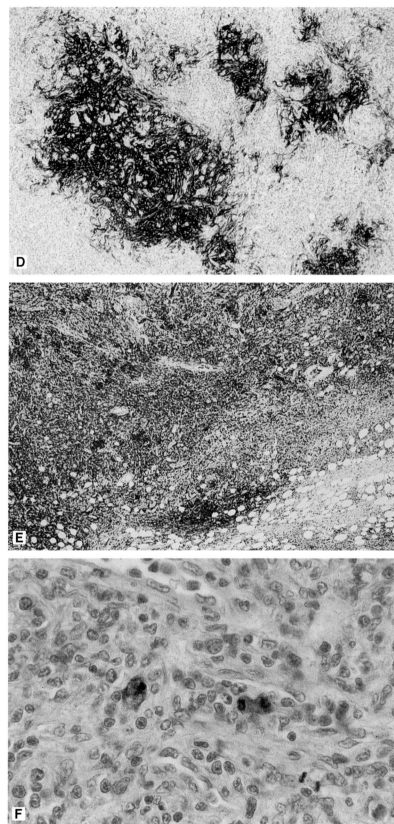

Figure 4–16. *D,* The follicular dendritic cells are CD21+ (immunoperoxidase technique on paraffin sections). *E,* The number of T cells (CD45RO+) is greatly increased compared to the earlier biopsy (immunoperoxidase technique on paraffin sections). *F,* A few immunoblasts (one in mitosis) express EBV-LMP (immunoperoxidase technique on paraffin sections). Although definitive diagnosis was not made on the basis of the biopsy specimen illustrated in Figure 4–15, in retrospect, the changes may represent an unusual pattern of early nodal involvement by AIL-TCL.

References

Anagnostopoulos I, Hummel M, Finn T, *et al*: Heterogeneous Epstein-Barr virus infection patterns in peripheral T-cell lymphoma of angioimmunoblastic lymphadenopathy type. Blood 80:1804–1812, 1992.

Feller A, Griesser H, Schilling C, *et al*: Clonal gene rearrangement patterns correlate with immunophenotype and clinical parameters in patients with angioimmunoblastic lymphadenopathy. Am J Pathol 133:549–556, 1988.

Frizzera G, Moran E, Rappaport H: Angioimmunoblastic lymphadenopathy with dysproteinemia. Lancet i:1070–1073, 1974.

Knecht H, Martius F, Bachman E, *et al*: A deletion mutant of the LMP1 oncogene of Epstein-Barr virus is associated with evolution of angioimmunoblastic lymphadenopathy into B immunoblastic lymphoma. Leukemia 9:458–465, 1995.

Pangalis GA, Moran EM, Rappaport H: Blood and bone marrow findings in angioimmunoblastic lymphadenopathy. Blood 51:71–83, 1978.

Siegert W, Agthe A, Griesser H, *et al*: Treatment of angioimmunoblastic lymphadenopathy (AILD)-type T-cell lymphoma using prednisone with or without the COPBLAM/IMVP-16 regimen. A multicenter study. Kiel Lymphoma Study Group. Ann Int Med 117:364–370, 1992.

Suchi T, Lennert K, Tu L-Y: Histopathology and immunohistochemistry of peripheral T-cell lymphomas: a proposal for their classification. J Clin Pathol 40:995–1015, 1987.

Weiss L, Jaffe E, Liu X, *et al*: Detection and localization of Epstein-Barr viral genomes in angioimmunoblastic lymphadenopathy and angioimmunoblastic lymphadenopathy-like lymphomas. Blood 79:1789–1795, 1992.

NASAL/NASAL-TYPE T/NK-CELL LYMPHOMA (ANGIOCENTRIC LYMPHOMA)

Synonyms and Related Disorders: Rappaport: not listed (diffuse poorly differentiated lymphocytic, mixed lymphocytic/histiocytic or histiocytic); Lukes-Collins: not listed (T-immunoblastic sarcoma); Kiel Classification: not listed (T, pleomorphic small, medium, and large cell); Working Formulation: not listed (diffuse small cleaved, mixed small and large cell, diffuse large cell, large cell immunoblastic); Other: angiocentric immunoproliferative lesion (Grades 2 and 3), polymorphic reticulosis, lethal midline granuloma, midline malignant reticulosis, nasal T-cell lymphoma, ? lymphomatoid granulomatosis (some cases).

Clinical Features

Nasal/nasal-type lymphoma is a rare disorder in the United States and Europe; it is more common in Asia and may be relatively common in parts of South America. A possible explanation for this geographic variation is the tendency of populations to be exposed to Epstein-Barr virus (EBV) at an early age in parts of the world where nasal/nasal-type lymphoma is more prevalent, since the pathogenesis of this lymphoma has been linked to EBV. It usually affects adults, but children are occasionally affected; there is a male preponderance. This lymphoma produces ulcerative, destructive lesions in extranodal sites—most often midline facial structures (nose and palate), but also skin, testis, gastrointestinal tract, and soft tissue. Cases that involve the central nervous system and the lungs may represent a different entity.

The clinical course is usually aggressive, and in most series, nasal/nasal-type lymphoma has been associated with a high mortality rate. A correlation between the clinical course and the number of large cells has been reported, but other studies have not confirmed that finding and have found that stage at presentation is a better prognostic indicator. In a study conducted at the Massachusetts General Hospital, patients with localized disease had a good response to radiation. Hemophagocytic syndromes may develop and are responsible for some of the fatalities in patients with nasal/nasal-type lymphoma.

Morphology

This disorder is characterized by an angioinvasive and angiodestructive infiltrate, usually composed of a mixture of normal-appearing small lymphocytes and variable numbers of small and large atypical lymphoid cells, along with plasma cells and, less often, eosinophils and histiocytes. The appearance of the neoplastic population varies from case to case. Obviously malignant large lymphoid cells predominate in some; small to intermediate-sized cells with subtle atypia, in others. The neoplastic cells may have distinct rims of clear cytoplasm. A characteristic feature is invasion of vascular walls by lymphoid cells with varying degrees of cytologic atypia usually with thrombosis and occlusion of lumina. The vascular occlusion is usually associated with prominent ischemic necrosis of both tumor cells and normal tissue and with fibrinoid change of the vascular wall. Karyorrhectic debris may be abundant. Occasionally, angioinvasion is not identified, although it is unclear whether this is caused by sampling artifact or the actual absence of angioinvasion in some cases; for this reason, the term nasal/nasal-type lymphoma is considered more appropriate than angiocentric lymphoma. Cytoplasmic azurophilic granules are often present when specimens from touch preparations are examined (Figs. 4–17 and 4–18).

Cases with features of pulmonary "lymphomatoid granulomatosis" (LyG) have traditionally been considered part of this category; however, studies suggest that many pulmonary cases may be EBV-associated B-cell proliferations and, therefore, a distinct disease category. Other pulmonary cases with the histologic appearance of LyG appear to be EBV-negative T-cell lymphomas that may also be distinct from nasal-type lymphoma (*see* the following section, "Lymphomatoid Granulomatosis").

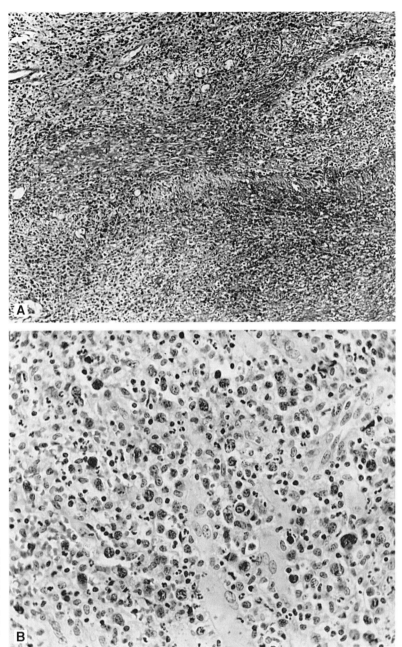

Figure 4–17. Nasal T/NK-cell (angiocentric) lymphoma. *A,* A dense diffuse infiltrate of atypical lymphoid cells is associated with invasion and destruction of a large blood vessel (H&E stain). *B,* This example shows large, atypical lymphoid cells with a prominent admixture of small lymphocytes and neutrophils (H&E stain). (From Ferry JA, Sklar J, Zukerberg LR, Harris NL: Nasal lymphoma. A clinicopathologic study with immunophenotypic and genotypic analysis. Am J Surg Pathol 15:268–279, 1991.)

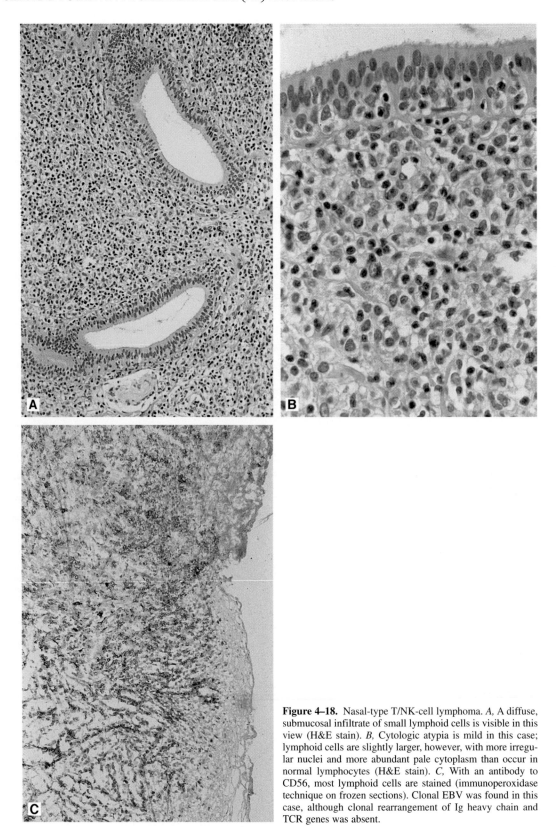

Figure 4–18. Nasal-type T/NK-cell lymphoma. *A,* A diffuse, submucosal infiltrate of small lymphoid cells is visible in this view (H&E stain). *B,* Cytologic atypia is mild in this case; lymphoid cells are slightly larger, however, with more irregular nuclei and more abundant pale cytoplasm than occur in normal lymphocytes (H&E stain). *C,* With an antibody to CD56, most lymphoid cells are stained (immunoperoxidase technique on frozen sections). Clonal EBV was found in this case, although clonal rearrangement of Ig heavy chain and TCR genes was absent.

Immunophenotype

Most cases are CD2+, CD45RO+, CD43+, CD56+, CD5−/+, CD7+/−, TCRαβ−, TCRγδ−. Surface CD3 is usually absent, but cytoplasmic CD3 may be detected on paraffin sections. Although the entire CD3 complex is not expressed by NK cells, the CD3 ε chain, which is recognized by paraffin section antibodies to CD3, may be found in NK cells. Neoplastic cells may be CD4+ or CD8+. Although they are typically CD56 (neural cell adhesion molecule [NCAM])+, they lack other NK-cell-associated antigens such as CD16 and CD57. EBV latent membrane protein may be expressed.

Genetic Features

TCR and Ig genes are usually germline; EBV genomes are present in the majority of cells in most cases and are clonal. Epstein Barr virus–encoded RNA (EBER) can be demonstrated in neoplastic cells in virtually all cases (Fig. 4–19).

In some cases of pulmonary LyG, clonal Ig gene rearrangement has been demonstrated, and EBV genomes are present in B cells, suggesting that this represents a different disease process.

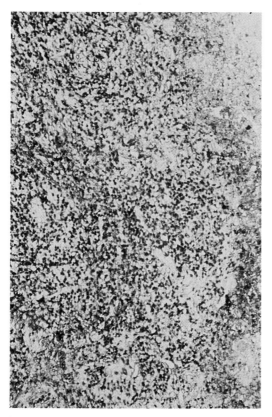

Figure 4–19. Nasal T/NK-cell lymphoma. Virtually all the neoplastic cells show staining for EBER (In situ hybridization on paraffin sections, performed by Dr. Douglas Kingma).

Postulated Normal Counterpart

? NK cell, ? unknown peripheral T-cell subset and may be related to cell of origin of NK-large granular lymphocyte leukemia.

Differential Diagnosis

1. Reactive/infectious process with extensive necrosis: The main difficulty in making a diagnosis of nasal-type T/NK-cell lymphoma is obtaining adequate viable tissue. In cases in which this type of lymphoma is a consideration, the surgeon must perform biopsies until diagnostic tissue is obtained.

   When the neoplastic cells are relatively small, the infiltrate may also be difficult to distinguish from an inflammatory process. When the cells in the infiltrate have nuclear atypia, rims of clear cytoplasm, mitotic activity, and demonstrable EBV, lymphoma is favored. Because CD56+ lymphocytes are typically found in very small numbers in reactive lymphoid infiltrates, the presence of many CD56+ cells supports a diagnosis of lymphoma.

2. Squamous cell carcinoma: Nasal lymphoma may be associated with marked hyperplasia of the overlying epithelium (Fig. 4–20). The atypia of the lymphoid infiltrate and a lack of significant atypia of the epithelial cells support a diagnosis of T-cell lymphoma.

References

Arber DA, Weiss LM, Albujar PF, et al: Nasal lymphomas in Peru. High incidence of T-cell immunophenotype and Epstein-Barr virus infection. Am J Surg Pathol 17:392–399, 1993.

Chan JKC, Tsang WYW, Lau W-H, et al: Aggressive T/natural killer cell lymphoma presenting as testicular tumor. Cancer 77:1198–1205, 1996.

Emile J-F, Boulland M-L, Haioun C, et al: CD5− CD56+ T-cell receptor silent peripheral T-cell lymphomas are natural killer cell lymphomas. Blood 87:1466–1473, 1996.

Ferry J, Sklar J, Zukerberg L, Harris N: Nasal lymphoma: a clinicopathologic study with immunophenotypic and genotypic analysis. Am J Surg Pathol 15:268–279, 1991.

Jaffe ES, Chan JKC, Su I-J, et al: Report of the workshop on nasal and related extranodal angiocentric T/natural killer cell lymphomas. Definitions, differential diagnosis, and epidemiology. Am J Surg Pathol 20:103–111, 1996.

Liang R, Todd D, Chan JK, et al: Treatment outcome and prognostic factors for primary nasal lymphoma. J Clin Oncol 13:666–670, 1995.

Lipford E, Margolich J, Longo D, et al: Angiocentric immunoproliferative lesions: a clinicopathologic spectrum of post-thymic T cell proliferations. Blood 5:1674–1681, 1988.

Myers JL, Kurtin PJ, Katzenstein A-L, et al: Lymphomatoid granulomatosis. Evidence of immunophenotypic diversity and relationship to Epstein-Barr virus infection. Am J Surg Pathol 19:1300–1312, 1995.

Nakamura S, Suchi T, Koshikawa T, et al: Clinicopathologic study of CD56 (NCAM)-positive angiocentric lymphoma occurring in sites other than upper and lower respiratory tract. Am J Surg Pathol 19:284–296, 1995.

Strickler JG, Meneses MF, Habermann TM, et al: Polymorphic reticulosis: a reappraisal. Hum Pathol 25:659–665, 1994.

Tsang WYW, Chan JKC, Ng CS, Pau MY: Utility of a paraffin section-reactive CD56 antibody (123C3) for characterization and diagnosis of lymphomas. Am J Surg Pathol 20(2):202–210, 1996.

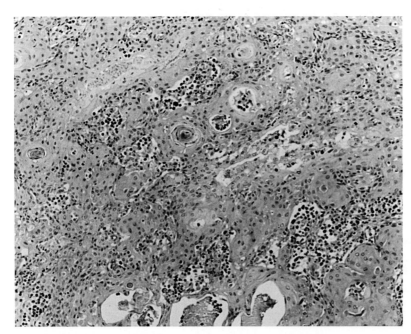

Figure 4–20. Nasal T/NK-cell lymphoma, showing marked pseudoepitheliomatous hyperplasia of the overlying squamous epithelium. Only small clusters of neoplastic lymphoid cells are present. This case was initially interpreted as squamous cell carcinoma (H&E stain). (From Ferry JA, Sklar J, Zukerberg LR, Harris NL: Nasal lymphoma. A clinicopathologic study with immunophenotypic and genotypic analysis. Am J Surg Pathol 15: 268–279, 1991.)

LYMPHOMATOID GRANULOMATOSIS (LyG)

Synonyms and Related Disorders: LyG-like lymphoma; angiocentric immunoproliferative lesion, some cases; angiocentric lymphoma, some cases.

Although many cases of lymphomatoid granulomatosis (LyG) appear to be B-cell lymphomas, and although it is not included as a separate category in the R.E.A.L. Classification, we discuss it following nasal/nasal-type T/NK-cell lymphoma because the two disorders historically have been considered together.

Lymphomatoid granulomatosis (LyG) was first described in 1972 by Liebow and associates. Although most, if not all, cases of LyG are today considered non-Hodgkin's lymphomas, at the time of its initial description, LyG was considered a form of angiitis and granulomatosis that was not clearly neoplastic. Subsequently, a number of similarities were noted between LyG and nasal-type T/NK-cell lymphoma (known previously as polymorphic reticulosis, lethal midline granuloma, or angiocentric lymphoma); these similarities included involvement of extranodal sites, angioinvasion, angiodestruction, extensive necrosis, and prominent inflammatory cell infiltrate with a large component of T cells. Because of these similarities, the two disorders were grouped together under the heading of angiocentric immunoproliferative lesions (AILs). AILs were subdivided into three grades, ranging from cases with few atypical cells (grade 1) to a predominance of atypical cells (grade 3) (Table 4–3). Both disorders were considered T-cell lymphomas, although the lineage of nasal and nasal-type lymphomas has since been shown to be most likely NK cell or

NK-like T cell. Many cases classified as LyG are B-lineage lymphomas (Fig. 4–21), some are T-cell lymphomas, and the lineage of others is uncertain. Some show evidence of EBV infection, although this has not been uniform. We reviewed a case of EBV-positive malignant lymphoma of probable NK lineage that had the classic clinical and histologic features of LyG (Fig. 4–22).

Thus, it is not clear whether LyG is a single entity, or whether the picture of LyG can be produced by lymphomas of more than one lineage; the latter seems more likely at this point. Because of the uncertainty concerning the nature of LyG, we recommend immunophenotyping all cases, especially on paraffin sections, and assigning the lineage only when the immunophenotype and (preferably) the clonality of the most atypical cells are clear. Evaluation for the presence of EBV is also recommended. In cases in which either the lineage is uncertain or the cytologic atypia is not sufficient for a definite diagnosis of lymphoma, obtaining molecular genetic analysis for B-cell, T-cell, and EBV clonality is optimal.

Clinical Features

Patients may present with LyG at any time from childhood to old age, but middle-aged patients are affected most often. There is a male preponderance (male:female ratio of 1.7:1 in the large series studied by Katzenstein and co-workers). Presenting complaints include fever, cough, malaise, weight loss, dyspnea, neurologic symptoms, or a combination of these. Rarely, patients are asymptomatic. Some patients have a history of non-Hodgkin's lymphoma,

Table 4–3
LYMPHOMATOID GRANULOMATOSIS (ANGIOCENTRIC IMMUNOPROLIFERATIVE LESION)
HISTOLOGIC FEATURES AND GRADE

Grade	Angiocentric, Angiodestructive	Small Lymphoid Cells	Large Lymphoid Cells	Other	Necrosis
1	Yes	Numerous typical small lymphocytes	Few; no cytologic atypia	Plasma cells, histiocytes, eosinophils +/−	Usually absent
2	Yes	Mild cytologic atypia	Occasional immuno-blasts or other large cells present; no marked cytologic atypia	As for grade 1	Often present
3 (Angiocentric lymphoma)	Yes	Marked cytologic atypia	Numerous; marked cytologic atypia; immunoblasts, occasional Reed-Sternberg-like cells	Inflammatory cells may be numerous at the periphery	Usually prominent

Hodgkin's disease, leukemia, autoimmune disease, HIV infection, or organ transplantation, suggesting that the pathogenesis in some cases may be related to an immunologic abnormality.

LyG most often affects the lungs, usually in the form of multiple nodules, with bilateral involvement being much more common than unilateral involvement. LyG also frequently involves the skin, the central nervous system, and the kidneys. Lymph nodes may be enlarged; they may show nonspecific reactive hyperplasia or involvement by LyG.

A minority of patients respond to corticosteroid therapy. Initial treatment with combination chemotherapy may yield better long-term survival. The mortality rate of LyG is high, and death is due most often to pulmonary insufficiency secondary to destruction of lung parenchyma. Other causes of death include sepsis, hemoptysis, CNS involvement, and complications of treatment with chemotherapy. A better prognosis has been associated with the absence of symptoms and of neurologic abnormalities at the time of diagnosis, unilateral lung disease, and the presence of a large proportion of small lymphocytes and histiocytes and a small proportion of atypical lymphoid cells.

Morphology

LyG is characterized by an angiocentric and angiodestructive lymphoid infiltrate, which is often associated with necrosis and with a variable admixture of plasma cells, histiocytes, and sometimes, eosinophils. Despite its name, LyG lacks true granulomas. In cases with extensive necrosis, viable cells may be found mainly around blood vessels. The degree of atypia of the lymphoid cells and the proportion of admixed inflammatory cells varies from case to case. A grading scheme has been suggested to subclassify angiocentric immunoproliferative lesions (including LyG): grade 1 lesions have no cytologic atypia and a polymorphous infiltrate of inflammatory cells; grade 3 lesions are monomorphous and show marked cytologic atypia. Grade 3 lesions have sufficient atypia to make a diagnosis of lymphoma; therefore, they have also been called angiocentric lymphoma (*see* Table 4–3). Although one might assume that the most atypical cells would be those infiltrating blood vessels, actually the most atypical lymphoid cells may be present as parenchymal nodules distant from vessels. The proportion of large cells and the grade often increase over time. Some patients develop diffuse high grade monomorphous lymphomas lacking features specific for LyG (*see* Figs. 4–21 and 4–22).

Immunophenotype and Genetic Features

Most lymphoid cells in LyG are T cells (predominantly CD4+); for this reason, LyG has long been considered a lymphoproliferative disorder of T cells. A study by Guinee and co-workers, however, demonstrated that, although the majority of small- to medium-sized cells were T cells (CD45RO+), the large cells, which represented the minority of the lymphoid population, were B cells (CD20+) in all ten cases studied. The B cells contained EBV genetic sequences. Using polymerase chain reaction technique, most cases were found to have clonal Ig heavy chain gene rearrangement. These researchers concluded that LyG is a disorder of B cells with numerous admixed reactive T cells. In a subsequent study of 17 cases of LyG by Myers and colleagues, although 11 cases appeared to be EBV-positive B-cell lymphomas, similar to those of Guinee and co-workers, 3 cases appeared to be EBV-negative T-cell lymphomas and 3 had indeterminate lineage, suggesting that LyG may be a heterogeneous disorder. Some cases may even have NK lineage, as suggested for nasal-type T/NK-cell lymphoma.

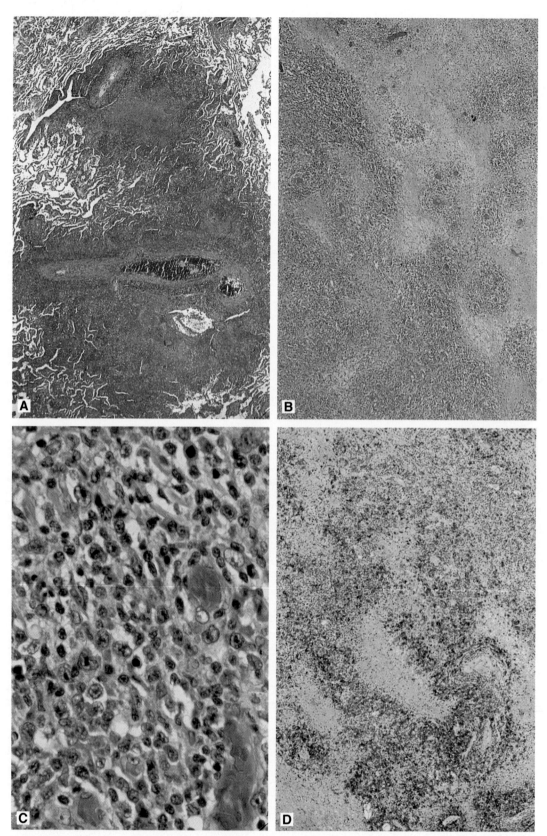

Figure 4–21. Diffuse large B-cell lymphoma (immunoblastic plasmacytoid) with features of lymphomatoid granulomatosis. Small *(A)* and large *(B)* pulmonary nodules show extensive necrosis, angioinvasion, and angiodestruction (H&E stain). *C,* In this area, immunoblasts predominate. Other areas had large numbers of small lymphocytes and histiocytes (H&E stain). *D,* Many cells are positive with an antibody to CD20 (L26), especially around necrotic areas and vessels (immunoperoxidase technique on paraffin sections).

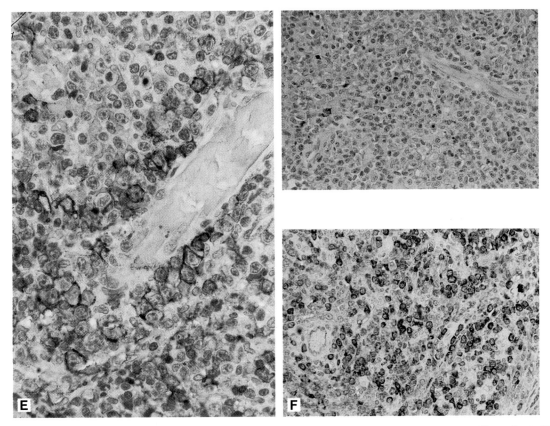

Figure 4–21. *E,* High power examination shows that the CD20+ cells are large cells (immunoperoxidase technique on paraffin sections). *F,* There is no staining for κ light chain *(top),* while many cells contain cytoplasmic λ *(bottom),* consistent with plasmacytic differentiation (immunoperoxidase technique on paraffin sections).

Differential Diagnosis

1. Wegener's granulomatosis (WG): WG contains more neutrophils and fewer lymphoid cells than LyG; in WG, the lymphoid cells are not atypical. Multinucleated histiocytic giant cells, palisading granulomas, and granulomatous vasculitis are features of WG, in contrast to LyG (Fig. 4–23).

2. Nasal-type T/NK-cell lymphoma: LyG does not have the predilection for Asian patients seen in nasal-type T/NK-cell lymphoma. Although the disease distribution is primarily extranodal in both LyG and nasal-type T/NK-cell lymphoma, the tissues preferentially involved are different. Most nasal-type T/NK-cell lymphomas produce midfacial disease and do not affect the lungs, CNS, or kidneys, whereas LyG affects the lungs in most cases and spares the upper respiratory tract and facial region. In viable areas of nasal-type lymphoma, the cellular infiltrate may consist of a relatively homogeneous (although often somewhat pleomorphic) population of T/NK cells. Non-neoplastic T cells may be found at the periphery of the lymphoma, but histiocytes usually are not prominent, whereas LyG may have a more truly heterogeneous composition. Immunoblasts and large atypical cells resembling Reed-Sternberg cells are said to occur more frequently in LyG.

3. Non-Hodgkin's lymphomas, non-LyG type, with pulmonary involvement: Lymphomas of many types involve the lung, and a variety of lymphomas invade blood vessels. Large B-cell lymphoma frequently invades blood vessels; follicle center lymphoma can invade blood vessels and may occasionally result in complete infarction of the involved lymph nodes. Low grade B-cell lymphoma of MALT may involve the lung, following the bronchovascular bundles, and although it occasionally shows angioinvasion, it is not angiodestructive. The distin-

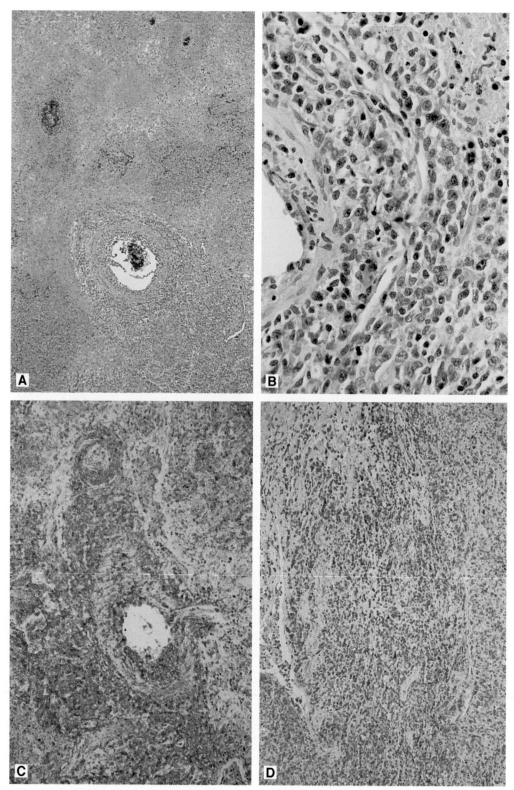

Figure 4–22. Large cell lymphoma of the lung of probable NK-cell lineage, with features of lymphomatoid granulomatosis. The patient had multiple lung nodules, as well as lesions in the central nervous system and kidneys. *A,* The lymphoma shows extensive necrosis, as well as angioinvasion and angiodestruction (H&E stain). *B,* In some areas, large atypical cells predominate, as seen here. In many other areas, small- and medium-sized lymphoid cells and histiocytes predominate (H&E stain). The large atypical cells are CD43+ *(C)* and CD56+ *(D)*. They also expressed CD30 and EBV-LMP, but were negative for other B- and T-cell-associated antigens, consistent with NK lineage (immunoperoxidase technique on paraffin sections).

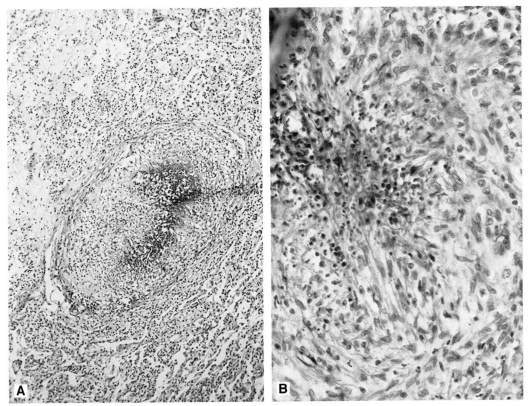

Figure 4–23. Wegener's granulomatosis. *A,* A destructive, necrotizing vasculitis involves a large blood vessel in this lung biopsy specimen (H&E stain). *B,* Some areas show well-formed palisading granulomas surrounding collections of neutrophils. Atypical lymphoid cells are absent (H&E stain).

guishing feature of LyG is its marked preference for an angiocentric distribution and its angiodestructive nature.
4. Hodgkin's disease (HD): Hodgkin's disease characteristically has an associated polymorphous inflammatory cell infiltrate and may show extensive necrosis. It lacks an angiocentric, angiodestructive pattern. LyG may have Reed-Sternberg-like cells, but diagnostic Reed-Sternberg cells are unusual. In LyG, small lymphoid cells are often atypical, having irregular, angulated nuclei, whereas in HD, the lymphocytes appear normal.

References

Guinee D, Jaffe ES, Kingma D, *et al*: Pulmonary lymphomatoid granulomatosis. Evidence for a proliferation of Epstein-Barr virus infected B lymphocytes with a prominent T cell component and vasculitis. Am J Surg Pathol 18:753–764, 1994.

Jaffe ES, Chan JKC, Su I-J, *et al*: Report of the workshop on nasal and related extranodal angiocentric T/natural killer cell lymphomas. Definitions, differential diagnosis, and epidemiology. Am J Surg Pathol 20:103–111, 1996.

Katzenstein A-LA, Carrington CB, Liebow AA: Lymphomatoid granulomatosis. A clinicopathologic study of 152 cases. Cancer 43:360–373, 1979.

Liebow AA, Carrington CRB, Friedman PJ: Lymphomatoid granulomatosis. Hum Pathol 3:457–558, 1972.

Lipford E, Margolich J, Longo D, *et al*: Angiocentric immunoproliferative lesions: a clinicopathologic spectrum of post-thymic T cell proliferations. Blood 5:1674–1681, 1988.

Myers JL, Kurtin PJ, Katzenstein A-L, *et al*: Lymphomatoid granulomatosis. Evidence of immunophenotypic diversity and relationship to Epstein-Barr virus infection. Am J Surg Pathol 19:1300–1312, 1995.

INTESTINAL T-CELL LYMPHOMA (ITL), WITH OR WITHOUT ENTEROPATHY

Synonyms: Rappaport: not listed (diffuse mixed lymphocytic-histiocytic, histiocytic); Lukes-Collins: not listed (T-immunoblastic sarcoma); Kiel: not listed (T, pleomorphic small, medium and large cell); Working Formulation: not listed (diffuse small cleaved cell, diffuse mixed small and large cell, diffuse large cell, large cell immunoblastic); Other: malignant histiocytosis of the intestine, ulcerative jejunitis.

Clinical Features

Intestinal T-cell lymphoma (ITL) occurs in adults, usually those with a history of celiac disease (gluten-sensitive enteropathy). This is an uncommon lymphoma, but it is seen with increased frequency in areas such as Wales and Ireland where celiac disease is more prevalent. The risk of developing ITL varies among different series; however, in one large study, the relative risk was 42.7 for developing lymphoma among patients with celiac sprue compared with the general population. The relative risk rose to 77.8 when a gluten-free diet was not observed, but there was no significant excess risk with a strict gluten-free diet in this and other studies. In some cases, a lymphoma with the distinctive features of ITL is encountered with no evidence of enteropathy.

The median age at diagnosis is 60 years; males are affected slightly more often than females. Patients frequently present with severe abdominal pain due to perfora-tion or obstruction. The course is aggressive, and death usu-ally occurs from multifocal intestinal perforation owing to refractory malignant ulcers.

Morphology

Gross examination reveals linear jejunal ulcers that are often multiple, circumferential, and associated with perfora-tion. The intestinal wall is frequently thickened only slightly in the area of the ulcers, and a discrete mass may or may not be apparent (Fig. 4–24). The lymphoma is composed of small, medium, or large cells, or a mixture of these. In some cases, tumor cells are anaplastic (Fig. 4–25). The adjacent mucosa shows villous atrophy, although not consistently, and often contains increased numbers of intraepithelial T cells. Early lesions may show mucosal ulceration with small numbers of atypical cells and numerous reactive histiocytes, which may be hemophagocytic.

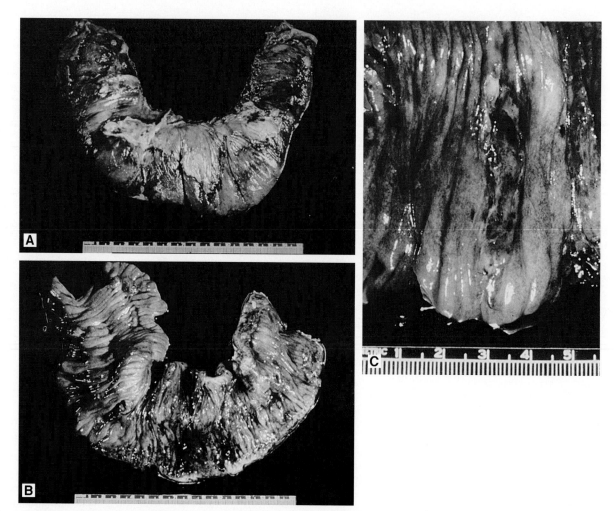

Figure 4–24. Intestinal (enteropathy-associated) T-cell lymphoma, gross appearance. *A,* Much of the serosal surface is covered by fibrinopurulent exudate. *B,* Multiple linear ulcers are oriented perpendicular to the long axis of the small intestine; one was associated with perforation. The wall of the bowel is not thickened significantly, and no discrete mass is seen. *C,* Close up view shows one linear ulcer, with necrotic tissue at its base. The surrounding mucosa is edematous and congested.

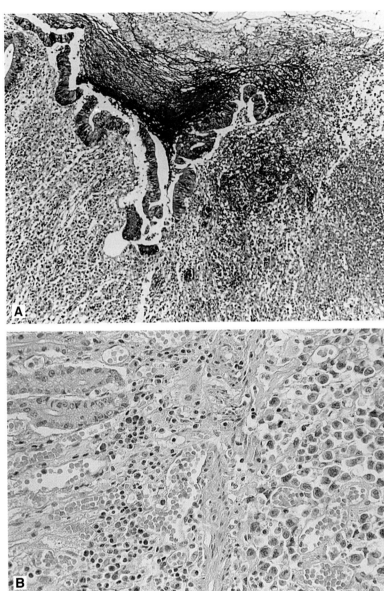

Figure 4–25. Intestinal (enteropathy-associated) T-cell lymphoma. *A,* A dense lymphoid infiltrate is associated with erosion of the overlying epithelium (H&E stain). *B,* Large bizarre lymphoid cells fill the submucosa (H&E stain).

Illustration continued on following page.

Rarely, patients with celiac sprue without lymphoma have markedly enlarged mesenteric lymph nodes (up to 8 cm) with cystification, so that all that remains of the node is a thickened fibrous capsule and a thin rim of lymphoid tissue enclosing clear or turbid fluid, probably lymph. This finding has been referred to as mesenteric lymph node cavitation. Because multiple lymph nodes are often affected, it is not practical to resect them, but in a study published in 1986, Holmes suggested treatment by aspiration of the fluid to decompress the lymph nodes.

Immunophenotype

Tumor cells are CD3+, CD7+, CD8+/−, CD4−, CD103+ (mucosal lymphocyte antigen [MLA] recognized by HML-1, LFG1, Bly7, Ber-ACT8).

Genetic Features

TCR genes are rearranged. Clonally integrated EBV has been identified in some cases.

Postulated Normal Counterpart

Intestinal intraepithelial T cell in various stages of transformation.

Differential Diagnosis

1. Non-neoplastic ulcers: The absence of prominent mural thickening on gross examination may raise the question

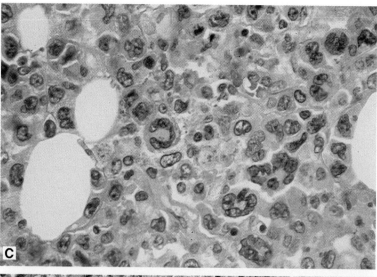

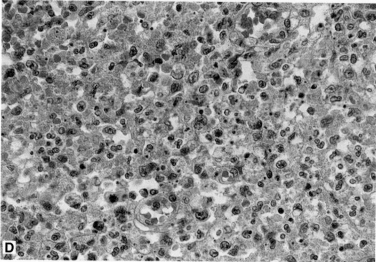

Figure 4–25. *Continued C,* In the same case, the neoplastic cells appear anaplastic (H&E stain). *D,* Another case shows a mixture of atypical lymphoid cells, histiocytes, granulocytes, and abundant debris, but no anaplastic large cells (H&E stain).

of a non-neoplastic disease. Reactive histiocytes and granulocytes may obscure the neoplastic population. Careful study of histologic sections usually discloses the lymphoma, although occasionally it is necessary to examine multiple sections to identify tumor cells.

2. B-cell lymphoma: The unusual location of the lymphoma, its distinctive gross and microscopic appearance, and its association with celiac sprue are features strongly associated with T lineage. Immunophenotyping, however, can resolve any uncertainty.

3. Nasal-type T/NK-cell/angiocentric lymphoma rarely involves the gastrointestinal tract, and in this site, may be difficult to distinguish from ITL. The presence of prominent villous atrophy, unequivocal T-antigen expression, and TCR gene rearrangement favor ITL.

References

Collin P, Reunala T, Pukkala E, *et al*: Coeliac disease–associated disorders and survival. (*See* comments.) Gut 35(9):1215–1218, 1994.

Holmes GKT: Mesenteric lymph node cavitation in celiac disease. Gut 27:728–733, 1986.

Holmes GKT, Prior P, Lane MR, *et al*: Malignancy in coeliac disease—effect of a gluten free diet. Gut 30:333–338, 1989.

Isaacson PG: Gastrointestinal lymphoma. Hum Pathol 25:1020–1029, 1994.

Murray A, Cuevas AC, Jones DB, Wright DH: Study of the immunohistochemistry and T cell clonality of enteropathy-associated T cell lymphoma. Am J Pathol 146:509–519, 1995.

Pan L, Diss TC, Peng H, *et al*: Epstein-Barr virus (EBV) in enteropathy-associated T cell lymphoma (EATL). J Pathol 170:137–143, 1993.

Spencer J, Cerf-Bensussan N, Jarry A, *et al*: Enteropathy-associated T-cell lymphoma is recognized by a monoclonal antibody (HML-1) that defines a membrane molecule on human mucosal lymphocytes. Am J Pathol 132:1–5, 1988.

ADULT T-CELL LYMPHOMA/LEUKEMIA (ATLL)

Synonyms: Rappaport: not recognized (diffuse poorly differentiated lymphocytic, mixed lymphocytic-histiocytic, or histiocytic); Lukes-Collins: not recognized (T-immunoblastic sarcoma); Kiel: pleomorphic small, medium, and large cell types (HTLV 1+); Working Formulation: not recognized (diffuse small cleaved cell, mixed small and large cell, diffuse large cell, large cell immunoblastic).

Clinical Features

Adult T-cell lymphoma/leukemia (ATLL) is a neoplasm caused by human T-cell lymphotrophic virus 1 (HTLV-1). Most patients are from Japan or the Caribbean where HTLV-1 is endemic, although occasional cases are found in the southeastern United States. Serologic studies are used to document exposure to HTLV-1.

Lymphoma/leukemia induced by HTLV-1 has a long incubation period: although infection typically occurs during infancy, ATLL virtually exclusively affects adults. In addition, ATLL arises in only about 1% of HTLV-1-infected individuals.

Several clinical forms of lymphoid neoplasia have been described. The most common, the acute form, is associated with hepatosplenomegaly, peripheral lymphadenopathy, cutaneous disease, hypercalcemia, bone lesions, numerous leukemic cells in the peripheral blood, and sometimes, profound immunodeficiency. Median survival time is less than 1 year. The rare lymphomatous form shows isolated lymphadenopathy or extranodal lymphoma without leukemia. A chronic form, with less marked lymphocytosis and without hypercalcemia or hepatosplenomegaly, has a slightly longer survival time. Rare cases of smoldering ATLL have mild lymphocytosis, which is demonstrably clonal, but an indolent course, which may be complicated by frequent infections. Both chronic and smoldering forms are associated with skin rashes, and both may progress to acute ATLL.

A high proportion of patients with the appearance of anaplastic large cell lymphoma (ALCL, *see* the next discussion) who are from areas endemic for HTLV-1 have clonally integrated proviral DNA. These patients have a prognosis similar to that for other ATLL patients, but a worse prognosis than for patients with ALCL without HTLV-1.

Morphology

In lymph nodes the lymphoma has a diffuse pattern; usually there is a mixture of pleomorphic small and large atypical cells (Figs. 4–26 and 4–27). Multinucleated giant cells reminiscent of Reed-Sternberg cells may be found in some cases. Cells with hyperlobated nuclei ("clover leaf" or "flower" cells) are common in the peripheral blood (Fig. 4–28). Marrow infiltration is diffuse and ranges from sparse to extensive.

Immunophenotype

Tumor cells have T-cell-associated antigens (CD2+, CD3+, CD5+), usually CD7−; most are CD4+, CD25+; rare CD8+ cases have been reported.

Genetic Features

TCR genes are rearranged; clonally integrated HTLV-1 genomes are found in all cases.

Postulated Normal Counterpart

Peripheral CD4+ T cell in various stages of transformation.

Differential Diagnosis

1. B-cell lymphoma: A lymph node involved by ATLL examined in isolation cannot be distinguished from a high grade B-cell lymphoma. Clinical information and review of a peripheral smear are important in making the correct diagnosis. Immunophenotyping confirms the diagnosis of a T-cell lymphoma. Demonstration of serum antibodies to HTLV-1 or clonally integrated HTLV-1 genomes is required to confirm the diagnosis.
2. Hodgkin's disease (HD): In the occasional case having Reed-Sternberg-like cells, evidence against HD and in favor of ATLL include atypia of smaller lymphoid cells, T-antigen expression by large cells, clonal TCR gene rearrangement, and monoclonal integration of HTLV-1 genomes.

References

Duggan D, Ehrlich G, Davey F, *et al*: HTLV-I induced lymphoma mimicking Hodgkin's disease. Diagnosis by polymerase chain reaction amplification of specific HTLV-I sequences in tumor DNA. Blood 71:1027–1032, 1988.

Jaffe E, Blattner W, Blayney D, Bunn P, *et al*: The pathologic spectrum of adult T-cell leukemia/lymphoma in the United States. Am J Surg Pathol 8:263–275, 1984.

Keufler PR, Bunn PA: Adult T-cell leukaemia/lymphoma. Clin Haematol 15:695–726, 1986.

Kikuchi M, Mitsui T, Takeshita M, *et al*: Virus associated adult T-cell leukemia (ATL) in Japan: clinical, histological and immunological studies. Hematol Oncol 4:67, 1987.

Ratner L, Griffith RC, Marselle L, *et al*: A lymphoproliferative disorder caused by human T-lymphotropic virus type I: demonstration of a continuum between acute and chronic adult T-cell leukemia/lymphoma. Am J Med 83:953–958, 1987.

Suchi T, Lennert K, Tu L-Y: Histopathology and immunohistochemistry of peripheral T-cell lymphomas: a proposal for their classification. J Clin Pathol 40:995–1015, 1987.

Takeshita M, Ohshima K, Akamatsu M, *et al*: CD30-positive anaplastic large cell lymphoma in a human T-cell lymphotropic virus-1 endemic area. Hum Pathol 26:614–619, 1995.

Tokunaga M, Sato E: Non-Hodgkin's lymphomas in a southern prefecture in Japan: an analysis of 715 cases. Cancer 46:1231–1239, 1980.

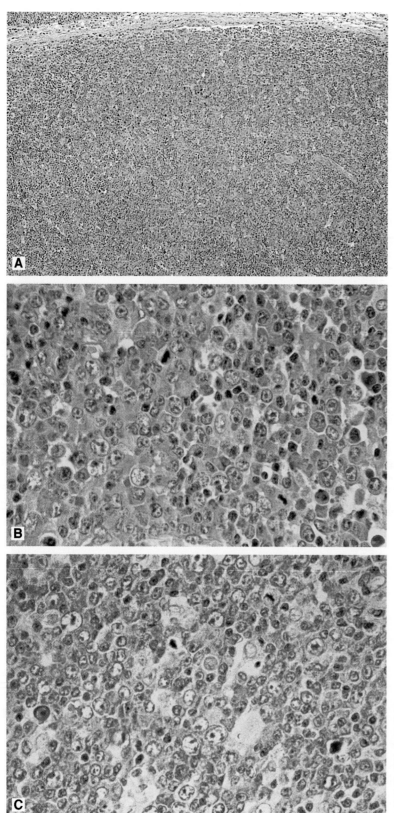

Figure 4–26. Adult T-cell lymphoma/leukemia, lymph node biopsy. *A,* Low power view shows diffuse obliteration of the nodal architecture (H&E stain). *B,* High power examination shows large- and occasionally medium-sized atypical lymphoid cells. Nuclear lobation from the lymph node specimen is not as striking as in peripheral blood specimens from this patient (*compare* to Fig. 4–28) (H&E stain). *C,* In other areas, small- and medium-sized neoplastic cells are slightly more numerous. A few tingible body macrophages are present; mitotic figures are frequent (Giemsa stain).

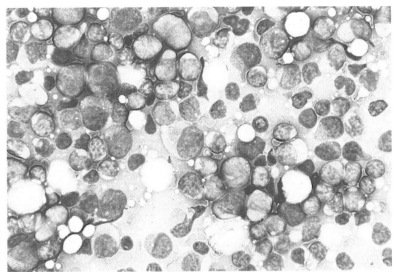

Figure 4–27. Adult T-cell lymphoma/leukemia, fine needle aspiration of a lymph node. This preparation shows cells of a range of sizes, from small to large, with predominantly round, occasionally lobated nuclei and light blue cytoplasm (Wright Giemsa stain).

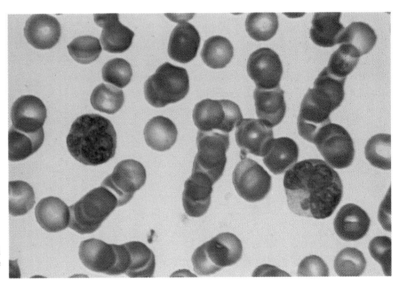

Figure 4–28. Adult T-cell lymphoma/leukemia, peripheral blood. Two flower cells with prominently lobated nuclei are present (H&E stain).

ANAPLASTIC LARGE CELL (CD30+) LYMPHOMA (ALCL) (T- AND NULL-CELL TYPES)

Synonyms: Rappaport: not listed (histiocytic, diffuse); Kiel: large cell anaplastic (T and null types); Lukes-Collins: T-immunoblastic sarcoma; Working Formulation: not listed (diffuse large cell immunoblastic); Possible other names: malignant histiocytosis, sinusoidal large cell lymphoma, regressing atypical histiocytosis.

Clinical Features

Anaplastic large cell lymphoma (ALCL) comprises about 5% of lymphomas in the United States and Europe. The age at onset ranges widely and is distributed bimodally, with an early peak in the second decade and a smaller peak after the seventh decade. The median age is about 40 years, and there is a slight male preponderance. ALCL represents one of the major subsets of childhood non-Hodgkin's lymphomas. It occurs in two forms: a primary systemic form and a primary cutaneous form.

In primary systemic ALCL, more than 80% of patients present with lymphadenopathy, and more than 40% have extranodal disease (with or without nodal disease), which most often involves the skin, followed by bone, soft tissue, and gastrointestinal tract. The marrow usually is not involved at presentation. The tumor is aggressive but potentially curable, similar to other high grade lymphomas. Some studies have suggested that the prognosis for ALCL is slightly better than for other high grade lymphomas.

Patients with primary cutaneous ALCL present with one or more nodules involving the dermis and, often, the subcutaneous tissue. If the lymphoma has not spread extracutaneously, the prognosis is excellent. In rare cases, spontaneous regression has been described. The entity that has been called regressing atypical histiocytosis may actually represent primary cutaneous ALCL.

Most cases of ALCL occur de novo, but lymphomas with anaplastic morphology may also develop in patients with a history of Hodgkin's disease, mycosis fungoides, and other T-cell and B-cell lymphomas.

Morphology

The designation of ALCL is reserved for cases of lymphoma with a distinctive morphology that have T- or null-cell phenotype and genotype. The designation of ALCL is not used for large T- or B-cell lymphomas with typical morphology that express CD30 or for B-cell lymphomas with anaplastic morphology. Prior to the recognition of ALCL, many cases were interpreted as malignant histiocytosis, lymphocyte-depleted Hodgkin's disease, regressing atyp-ical histiocytosis, metastatic carcinoma, or malignant melanoma.

ALCL may completely or partially involve lymph nodes. In the partially involved case, the lymphoma may spread in an interfollicular pattern or preferentially invade the sinuses. The neoplastic cells are usually larger than those of diffuse large B-cell lymphoma or peripheral T-cell lymphoma; they are often bizarre or multinucleate, resembling Reed-Sternberg cells. Some have described the nuclei as embryo-, jellyfish-, or wreath-like. Nuclei are vesicular; nucleoli are prominent. Cytoplasm is abundant and may be pale, eosinophilic, or basophilic. A prominent hof may be seen. Tumor cells may appear cohesive. The mitotic rate is high, and tingible body macrophages and areas of necrosis may be visible (Figs. 4–29 and 4–30). The tumor may be associated with fibrosis; in fibrotic areas, tumor cells may assume a spindled shape. Reactive cells, including eosinophils and plasma cells, may be present, although typically in smaller numbers than in Hodgkin's disease.

In the primary cutaneous form, sheets of neoplastic cells occur in the dermis, and usually, the subcutaneous tissue, along with few interspersed inflammatory cells. The epidermis is usually spared by the tumor cells, although pseudoepitheliomatous hyperplasia may exist (Fig. 4–31).

Two variants have been described: a small cell variant (Fig. 4–32) and a histiocyte-rich variant (lymphohistiocytic T-cell lymphoma (Fig. 4–33), in which many of the neoplastic cells may be smaller than classic ALCL cells. These variants may be more common in children and adolescents.

The small cell variant of ALCL most often affects skin and lymph nodes. On microscopic examination, there is an infiltrate of small lymphoid cells with irregular nuclei and slightly more pale cytoplasm than a normal lymphocyte. Scattered among the small cells are small numbers of large cells. Both small and large cells are T cells, but usually only the large cells are CD30+.

In the histiocyte-rich variant of ALCL (lymphohistiocytic T-cell lymphoma), the predominant cell is a histiocyte with an eccentric nucleus and abundant, finely granular eosinophilic cytoplasm. The appearance of these histiocytes is distinctive; their shape is reminiscent of a large plasma cell. Scattered among the reactive histiocytes are isolated, occasionally clustered, CD30+, atypical T-lymphoid cells that are usually large, although not as large as the classic anaplastic large cell. A neutrophil-rich variant has also been described in which anaplastic large cells are interspersed with intact neutrophils (Fig. 4–34).

Bone marrow involvement in cases of ALCL may be focal or extensive and is occasionally quite subtle; some investigators have suggested that subjecting staging bone marrow biopsy specimens to immunostaining with antibodies to CD30 could be helpful in identifying a small population of tumor cells.

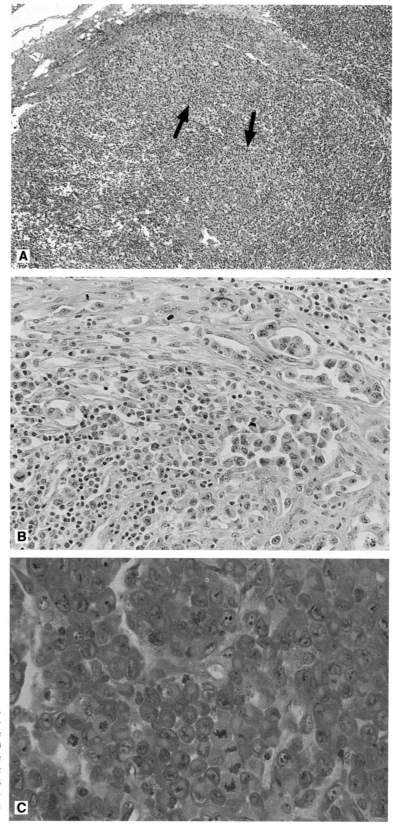

Figure 4–29. Anaplastic large cell lymphoma, lymph node. *A,* The lymph node is partially involved with lymphoma, represented by the broad subcapsular eosinophilic band and the large, poorly delimited nodule deeper in the node *(arrows)* (H&E stain). *B,* Cohesive aggregates of neoplastic cells are present in small vascular spaces in and beneath the fibrotic capsule (H&E stain). *C,* High power view shows large cells with vesicular, sometimes eccentric nuclei, prominent nucleoli, abundant basophilic cytoplasm, and prominent Golgi regions. Mitoses are frequent (Giemsa stain).

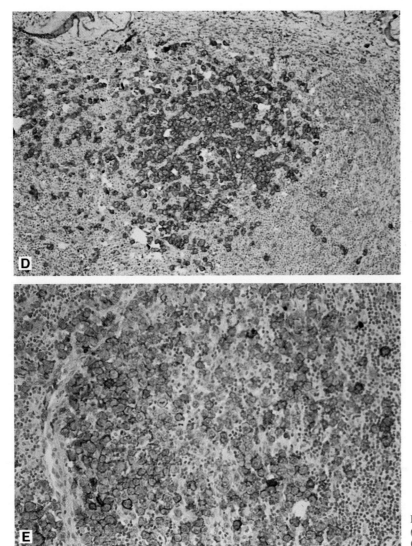

Figure 4–29. Immunostaining with antibodies to CD30. *(D)* and EMA *(E)* highlights aggregates of neoplastic cells (immunoperoxidase technique on paraffin sections).

Immunophenotype

In the systemic form of ALCL, tumor cells are CD30+, CD45+/−, CD25+/−, EMA+/−, CD15−/+, CD3−/+, CD43+/−, CD45RO+/−, other T-cell-associated antigens variable, CD68− (when studied using PGM1; KP1 may stain some cases), and lysozyme-negative (Fig. 4–29, *D* and *E*). Primary cutaneous cases typically lack EMA and express the cutaneous lymphocyte antigen (CLA, HECA-452). CD30, a transmembrane protein expressed in nearly all cases of ALCL, is believed to be a member of the tumor necrosis factor receptor superfamily.

Genetic Features

TCR genes are rearranged in 50% to 60% of cases; 40% to 50% have no rearrangement of TCR genes or Ig genes. Cytogenetic studies show that some cases of the systemic (but not the cutaneous) form of ALCL have t(2;5)(p23;q35). The reported frequency varies; it appears to be more common in primary T- or null-cell ALCL in young patients. The locus on chromosome 2 involved in the translocation is thought to code for a novel anaplastic lymphoma kinase (alk); 5q35 is believed to contain the gene for nucleophosmin (npm), a protein thought to play a role in ribosomal pro-

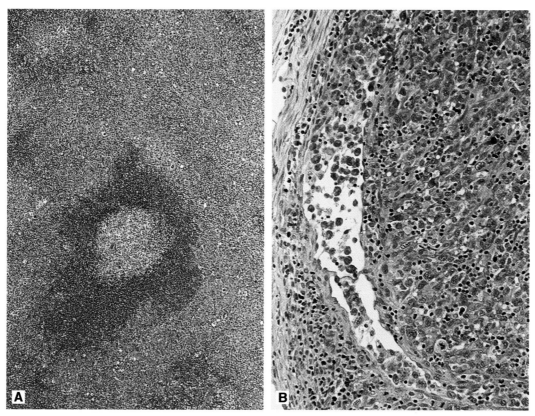

Figure 4–30. Anaplastic large cell lymphoma, involving the femoral lymph node of an 11-year-old boy. *A,* Low power examination shows lymphoma surrounding a reactive lymphoid follicle (H&E stain). *B,* Invasion of sinuses by neoplastic cells (H&E stain).

tein assembly and nuclear/cytoplasmic transport. The npm-alk fusion product has tyrosine kinase activity and may contribute to malignant transformation in cases of ALCL.

Postulated Normal Counterpart

Extrafollicular CD30+ blasts.

Differential Diagnosis

1. Hodgkin's disease (HD): HD is the entity most commonly included in the differential diagnosis of ALCL. Table 4–4 lists features that help in distinguishing the two. There appears to be a continuum between HD and ALCL, and some cases cannot be clearly subclassified as one or the other. The provisional entity of Hodgkin's-related ALCL (*see* Chapter 5) is an example of the borderline between ALCL and HD. In morphologically borderline cases, the immunophenotype can be helpful. If the immunophenotype is classic for HD, we generally make a diagnosis of HD; if there is clear-cut T-antigen expression and lack of CD15, a diagnosis of ALCL is made. If both morphology and immunophenotype are borderline, the case is considered unclassifiable.

2. Non-lymphoid neoplasia: The tendency of ALCL to involve nodal sinuses and its abundant cytoplasm, cohesive growth, highly atypical nuclei, and frequent CD45 negativity and EMA positivity often raise the question of metastatic carcinoma or melanoma. Primary cutaneous cases may be misdiagnosed as melanoma. ALCL may contain spindle cells and mimic sarcoma. The key to avoiding misdiagnosing ALCL as a nonlymphoid tumor is remembering to include ALCL in the differential diagnosis of undifferentiated large cell neoplasms, especially in those patients who present with disease in skin or in lymph nodes without a known primary tumor. Immunohistochemistry assists greatly in establishing a diagnosis:

   ALCL: CD30+, CD45+/−, EMA+/−, T- antigen+/−, keratin− (although there are rare reports of keratin expression, usually with a dot-like paranuclear pattern).

   Carcinoma: keratin+, CD30− (a few carcinomas, especially embryonal carcinoma, may be CD30+), CD45−, T- and B-antigen−.

   Melanoma: S-100+, HMB-45+, CD45−, CD30− (rare reports describe weak CD30 expression), T- and B-antigen−.

Table 4–4
ANAPLASTIC LARGE CELL LYMPHOMA (ALCL) VS. HODGKIN'S DISEASE (HD)

	ALCL	HD
Clinical Features		
Young age	Frequent	Frequent
Bimodal age distribution	Present	Present
Mediastinal mass	Infrequent	Frequent
Noncontiguous nodal disease	Frequent	Rare
Inguinal adenopathy	Frequent	Infrequent
Skin involvement	Frequent	Rare
GI tract	Occasional	Rare
Stage I/II disease	Minority	Majority
Histologic Features		
Partial nodal involvement	Frequent	Frequent
Pattern	Diffuse/sinus	Diffuse/nodular
Sclerosis	Inconspicuous	Prominent, band-like in NS
RS cells, lacunar cells	Rare	Present
Histiocytes, granulomas	Rare	Frequent
Phagocytic tumor cells	Infrequent	Absent
Immunophenotype		
Classic	CD30+, CD45+, CD15−, EMA+, T>null	CD15+, CD30+, CD45−, EMA−, T-antigen−, B-antigen−
Variations	CD45−, CD15+, EMA−	CD45+, B-antigen+, rarely T-antigen+
Genotype	Clonal TCR> germline TCR & Ig	Germline TCR and Ig> clonal Ig>clonal TCR
t(2;5)	Frequent	Rare or absent
EBV DNA, RNA, LMP	Minority	Approximately 1/2

Abbreviations: NS, nodular sclerosis Hodgkin's disease; RS, Reed-Sternberg; TCR, T-cell receptor genes; Ig, immunoglobulin genes; EBV, Epstein-Barr virus.

3. Reactive hyperplasia vs. systemic form of ALCL: Florid reactive lymphoid hyperplasia with large numbers of paracortical or sinusoidal immunoblasts may give rise to a differential diagnosis of partial nodal involvement by ALCL. Features in favor of ALCL are marked cytologic atypia, pleomorphism, and cohesiveness of the large cells, with strong diffuse CD30 expression and T-cell antigen and EMA expression. In favor of reactive hyperplasia are clinical or serologic evidence of an inciting agent (especially infectious mononucleosis), lack of marked atypia, B-antigen expression, and lack of EMA in the large cells. Genotyping may be required to establish a diagnosis in some cases.

4. Reactive hyperplasia vs. small cell and histiocyte-rich variants of ALCL: In both the small cell and the histiocyte-rich variant, the most common error in diagnosis is failure to recognize these entities as neoplastic. In the histiocyte-rich variant, only small numbers of tumor cells are present, and they are easily overlooked because of the extensive histiocytic infiltrate. In the small cell variant,

the cytologic atypia of the small cells is somewhat subtle, and only a few large atypical cells may be present. For both of these variants, familiarity with their distinctive appearance, combined with supportive immunohistochemical findings, will lead to the correct diagnosis.

5. Malignant histiocytosis (MH): Most cases previously classified as MH are now believed to represent non-Hodgkin's lymphomas, most often ALCL. A diagnosis of MH should be made with extreme caution and only if there is unequivocal evidence of histiocytic differentiation (e.g., lysozyme expression, and lack of evidence for B- or T-cell differentiation). True cases of MH are rare.

6. Lymphomatoid papulosis (LyP): LyP consists of multiple small papules that often have a regional or generalized distribution in the skin, whereas cutaneous ALCL usually forms large nodules that may be solitary, or if multiple, have a localized distribution. LyP has large numbers of inflammatory cells and only scattered CD30+ large cells. Borderline cases, however, may be difficult to subclassify.

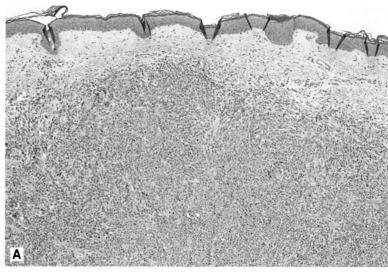

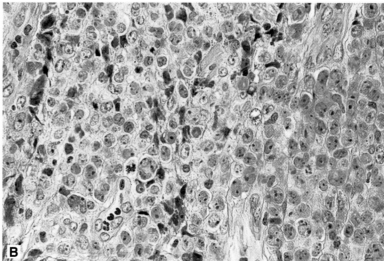

Figure 4–31. Primary cutaneous anaplastic large cell lymphoma. *A,* Low power view shows a dense dermal infiltrate that spares the epidermis (H&E stain). *B,* High power view shows large cells that have oval nuclei, prominent nucleoli, and a moderate amount of cytoplasm. Binucleated and trinucleated cells are present (H&E stain).

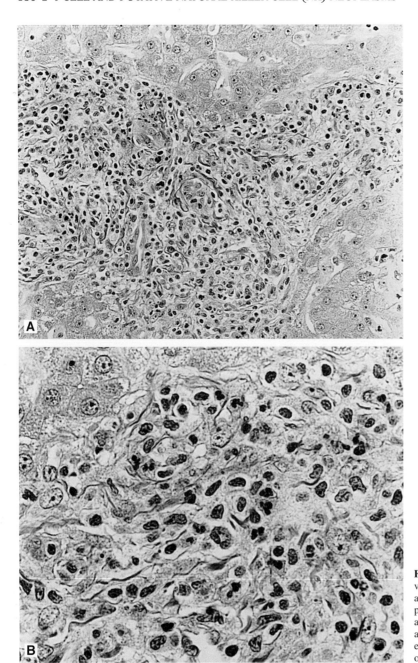

Figure 4–32. Anaplastic large cell lymphoma, small cell variant, involving the liver of a young man. *A,* Portal triads are infiltrated by neoplastic cells (H&E stain). *B,* Most neoplastic cells are small, having irregular nuclei and a moderate amount of clear cytoplasm; only a few large cells appear. (One large cell with a nearly circular nucleus is present centrally.) Both small and large cells were T cells, but only the large cells were CD30+ (H&E stain).

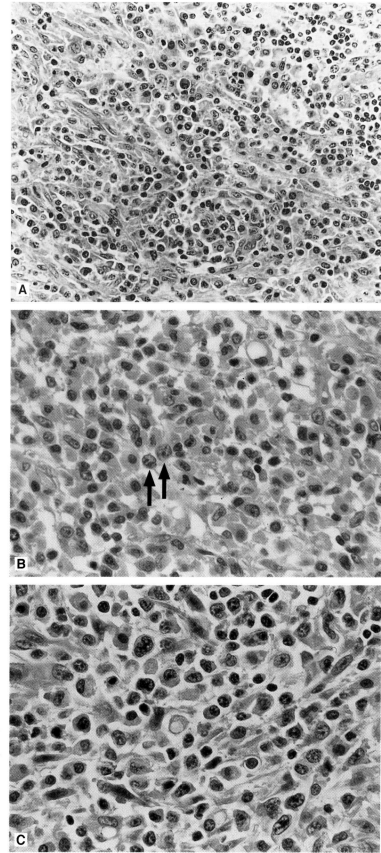

Figure 4–33. Anaplastic large cell lymphoma, histiocyte-rich (lymphohistiocytic T-cell lymphoma). *A,* This specimen shows a polymorphous infiltrate of lymphocytes, plasma cells, and many histiocytes; large lymphoid cells are inconspicuous (H&E stain). *B,* On higher power examination, histiocytes having round nuclei, fine chromatin, abundant finely granular, eccentrically placed cytoplasm, and ill-defined cell borders predominate. Rare large lymphoid cells are present *(arrows)* (H&E stain). *C,* In other areas, large and small atypical cells are more numerous, although reactive cells are still relatively abundant (H&E stain).

Illustration continued on following page.

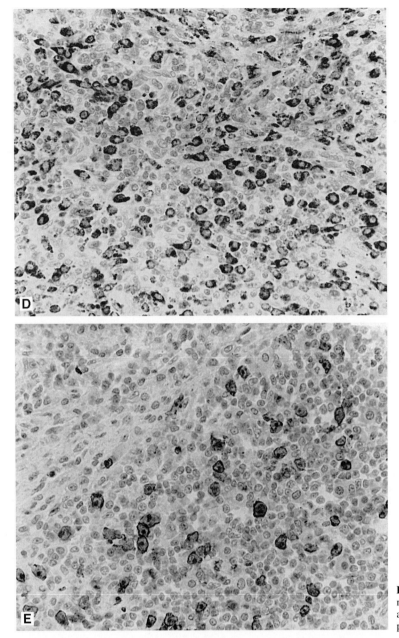

Figure 4–33. *Continued D,* The histiocytes are CD68+ (immunoperoxidase technique on paraffin sections). *E,* The large atypical cells are CD30+ (immunoperoxidase technique on paraffin sections).

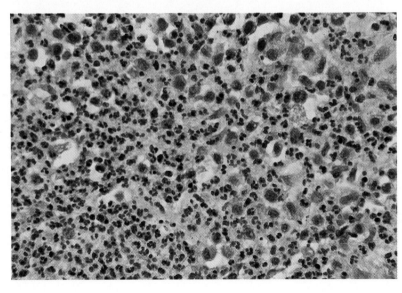

Figure 4–34. CD30+ T-cell lymphoma, neutrophil-rich. The lymphoma consists of relatively small numbers of atypical lymphoid cells that were CD30+ in a background of numerous neutrophils. The neoplastic cells in this case are relatively small, suggesting a relationship to the small cell variant of ALCL (H&E stain).

References

Agnarsson B, Kadin M: Ki-1 positive large cell lymphoma: a morphologic and immunologic study of 19 cases. Am J Surg Pathol 12:264–274, 1988.

Chott A, Kaserer K, Augustin I, *et al*: Ki-1 positive large cell lymphoma. A clinicopathologic study of 41 cases. Am J Surg Pathol 14:439–448, 1990.

Elmberger PG, Lozano MD, Weisenburger DD, *et al*: Transcripts of the npm-alk fusion product gene in anaplastic large cell lymphoma, Hodgkin's disease and reactive lymphoid lesions. Blood 86:3517–3521, 1995.

Ferreiro JA: Ber-H2 expression in testicular germ cell tumors. Hum Pathol 25:522–524, 1994.

Fraga M, Brousset P, Schlaifer D, *et al*: Bone marrow involvement in anaplastic large cell lymphoma. Immunohistochemical detection of minimal disease and its prognostic significance. Am J Clin Pathol 103:82–89, 1995.

Gustmann C, Altmannsberger M, Osborn M, *et al*: Cytokeratin expression and vimentin content in large cell anaplastic lymphomas and other non-Hodgkin's lymphomas. Am J Pathol 138:1413–1422, 1991.

Herbst H, Tippelmann G, Anagnostopoulos I, *et al*: Immunoglobulin and T cell receptor gene rearrangements in Hodgkin's disease and Ki-1-positive anaplastic large cell lymphoma: dissociation between phenotype and genotype. Leuk Res 13:103–116, 1989.

Kadin ME: Ki-1-positive anaplastic large-cell lymphoma: a distinct clinicopathologic entity. Ann Oncol 5(Suppl.1):S25–S30, 1994.

Kadin ME: Ki-1/CD30+ (anaplastic) large-cell lymphoma: maturation of a clinicopathologic entity with prospects of effective therapy (Editorial.) J Clin Oncol 12:884–887, 1994.

Kinney M, Collins R, Greer J, *et al*: A small-cell-predominant variant of primary Ki-1 (CD30)+ T-cell lymphoma. Am J Surg Pathol 17:859–868, 1993.

Lopategui JR, Sun LH, Chan JK, *et al*: Low frequency association of the t(2;5)(p23;q35) chromosomal translocation with CD30+ lymphomas from American and Asian patients. A reverse transcriptase-polymerase chain reaction study. Am J Pathol 146:323–328, 1995.

Mann KP, Hall B, Kamino H, *et al*: Neutrophil-rich, Ki-1-positive anaplastic large-cell malignant lymphoma. Am J Surg Pathol 19:407–416, 1995.

Mason D, Bastard C, Rimokh R, *et al*: CD30-positive large cell lymphomas ("Ki-1 lymphoma") are associated with a chromosomal translocation involving 5q35. Br J Haematol 74:161–168, 1990.

Pileri S, Falini B, Delsol G, *et al*: Lymphohistiocytic T-cell lymphoma (anaplastic large cell lymphoma CD30+/Ki1+) with a high content of reactive histiocytes. Histopathology 16:383–391, 1990.

Piris M, Brown D, Gatter K, Mason D: CD30 Expression in non-Hodgkin's lymphoma. Histopathology 17:211–218, 1990.

Schwarting R, Gerdes J, Dürkop H, *et al*: BER-H2: a new anti-Ki-1 (CD30) monoclonal antibody directed at a formol-resistant epitope. Blood 74:1678–1689, 1989.

Segal GH, Kjeldsberg CR, Smith GP, Perkins SL: CD30 antigen expression in florid immunoblastic proliferations. A clinicopathologic study of 14 cases. Am J Clin Pathol 102:292–298, 1994.

Stein H, Mason D, Gerdes J, *et al*: The expression of the Hodgkin's disease associated antigen Ki-1 in reactive and neoplastic lymphoid tissue: evidence that Reed-Sternberg cells and histiocytic malignancies are derived from activated lymphoid cells. Blood 66:848–858, 1985.

Waggott W, Lo YM, Bastard C, *et al*: Detection of NPM-ALK DNA rearrangement in CD30 positive anaplastic large cell lymphoma. Br J Haematol 89:905–907, 1995.

CHAPTER 5

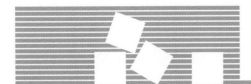

Hodgkin's Disease

Lymphocyte Predominance Hodgkin's Disease (LPHD)

The classification of Hodgkin's disease (HD) in the R.E.A.L. Classification is similar to that in the Rye Classification, with several modifications. Lymphocyte predominance HD is considered an entity distinct from the other types of HD—nodular sclerosis, mixed cellularity, and lymphocyte depletion. The latter have been grouped together under the heading of classic HD. In addition, two provisional entities have been proposed: lymphocyte-rich classic HD and anaplastic large cell lymphoma, Hodgkin's-like or Hodgkin's-related (Table 5–1).

Synonyms: Lukes and Butler: lymphocytic and/or histiocytic, nodular; lymphocytic and/or histiocytic, diffuse (some cases); Lennert and Mohri: paragranuloma, nodular or diffuse.

Clinical Features

Lymphocyte predominance Hodgkin's disease (LPHD) constitutes 6% of cases of HD. Unlike the bimodal age distribution of other types of HD, LPHD has a single peak in the fourth decade. Men are affected more often than women. A few patients have a prior history of lymphadenopathy with progressive transformation of germinal centers. Patients with LPHD most often present with cervical or axillary lymphadenopathy that spares the mediastinum. Presentation with extranodal disease is rare; LPHD is usually localized at diagnosis, but may be disseminated. Survival time for localized cases is long, with or without treatment. Late relapses are reportedly more common than in other types of HD. A small proportion of cases (approximately 5%) may be associated with, or progress to, large B-cell lymphoma.

Table 5–1
CLASSIFICATION OF HODGKIN'S DISEASE

Lymphocyte predominance Hodgkin's disease (LPHD)
Classic Hodgkin's disease (HD)
    Nodular sclerosis Hodgkin's disease (NSHD)
    Mixed cellularity Hodgkin's disease (MCHD)
    Lymphocyte depletion Hodgkin's disease (LDHD)
    Lymphocyte-rich, classic Hodgkin's disease (provisional entity)
    Anaplastic large cell lymphoma, Hodgkin's-like (provisional entity)

Morphology

LPHD usually has a nodular growth pattern with or without diffuse areas; it is rarely, if ever, purely diffuse. The atypical cells—called L and H cells (lymphocytic and/or histiocytic) or "popcorn" cells—have vesicular, polylobated nuclei, small nucleoli, and scant to moderate amounts of pale cytoplasm. They may be very numerous, but diagnostic Reed-Sternberg cells (RSC) are rare or absent. The background cells are small lymphocytes, which often look normal, but may have slightly larger nuclei, occasional nucleoli, or slightly irregular or indented nuclei (Fig. 5–1). Typical cleaved cells (centrocytes) are not seen. Residual lymphoid follicles, which sometimes have progressively transformed germinal centers, may be present. Epithelioid histiocytes may be prominent, distributed throughout the node either diffusely or in clusters. Occasionally, small aggregates of epithelioid histiocytes encircle the nodules of LPHD. The admixture of granulocytes and plasma cells seen in other types of HD is inconspicuous or absent. Necrosis does not occur in this variant; fibrosis is minimal or absent.

Associated large B-cell lymphomas may be indistinguishable from de novo large cell lymphoma or may be composed

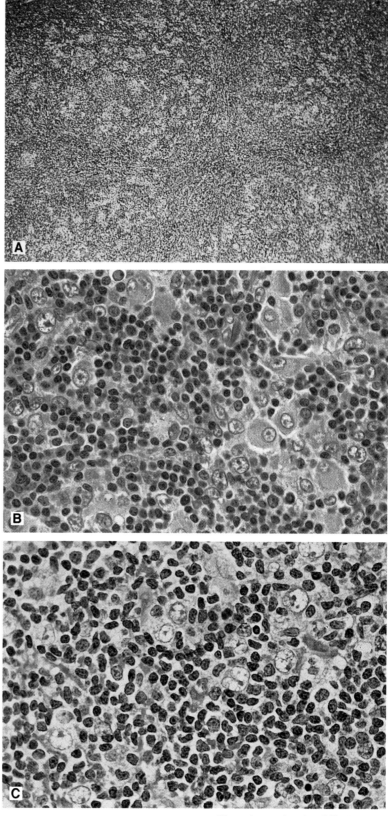

Figure 5–1. Nodular lymphocyte predominance Hodgkin's disease (LPHD). *A,* Four crowded, ill-defined, mottled pink and blue nodules obliterate the normal nodal architecture (H&E stain). *B,* Viewed at higher power, the nodules consist of a mixture of small lymphocytes and histiocytes (H&E stain). *C,* Some areas show L and H cells (popcorn cells), which have large, vesicular, round to lobated nuclei, small nucleoli, and scant cytoplasm (H&E stain).

Illustration continued on following page.

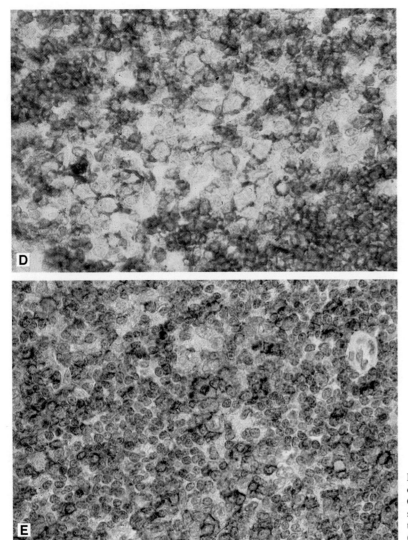

Figure 5–1. *Continued D,* The L and H cells as well as most of the surrounding small lymphocytes stain with an anti-CD20 antibody (immunoperoxidase technique on paraffin sections). *E,* Large numbers of lymphocytes, including those immediately around the L and H cells, are CD57+ (immunoperoxidase technique on paraffin sections).

of cells resembling L and H cells (Fig. 5–2). In almost all instances, the large cell lymphoma has a diffuse pattern, although we have reviewed an unusual case in which the large cell lymphoma maintained the nodular architecture of the underlying LPHD (Fig. 5–3).

Immunophenotype

The atypical cells are CD45+, CD20+, CDw75+, EMA+/−, CD30−/+, CD15−, J-chain+ (Fig. 5–1D). Although L and H cells are usually described as Ig−, monotypic Ig expression has been reported (virtually always κ) in some cases. The background population consists of B cells expressing polytypic Ig with an admixture of variable numbers of T cells. A relative increase in CD57+ T cells has been described; these cells may form a collarette around individual L and H cells (Fig. 5–1E). In other instances, L and H cells are surrounded by a collarette of CD57-negative T cells.

Genetic Features

Immunoglobulin (Ig) and T-cell receptor (TCR) genes have been reported as germline using Southern blot hybridization, but one study has found clonal Ig heavy chain gene rearrangements in 67% of cases using polymerase chain reaction (PCR). When isolated L and H cells were evaluated by PCR in one report, they were clonal B cells; in another, they were polyclonal B cells. Using in situ hybridization, monoclonal light chain mRNA has been described in the L and H cells. L and H cells are almost always EBV-negative. These data suggest that L and H cells are derived from B lymphocytes. It is possible that they are clonal in some instances and polyclonal in others.

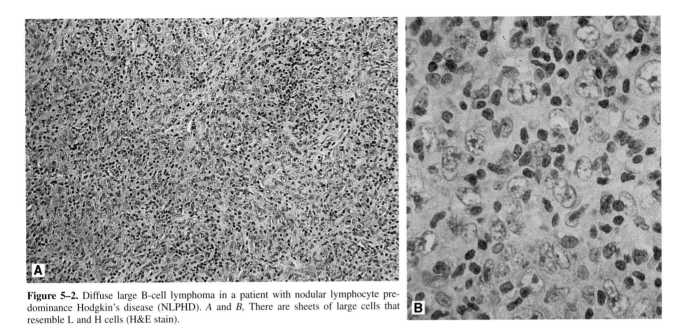

Figure 5–2. Diffuse large B-cell lymphoma in a patient with nodular lymphocyte predominance Hodgkin's disease (NLPHD). *A* and *B,* There are sheets of large cells that resemble L and H cells (H&E stain).

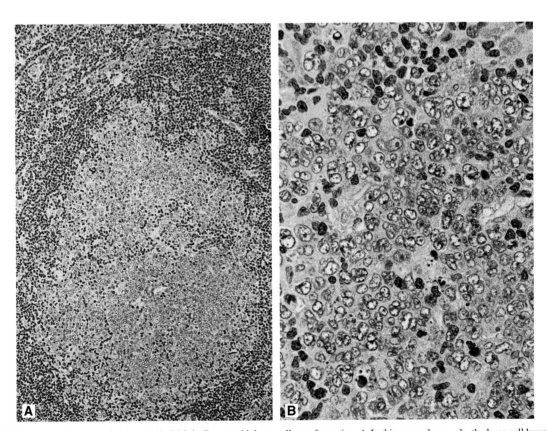

Figure 5–3. Nodular lymphocyte predominance Hodgkin's disease with large cell transformation. *A,* In this unusual example, the large cell lymphoma maintains a nodular pattern (Giemsa stain). *B,* High power view shows large lymphoid cells with vesicular, round, or lobated nuclei (Giemsa stain).

Postulated Normal Counterpart

Undefined peripheral B cell, possibly an altered centro-blast.

Differential Diagnosis (See also Table 5–2)

1. Reactive hyperplasia: The appearance of the nodules in nodular LPHD may be similar to that of progressively transformed germinal centers (PTGC). In general, the nodal architecture is effaced in LPHD and the nodules contain L and H cells. In reactive hyperplasia with PTGCs, the nodal architecture is intact and PTGCs are usually scattered among typical-appearing reactive follicles. Residual follicle center cells are often identifiable in PTGC.

2. Small lymphocytic lymphoma/chronic lymphocytic leukemia (CLL): CLL with or without pseudofollicles may be included in the differential diagnosis of LPHD that is predominantly nodular or diffuse respectively. CLL lacks L and H cells, contains prolymphocytes and paraimmunoblasts, and is composed of CD5+ B cells expressing monotypic Ig. Histiocytes are not a prominent feature.

3. Follicle center lymphoma, follicular (FCL): The follicles of FCL are usually more discrete than the nodules of nodular LPHD and contain centrocytes (small cleaved cells) and centroblasts (large noncleaved cells) rather than small lymphoid cells and L and H cells. Neoplastic cells express monotypic Ig.

4. T-cell-rich large B-cell lymphoma (TCR-BCL): TCR-BCL is part of the differential diagnosis of LPHD with prominent diffuse areas (and also of mixed cellularity and lymphocyte-rich classic HD). TCR-BCL is usually described as a diffuse large B-cell lymphoma with numerous admixed small lymphocytes of T-lineage. Epithelioid histiocytes may be prominent (and for this reason, similar cases have been called histiocyte-rich B-cell lymphoma). Granulocytes and plasma cells may be present but are usually sparse. The large cells may have the appearance of mononuclear Reed-Sternberg variants of the classic type, although diagnostic Reed-Sternberg cells occur infrequently. Lacunar cells are infrequent or absent, whereas L and H cells usually are not prominent. The large cells are CD45+, CD20+, EMA+/−, CD15−, CD30−/+. CD57+ cells are infrequent, and they do not form collarettes around the neoplastic cells.

Monotypic immunoglobulin expression by the large cells of TCR-BCL is sometimes demonstrated, although this may be technically difficult on paraffin sections. Identification of the few neoplastic cells on frozen sections may make interpretation problematic.

Patients with TCR-BCL, in contrast to those with HD, tend to present with advanced stage disease that fre-

---

Table 5–2
LYMPHOCYTE PREDOMINANCE HODGKIN'S DISEASE: DIFFERENTIAL DIAGNOSIS

	NLPHD	DLPHD*	B-CLL	FCL	TCR-BCL	Classic HD
Pattern	Nodular +/− diffuse areas	Diffuse	Diffuse +/− pseudofollicles	Nodular +/− diffuse	Diffuse	Diffuse or nodular
Large cells	L&H cells: CD20+, CD45+, CD15−, CD30−/+, EMA+/−, Ig− or polytypic, (rarely, monotypic)	As for NLPHD	Paraimmunoblasts, prolymphocytes: CD20+, CD45+, CD15−, CD30−, monotypic Ig+	Centroblasts (large noncleaved cells): CD20+, CD45+, CD15−, CD30−, monotypic Ig+	Centroblasts & immunoblasts; few L&H cells: CD20+, CD45+, EMA+/−; monotypic Ig+/−	Diagnostic RSCs, mononuclear variants: CD15+, CD30+, CD20−/+, CD45−, EMA−, Ig−
Small cells	Small lymphocytes: polytypic B cells & variable number of T cells	Polytypic B cells & many T cells	Small lymphocytes: monotypic B cells	Small cleaved cells: monotypic B cells	Small lympho-cytes: T cells	Small lymphocytes: T cells
CD57+ cells	Many; may form collarette around L&H cells	Fewer than in NLPHD	Fewer than in NLPHD; No collarette	No collarette	Fewer than in NLPHD; no collarette	Fewer than in NLPHD; no collarette
Histiocytes	Usually prominent	Usually prominent	Uncommon	Uncommon	May be prominent	Often prominent
Stage at presentation	Usually localized	Usually localized	Usually disseminated	Often disseminated, sometimes localized	Usually disseminated	Majority localized
Fibrosis	Occasional	Occasional	Rare	Common	Occasional	Common
Necrosis	Rare	Rare	Rare	Unusual	Occasional	Common

NLPHD, nodular lymphocyte predominance Hodgkin's disease; DLPHD, diffuse LPHD; B-CLL, B-cell chronic lymphocytic leukemia; FCL, follicle center lymphoma; TCR-BCL: T-cell-rich large B-cell lymphoma; RSC, Reed-Sternberg cell.
*The existence of a completely diffuse form of LPHD has been questioned.

quently involves the bone marrow and spleen. TCR-BCL may also involve sites virtually never affected by HD, such as mesenteric lymph nodes and CNS.

In cases in which the morphologic features are equivocal or the clinical features are unusual for HD, immunophenotyping is recommended to investigate the possibility of TCR-BCL since affected patients may not respond well to treatment regimens directed against HD.

5. Other forms of HD (classic HD): LPHD with fibrosis may resemble nodular sclerosis Hodgkin's disease (NSHD). NSHD lacks L and H cells and contains lacunar cells and diagnostic Reed-Sternberg cells with the immunophenotype of RSCs in classic (non-LP) HD (CD15+, CD30+, CD45−, B- and T-cell associated antigen−). Some forms of HD have RSCs with the morphology and immunophenotype of classic HD in a background composed predominantly of lymphocytes. These cases fit best in the provisional category of lymphocyte-rich classic HD. In the differential diagnosis with other types of HD, immunophenotyping is crucial; expression of CD15 and CD30 strongly favors classic HD.

References

Burns B, Colby T, Dorfman R: Differential diagnostic features of nodular L&H Hodgkin's disease, including progressive transformation of germinal centers. Am J Surg Pathol 8:253–261, 1984.

Delabie J, Tierens A, Wu G, et al: Lymphocyte predominance Hodgkin's disease: lineage and clonality determination using a single-cell assay. Blood 84:3291–3298, 1994.

Hansmann M, Stein H, Fellbaum C, et al: Nodular paragranuloma can transform into high-grade malignant lymphoma of B type. Hum Pathol 20:1169–1175, 1989.

Kuppers R, Rajewsky K, Zhao M, et al: Hodgkin disease: Hodgkin and Reed-Sternberg cells picked from histological sections show clonal immunoglobulin gene rearrangements and appear to be derived from B cells at various stages of development. Proc Natl Acad Sciences USA 91:10962–10966, 1994.

Lukes R, Butler J, Hicks E: Natural history of Hodgkin's disease as related to its pathological picture. Cancer 19:317–344, 1966.

McBride JA, Rodriguez J, Luthra R, et al: T-cell-rich B large-cell lymphoma simulating lymphocyte-rich Hodgkin's disease. Am J Surg Pathol 20(2):193–201, 1996.

Medeiros LJ, Greiner TC: Hodgkin's disease. Cancer 75(Suppl 1):357–369, 1995.

Pinkus G, Said J: Hodgkin's disease, lymphocyte predominance type, nodular—further evidence for a B cell derivation: L&H variants of Reed-Sternberg cells express L26, a pan B cell marker. Am J Pathol 133:211–217, 1988.

Regula D, Hoppe R, Weiss L: Nodular and diffuse types of lymphocyte predominance Hodgkin's disease. N Engl J Med 318:214–219, 1988.

Said J, Sassoon A, Shintaku I, et al: Absence of bcl-2 major breakpoint region and Jh gene rearrangement in lymphocyte predominance Hodgkin's disease: results of Southern blot analysis and polymerase chain reaction. Am J Pathol 138:261–264, 1991.

Schmid C, Sargent C, Isaacson P: L and H cells of nodular lymphocyte predominant Hodgkin's disease show immunoglobulin light-chain restriction. Am J Pathol 139:1281–1289, 1991.

Siebert JD, Steickey JH, Kurtin PJ, Banks PM: Extranodal lymphocyte predominance Hodgkin's disease. Clinical and pathological features. Am J Clin Pathol 103:485–491, 1995.

Stoler MH, Nichols GE, Symbula M, Weiss LM: Lymphocyte-predominance Hodgkin's disease. Evidence for a kappa light chain–restricted monotypic B-cell neoplasm. Am J Pathol 146:812–818, 1995.

Tamaru J, Hummel M, Zemlin M, et al: Hodgkin's disease with a B-cell phenotype often shows a VDJ rearrangement and somatic mutations in the VH genes. Blood 84:708–715, 1994.

Classic Hodgkin's Disease

NODULAR SCLEROSIS HODGKIN'S DISEASE (NSHD)

Clinical Features

Nodular sclerosis Hodgkin's disease (NSHD) is the most common type of HD (constituting approximately 58% of all cases). It occurs most often in adolescents and young adults, with an equal sex ratio. Patients commonly present with cervical or supraclavicular lymphadenopathy. The mediastinum is involved frequently, and most patients have stage I or II disease at presentation. The prognosis is good in most cases.

Morphology

NSHD is characterized by fibrous bands dividing the tumor into nodules. The cellular composition within the nodules varies, ranging from predominantly lymphocytes with only a few Reed-Sternberg cells (RSCs) to predominantly neoplastic cells with few reactive cells. The characteristic lacunar cell is a variant of the RSC, having a lobated nucleus, a nucleolus smaller than that of a typical RSC, and an abundant pale cytoplasm that retracts in formalin-fixed tissue (Figs. 5–4 and 5–5). A variable number of histiocytes, granulocytes, or plasma cells are seen. Areas with a diffuse pattern of growth and necrosis may appear. "Cellular phase" of NSHD refers to cases without fibrous bands, presumably representing early involvement of the affected tissue. "Syncytial variant" refers to cases in which neoplastic cells grow in cohesive sheets (Fig. 5–6).

The proportion of neoplastic cells varies greatly from case to case, and attempts have been made to grade NSHD to identify cases that would be expected to carry a better or worse prognosis. Cases without an excessive number of

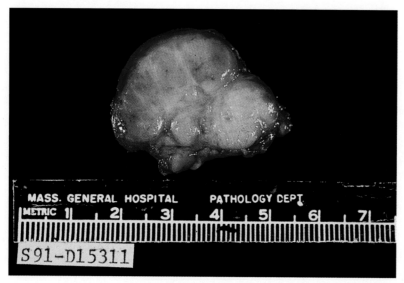

Figure 5–4. Nodular sclerosis Hodgkin's disease. On gross examination, white fibrous bands divide the lymph node into tan-yellow nodules.

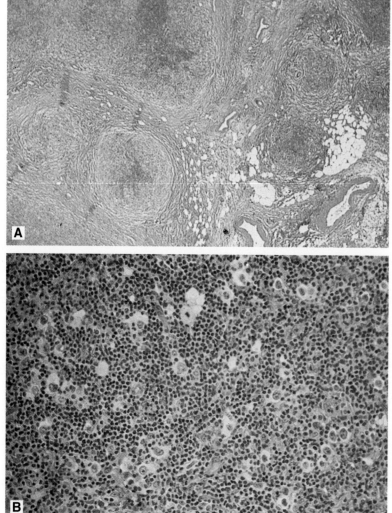

Figure 5–5. Nodular sclerosis Hodgkin's disease. *A,* On microscopic examination, broad, well-defined fibrous bands surround cellular nodules (H&E stain). *B,* Higher power examination shows scattered lacunar cells in a background of small lymphocytes (H&E stain).

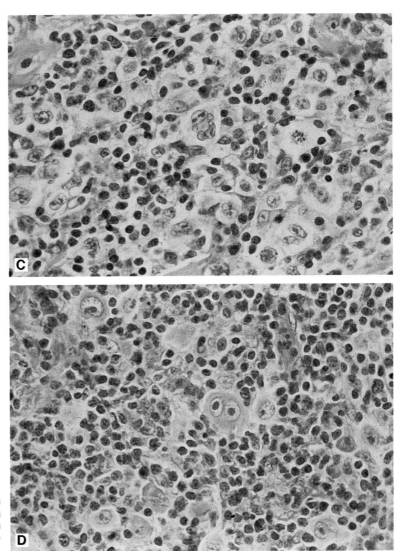

Figure 5–5. *C,* Lacunar cells have oval to lobated pale nuclei with small red nucleoli and abundant pale cytoplasm that retracts in formalin-fixed tissue (H&E stain). *D,* In addition to lacunar cells, occasional diagnostic Reed-Sternberg cells are visible *(center)* (H&E stain).

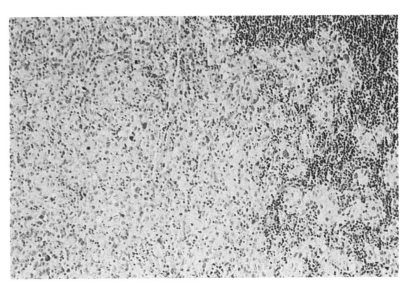

Figure 5–6. Nodular sclerosis Hodgkin's disease (NSHD), lymphocyte-depleted subtype. Sheets of Reed-Sternberg cells and variants are visible, consistent with NSHD, grade 2 (NS2, lymphocyte-depleted subtype) or syncytial variant (H&E stain).

tumor cells have been designated NS1; those with prominent areas of lymphocyte depletion have been called NS2 (*see* Fig. 5–6). When the outcomes of NS1 and NS2 patients have been compared, NS2 patients appeared to have a worse prognosis in older studies and in series in which they had been treated in a conservative manner. In more recent series, no difference has been apparent in the outcomes of NS1 and NS2 patients. This finding suggests that a difference does exist in the natural history of NS1 and NS2, but it can be eliminated with the use of optimal, or aggressive, therapy.

Immunophenotype

Tumor cells are CD15+/−, CD30+, CD45− (may be positive in frozen sections); B antigen −/+, T antigen−−/+, EMA−. CD30 is usually more weakly expressed than in ALCL. EBV latent membrane protein (LMP) is expressed by the tumor cells in fewer than half of cases.

Genetic Features

Immunoglobulin (Ig) and T-cell receptor (TCR) genes are usually germline, but rearrangements of Ig genes are reported in some cases using Southern blot hybridization, usually with faint bands. Using the polymerase chain reaction (PCR) to evaluate Ig heavy chain genes has shown that up to half of cases have clonal gene rearrangements. Among cases in which RSCs express B-lineage antigens, the majority show clonal Ig rearrangement. Single RSCs studied using PCR have shown Ig gene rearrangements in some cases but not in others. In one such study, reported by Hummel and co-workers, some cases contained individual RSCs with identical Ig gene rearrangements (monoclonal), but other cases contained different rearrangements (polyclonal) or a mixture of polyclonal and monoclonal RSCs. The results of this study suggest that in some cases, Reed-Sternberg cells are not derived from a single progenitor cell and may be clonally unrelated. This finding contrasts with our usual concept of a malignant tumor being derived from a single progenitor cell. These results, however, should be confirmed in larger studies from other institutions before firm conclusions are drawn. Tumor cells are EBV+ in about 40% of the cases.

Postulated Normal Counterpart

Unknown; ?activated lymphoid cell of a B-cell or T-cell subset not yet identified or a primitive lymphoid cell.

Differential Diagnosis

1. Anaplastic large cell lymphoma (ALCL), especially Hodgkin's-related ALCL: NSHD, particularly cases with a high proportion of neoplastic cells, as in the syncytial variant, may be difficult to distinguish from non-Hodgkin's lymphoma, especially ALCL (*see* Table 4–4).
2. Lymphocyte predominance Hodgkin's disease (LPHD): *see* preceding discussion.
3. Mixed cellularity Hodgkin's disease (MCHD) or lymphocyte depletion Hodgkin's disease (LDHD): MCHD and LDHD may have irregular fibrosis, but they do not have well-formed fibrous bands or prominent lacunar cells. In cases of the cellular phase of NSHD, fibrous bands are absent, but lymph nodes may have fibrous thickening of the capsule, perivascular fibrosis, and vague nodularity.

References

Ferry J, Linggood R, Convery K, *et al*: Hodgkin's disease, nodular sclerosis type: implications of histologic subclassification. Cancer 71:457–463, 1993.

Haybittle JL, Easterling MJ, Bennett MH, *et al*: Review of British National Lymphoma Investigation studies of Hodgkin's disease and development of prognostic index. Lancet 1:967–972, 1985.

Herbst H, Dallenbach F, Hummel M, *et al*: Epstein-Barr virus latent membrane protein expression in Hodgkin and Reed-Sternberg cells. Proc Natl Acad Sci USA 88:4766–4770, 1991.

Hess JL, Bodis S, Pinkus G, *et al*: Histopathologic grading of nodular sclerosis Hodgkin's disease. Lack of prognostic significance in 254 surgically staged patients. Cancer 74:708–714, 1994.

Hummel M, Ziemann K, Lammert H, *et al*: Hodgkin's disease with monoclonal and polyclonal populations of Reed-Sternberg cells. N Engl J Med 333:901–906, 1995.

Jacobson J, Wilkes B, Harris N: T cell receptor genes are polyclonally rearranged in Hodgkin's disease: implications for diagnosis. Mod Pathol 4:172–177, 1991.

Kamel OW, Chang PP, Hsu FJ, *et al*: Clonal VDJ recombination of the immunoglobulin heavy chain gene by PCR in classical Hodgkin's disease. Am J Clin Pathol 104:419–423, 1995.

Kuppers R, Rajewsky K, Zhao M, *et al*: Hodgkin disease: Hodgkin and Reed-Sternberg cells picked from histological sections show clonal immunoglobulin gene rearrangements and appear to be derived from B cells at various stages of development. Proc National Acad Sciences USA 91:10962–10966, 1994.

Lukes R, Butler J, Hicks E: Natural history of Hodgkin's disease as related to its pathological picture. Cancer 19:317–344, 1966.

MacLennan KA, Bennett MH, Tu A, *et al*: Relationship of histopathologic features to survival and relapse in nodular sclerosing Hodgkin's disease. Cancer 64:1686–1693, 1989.

Medeiros LJ, Greiner TC: Hodgkin's disease. Cancer 75(Suppl 1): 357–369, 1995.

Orazi J, Jiang B, Lee C-H, *et al*: Correlation between presence of clonal rearrangements of immunoglobulin heavy chain genes and B-cell antigen expression in Hodgkin's disease. Am J Clin Pathol 104:413–418, 1995.

Roth J, Daus H, Trumper L, *et al*: Detection of immunoglobulin heavy-chain gene rearrangement at the single-cell level in malignant lymphomas: no rearrangement is found in Hodgkin's and Reed-Sternberg cells. Int J Cancer 57:799–804, 1994.

Strickler J, Michie S, Warnke R, Dorfman R: The "syncytial variant" of nodular sclerosing Hodgkin's disease. Am J Surg Pathol 10:470–477, 1986.

Tamaru J, Hummel M, Zemlin M, *et al*: Hodgkin's disease with a B-cell phenotype often shows a VDJ rearrangement and somatic mutations in the VH genes. Blood 84:708–715, 1994.

MIXED CELLULARITY HODGKIN'S DISEASE (MCHD)

Clinical Features

Patients are usually adults; among patients over 50, MCHD is the most common type of HD. The male:female ratio is approximately 2:1. The stage may be more advanced than in nodular sclerosis (NSHD) or lymphocyte predominance (LPHD) types. The course is moderately aggressive, but patients are often cured.

Morphology

The infiltrate is usually diffuse and lacks sclerotic bands, although irregular areas with fine interstitial fibrosis may be present. Reed-Sternberg cells are the classic type. Lacunar cells are not prominent. Tumor cells are scattered among a mixture of lymphocytes, histiocytes, eosinophils, neutrophils, and plasma cells (Fig. 5–7).

Immunophenotype

Tumor cells have the same immunophenotype as NSHD (see preceding discussion). Expression of Epstein-Barr virus latent membrane protein (EBV-LMP) occurs in cases with EBV genomic material (Fig. 5–7, C and D).

Genetic Features

Ig heavy and light chain genes and T-cell receptor (TCR) genes are usually germline, as for NSHD. Results of polymerase chain reaction (PCR) studies are similar to those described earlier for NSHD. Tumor cells are EBV+ in the majority of the cases (60% to 70%).

Attention has focused on a mutation near the 3' end of the gene for EBV-LMP that has been found in a small number of cases of HD. Although the cases of HD reported to have this mutation are few, a correlation with the mutation and certain clinical and pathologic features has been suggested. In one report of five patients with the deletion mutant, all were mixed cellularity type; all had numerous RSCs; three had bizarre, anaplastic RSCs; and three presented with advanced stage disease. Although follow-up was available for only three patients, they showed an apparent tendency for poor response to therapy. The explanation for these observations is not certain, but LMP is reported to have transforming capacity in vitro, and the deletion mutant may confer a longer half-life on LMP, possibly leading to a survival advantage for tumor cells with the mutation. Alternatively, the LMP-derived from the mutated gene may be less immunogenic, leading to less effective immune response of patients with EBV+ HD carrying this mutation.

Postulated Normal Counterpart

Unknown; ?activated lymphoid cell of a B-cell or T-cell subset not yet identified or a primitive lymphoid cell.

Differential Diagnosis

1. Nodular sclerosis Hodgkin's disease (NSHD): See preceding discussion.
2. Anaplastic large cell lymphoma (ALCL): See Table 4–4.
3. Lymphocyte predominance Hodgkin's disease (LPHD): The presence of granulocytes and plasma cells in the background infiltrate, necrosis, and RSCs and their variants having the classic morphology and immunophenotype favor a diagnosis of MCHD. See also Table 5–2.
4. T-cell-rich large B-cell lymphoma (TCR-BCL): Cells with the appearance of diagnostic Reed-Sternberg cells are absent or present in very small numbers. Large cells are typically CD45+, CD20+, Ig+/−, CD15−, in contrast to the CD15+/−, CD45−, CD20−, Ig− neoplastic cells in MCHD. See also Table 5–2.

References

Brousset P, Chittal S, Schlaifer D, et al: Detection of Epstein-Barr virus messenger RNA in Reed-Sternberg cells of Hodgkin's disease by in situ hybridization with biotinylated probes on specially processed modified acetone methyl benzoate xylene (ModAMeX) sections. Blood 77:1781–1786, 1991.
Herbst H, Dallenbach F, Hummel M, et al: Epstein-Barr virus latent membrane protein expression in Hodgkin and Reed-Sternberg cells. Proc Natl Acad Sci USA 88:4766–4770, 1991.
Knecht H, Bachmann E, Brousset P, et al: Deletions within the LMP1 oncogene of Epstein-Barr virus are clustered in Hodgkin's disease and identical to those observed in nasopharyngeal carcinoma. Blood 82:2937–2942, 1993.
Lukes R, Butler J, Hicks E: Natural history of Hodgkin's disease as related to its pathological picture. Cancer 19:317–344, 1966.
Medeiros LJ, Greiner TC: Hodgkin's disease. Cancer 75(Suppl 1):357–369, 1995.
Weiss L, Chen Y, Liu X, Shibata D: Epstein-Barr virus and Hodgkin's disease: a correlative in situ hybridization and polymerase chain reaction study. Am J Pathol 139:1259–1265, 1991.

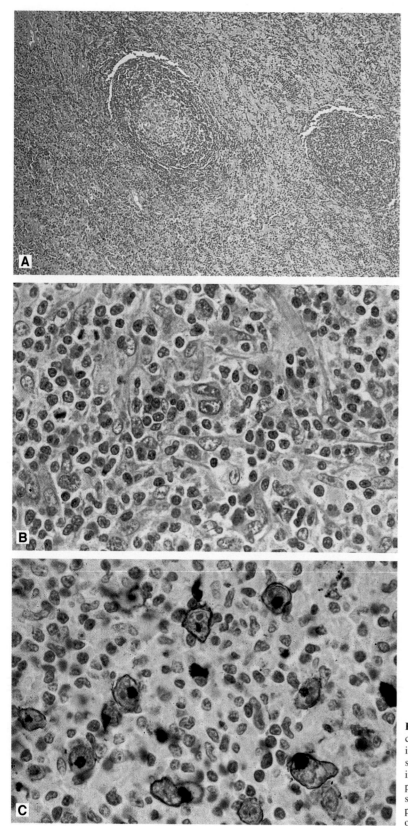

Figure 5–7. Hodgkin's disease, mixed cellularity. *A,* This case shows a few residual reactive lymphoid follicles and an interfollicular infiltrate with a mottled appearance (H&E stain). *B,* Occasional diagnostic Reed-Sternberg cells are set in a background of lymphocytes, histiocytes, and eosinophils (H&E stain). *C,* Reed-Sternberg cells and variants show the classic pattern of reactivity for CD15: intense plasma membrane and Golgi region staining (immunoperoxidase technique on paraffin sections).

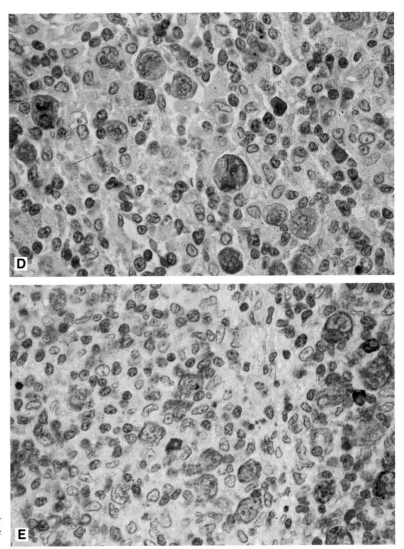

Figure 5–7. *D* and *E* show diffuse cytoplasmic staining for CD30 *(D)* and EBV-LMP *(E)* (immunoperoxidase technique on paraffin sections).

LYMPHOCYTE DEPLETION HODGKIN'S DISEASE (LDHD)

Clinical Features

This is the least common variant of HD (approximately 4%) and occurs most frequently in older people, in HIV+ individuals, and in people of nonindustrialized countries. The number of male patients slightly exceeds that of female patients. Patients with LDHD arising de novo tend to present with abdominal lymphadenopathy and involvement of the spleen, liver, and bone marrow, without peripheral lymphadenopathy. The stage is usually advanced at diagnosis; however, response to treatment is similar to that of other subtypes. Relapsed HD of the nodular sclerosis or mixed cellularity types occasionally has the appearance of LDHD.

Morphology

LDHD has a diffuse pattern, often with extensive fibrosis and necrosis. Reed-Sternberg cells (RSCs) are numerous; their morphology may be typical, or they may have a bizarre "sarcomatous" appearance. Reactive cells are relatively scarce. Two patterns occur: (1) diffuse fibrosis, in which neoplastic cells are scattered in loose connective tissue (Fig. 5–8), and (2) a reticular variant (Hodgkin's sarcoma), in which neoplastic cells appear in confluent sheets (Fig. 5–9). The borderline between the reticular variant and anaplastic large cell lymphoma (ALCL) is not sharp and may be a matter of definition. Further studies are required to resolve this issue.

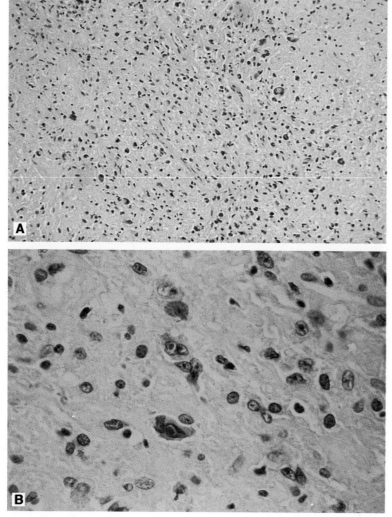

Figure 5–8. Hodgkin's disease, lymphocyte depleted, diffuse fibrosis subtype. *A,* The neoplasm is hypocellular, having large atypical cells in a background of disorganized collagen (H&E stain). *B,* On higher power examination, occasional diagnostic Reed-Sternberg cells are visible (H&E stain).

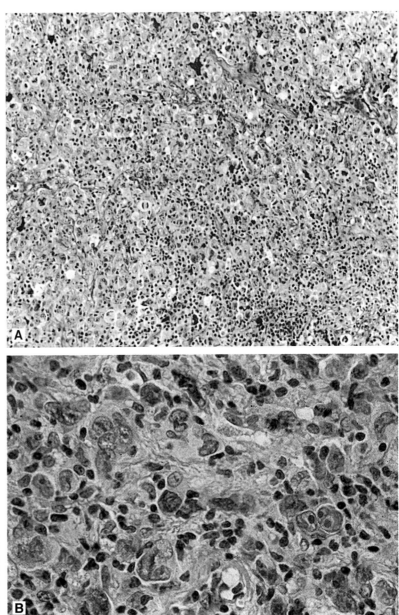

Figure 5–9. Hodgkin's disease (HD), lymphocyte depleted, reticular subtype, involving para-aortic lymph nodes of a 60-year-old man. *A,* Low power examination shows sheets of large neoplastic cells and scattered small lymphocytes (H&E stain). *B,* High power view shows a predominance of Reed-Sternberg cells and variants. Immunohistochemical studies supported the diagnosis of HD (H&E stain).

Immunophenotype

Tumor cells are CD15+/−, CD30+, CD45−, B- and T-cell-associated antigens−, EMA−. Since the differential diagnosis often includes non-Hodgkin's lymphoma, the absence of T- and B-cell markers is usually required for diagnosis.

Genetic Features

Ig heavy and light chain genes and T-cell receptor (TCR) genes are germline. (If rearrangements are found, the tumor is usually classified as a B-cell or T-cell lymphoma.)

Postulated Normal Counterpart

Unknown; ?activated lymphoid cell of a B-cell or T-cell subset not yet identified or a primitive lymphoid cell.

Differential Diagnosis

1. Non-Hodgkin's lymphoma: Diffuse large cell lymphoma is often in the differential diagnosis of LDHD. Features that favor a diagnosis of LDHD include neoplastic cells with the appearance of Reed-Sternberg cells, CD15 expression, absence of B-cell or T-cell antigen expression, and absence of clonal Ig or TCR genes. For the dif-

ferential diagnosis with anaplastic large cell lymphoma (ALCL), *see* Table 4–4.

2. Nodular sclerosis Hodgkin's disease (NSHD): Well-formed fibrous bands and neoplastic cells with the morphology of lacunar cells favor NSHD.

References

Kant J, Hubbard S, Longo D, *et al*: The pathologic and clinical heterogeneity of lymphocyte-depleted Hodgkin's disease. J Clin Oncol 4:284–294, 1986.

Lukes R, Butler J, Hicks E: Natural history of Hodgkin's disease as related to its pathological picture. Cancer 19:317–344, 1966.

Medeiros LJ, Greiner TC: Hodgkin's disease. Cancer 75(Suppl 1): 357–369, 1995.

Pelstring R, Zellmer R, Sulak L, *et al*: Hodgkin's disease in association with human immunodeficiency virus infection. Cancer 67:1865–1873, 1991.

Stein H, Herbst H, Anagnostopoulos I, *et al*: The nature of Hodgkin and Reed-Sternberg cells, their association with EBV, and their relationship to anaplastic large-cell lymphoma. Ann Oncol 2 (Suppl 2):33–38, 1991.

PROVISIONAL CATEGORY: LYMPHOCYTE-RICH CLASSIC HODGKIN'S DISEASE

Synonyms: Lukes and Butler: subset of diffuse lymphocyte predominance; Lennert and Mohri: lymphocyte predominant, mixed cellularity.

Morphology

The designation applies to cases of Hodgkin's disease (HD) in which the morphology and immunophenotype of the neoplastic cells is that of HD of the usual type, rather than L and H cells, with a background of small lymphocytes and only a few admixed eosinophils or plasma cells. RSCs are not abundant. The pattern is diffuse. Cases in this category overlap with diffuse lymphocyte predominance, the cellular phase of nodular sclerosis, and mixed cellularity. The clinical features, immunophenotype, and genetic features are similar to those of nodular sclerosis and mixed cellularity HD (Fig. 5–10).

References

Lennert K, Mohri N: Histologische Klassifizierung und Vorkommen des M. Hodgkin. Internist 15:57–65, 1974.

Lukes R, Butler J, Hicks E: Natural history of Hodgkin's disease as related to its pathological picture. Cancer 19:317–344, 1966.

PROVISIONAL CATEGORY: ANAPLASTIC LARGE CELL LYMPHOMA, HODGKIN'S-LIKE (HODGKIN'S-RELATED)

Clinical Features

Patients are usually young adults with lymph node involvement and, often, a large mediastinal mass. Wide-spread (stage III and IV) disease is less common than in cases of classic anaplastic large cell lymphoma (ALCL). Patients may do poorly with therapy for HD, but may have a good response to aggressive chemotherapeutic regimens used for high grade non-Hodgkin's lymphomas. Further study is needed to clarify the relationship of this entity to both HD and classic ALCL.

Morphology

This tumor has features intermediate between HD and ALCL. As in classic ALCL, there is cohesive growth of large, bizarre neoplastic cells, although intrasinusoidal spread may be less striking. Architectural features resemble Hodgkin's disease, nodular sclerosis type (NSHD), including capsular thickening, nodular growth of tumor cells, and sclerotic bands. Admixed reactive cells (histiocytes, lymphocytes, plasma cells, and granulocytes) are often present, but in contrast to most cases of HD, compose a minority of the cellular population (Fig. 5–11). Some cases classified as NSHD (syncytial, lymphocyte-depleted, or NS2 type) or LDHD (reticular type) may represent cases of ALCL, Hodgkin's-like (Fig. 5–12).

Immunophenotype

The immunophenotype is heterogeneous. It is often identical to classic ALCL, but in some cases, it may be intermediate between HD and classic ALCL. In a minority of cases, neoplastic cells express B-cell-associated antigens. Tumors are usually EBV-negative.

Genetic Features

These are not known.

Postulated Normal Counterpart

Not known (as for ALCL or NSHD).

Differential Diagnosis

This is as for HD and classic ALCL (*see* preceding discussion).

References

Pileri S, Bocchia M, Baroni C, *et al*: Anaplastic large cell lymphoma (CD30+/Ki-1+): results of a prospective clinicopathologic study of 69 cases. Br J Haematol 86:513–523, 1994.

Rosso R, Paulli M, Magrini U, *et al*: Anaplastic large cell lymphoma, CD30/Ki-1 positive, expressing the CD15/Leu-M1 antigen. Immunohistochemical and morphological relationships to Hodgkin's disease. Virchow's Arch [A] 416:229–235, 1990.

Stein H, Herbst H, Anagnostopoulos I, *et al*: The nature of Hodgkin and Reed-Sternberg cells, their association with EBV, and their relationship to anaplastic large-cell lymphoma. Ann Oncol 2 (Suppl 2):33–38, 1991.

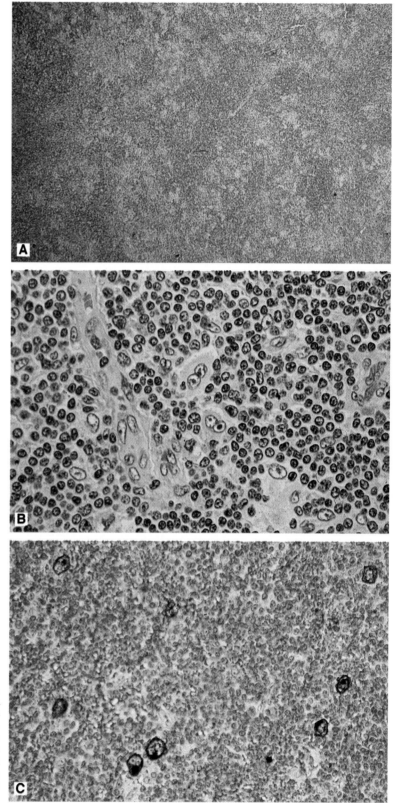

Figure 5–10. Lymphocyte-rich classic Hodgkin's disease. *A,* Low power examination shows nodal effacement by a mottled infiltrate of lymphocytes and histiocytes in a diffuse pattern (Giemsa stain). *B,* The large cells have round, vesicular nuclei and prominent nucleoli, resembling classic Reed-Sternberg cells and variants rather than L and H cells. The background infiltrate is composed of small lymphocytes and a few histiocytes, but no granulocytes (Giemsa stain). *C,* The large cells are CD15+, like classic Reed-Sternberg cells (immunoperoxidase technique on paraffin sections).

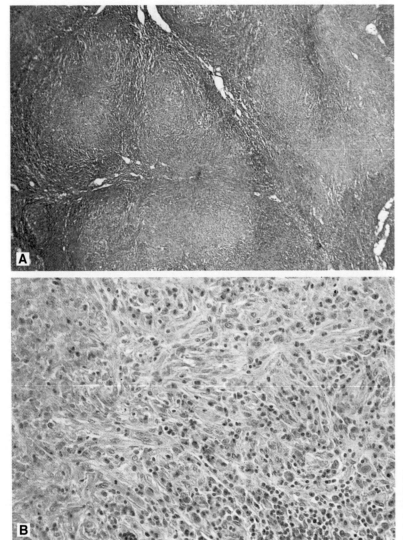

Figure 5–11. Anaplastic large cell lymphoma, Hodgkin's-like. In some areas, the appearance is reminiscent of Hodgkin's disease, with a nodular pattern at low power examination *(A)*, and a mixed inflammatory cell infiltrate with scattered neoplastic cells at high power *(B)* (H&E stain).

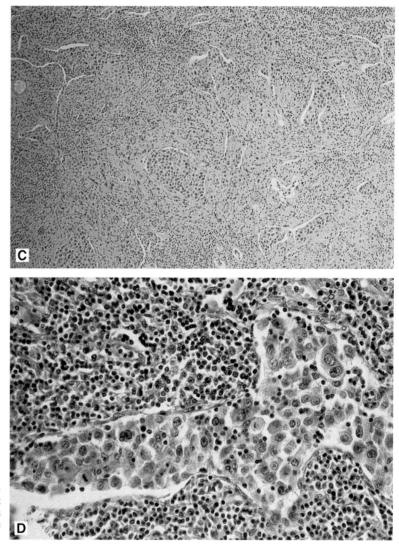

Figure 5–11. *C,* In other areas of the same specimen, vascular spaces are invaded extensively (H&E stain). *D,* At higher power examination, neoplastic cells within a sinus are large and have abundant cytoplasm and a cohesive growth pattern (H&E stain).

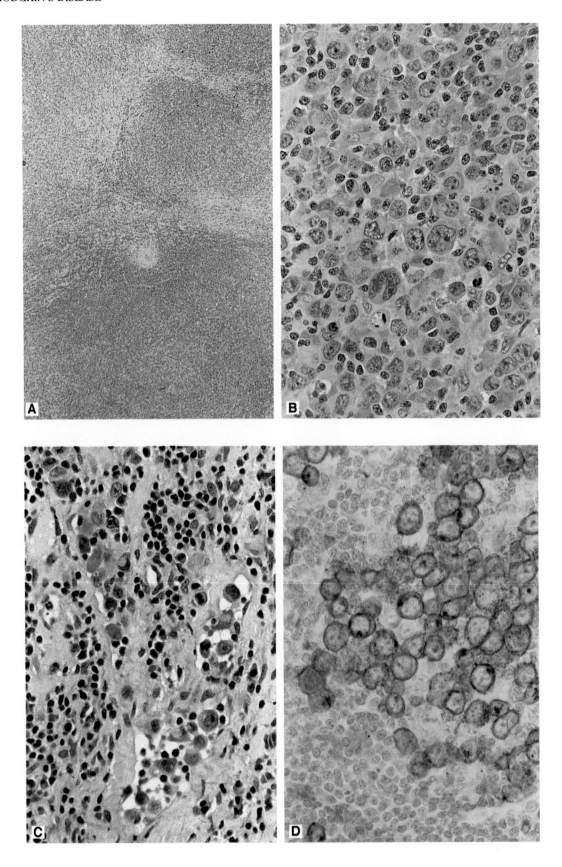

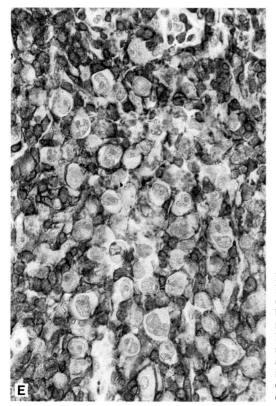

Figure 5–12. Malignant lymphoma, consistent with anaplastic large cell lymphoma, Hodgkin's-like. The histologic features border on nodular sclerosis Hodgkin's disease (NSHD), syncytial variant. Immunophenotyping studies do not distinguish definitively between Hodgkin's disease and non-Hodgkin's lymphoma. *A,* Large, well-defined tumor nodules replace the lymph node (H&E stain). *B,* Higher power examination shows sheets of large bizarre cells, some of which have an appearance like Reed-Sternberg cells (H&E stain). *C,* This specimen shows sinus invasion by tumor cells (H&E stain). *D,* Tumor cells are strongly CD30+, as shown here. A few were also CD15+ and EMA+ (immunoperoxidase technique on paraffin sections). *E,* With antibodies to CD45RO, there is a suggestion of staining of large cells, although this is difficult to evaluate because of the large numbers of admixed small T cells (immunoperoxidase technique on paraffin sections).

Staging of Hodgkin's Disease

Hodgkin's disease (HD) is staged according to the Ann Arbor system (Table 5–3). Staging of HD requires a bone marrow biopsy and, in some cases, a staging laparotomy, including splenectomy, abdominal lymph node sampling, and liver biopsy.

1. Lymph nodes: Criteria for determining involvement of lymph nodes by HD are the same as those for a primary diagnosis—diagnostic Reed-Sternberg cells (RSCs) and variants must be found in the appropriate background.
2. Spleen: A diagnosis of splenic involvement by HD is made employing the same criteria as those applied to lymph nodes. Splenic involvement has the appearance of one or more pale yellow nodules that may be tiny, resembling normal white pulp, or quite large (Figs. 5–13 and 5–14).

Table 5–3
HODGKIN'S DISEASE: STAGING

Stage		Definition
I		Single lymph node or group of nodes involved
II		Two or more lymph node groups on same side of diaphragm involved
	II$_S$	One or more subdiaphragmatic lymph node groups and spleen involved
III		Lymph node involvement on both sides of diaphragm
	III$_S$	Lymph nodes above diaphragm and spleen involved with or without subdiaphragmatic lymph node involvement
IV		Any of the above, plus extranodal disease (such as bone marrow, bone, liver, lung). Direct extension into extranodal tissue from involved lymph nodes is not included as stage IV
I$_E$, II$_E$, III$_E$		Stage I, II, or III disease with direct extension into extranodal tissue

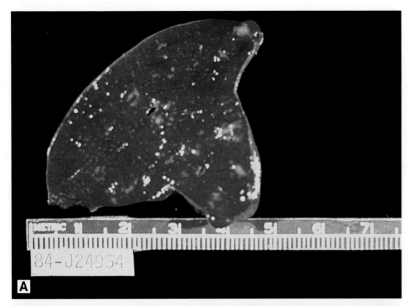

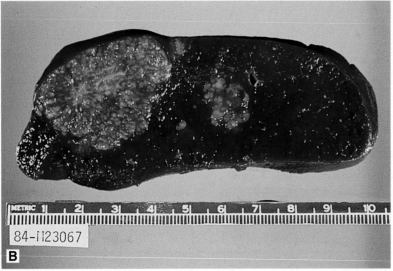

Figure 5–13. Hodgkin's disease, splenic involvement. *A,* In this case, splenic involvement is subtle on gross examination. Several tan-yellow nodules, only slightly larger than the normal white pulp, proved to be Hodgkin's disease on microscopic examination. *B,* In a specimen from another case, one large and several smaller foci of Hodgkin's disease occur in the spleen.

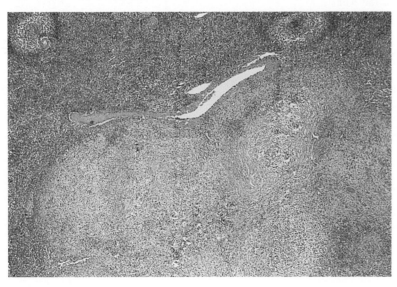

Figure 5–14. Spleen with Hodgkin's disease (HD). A large, irregular multinodular focus with fibrosis and a mixed inflammatory cell infiltrate proved to be HD. Two foci of white pulp *(top)* are much smaller than the nodule with HD (H&E stain).

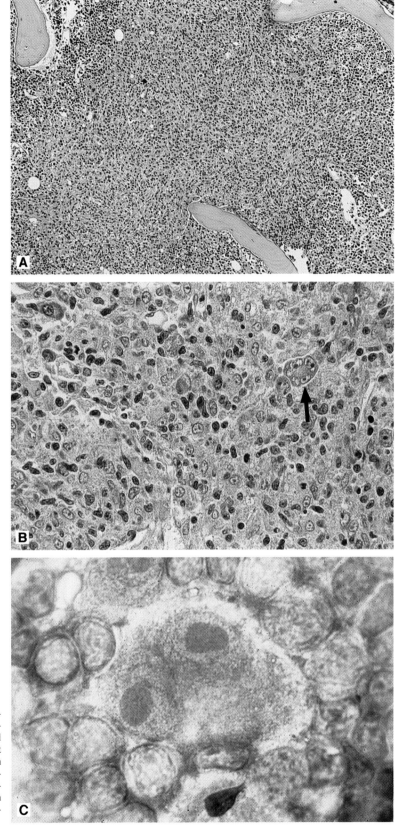

Figure 5–15. Hodgkin's disease, bone marrow involvement. *A,* On low power examination, a polymorphous infiltrate has filled much of the marrow space. A few residual hematopoietic precursors and hematopoietic cells appear at the periphery (H&E stain). *B,* Higher power examination shows lymphocytes, histiocytes, plasma cells, and occasional atypical cells, including one multinucleated Reed-Sternberg cell *(arrow)* (Giemsa stain). *C,* Touch preparation of a bone marrow biopsy shows a binucleated Reed-Sternberg cell (Wright-Giemsa stain).

3. Bone marrow: Because a bone marrow biopsy yields only a small amount of tissue for microscopic examination, it is permissible to make a diagnosis of marrow involvement by HD in a patient with a previously established diagnosis of HD if the marrow shows RSC variants in the appropriate background, even if no diagnostic RSCs are identified. Marrow involvement in HD is usually recognizable on low power examination as a zone with a mixed infiltrate of lymphocytes, plasma cells, histiocytes, or eosinophils, with variable numbers of large atypical cells. The abnormal area often appears fibrotic. If initial sections of the biopsy sample show only a mixed inflammatory infiltrate with or without fibrosis, additional levels should be examined to search for neoplastic cells (Fig. 5–15).

Areas involved by HD are difficult to aspirate, and RSCs are only rarely identified on aspirate smear specimens. Occasionally, examination of touch preparations of the core biopsy specimen reveals RSCs (Fig. 5–15C).

A primary diagnosis of HD is rarely made on the basis of the bone marrow biopsy alone; in this situation, RSCs (not just mononuclear variants) must be identified to establish a diagnosis. Subclassification of HD based on the appearance in the bone marrow is not recommended.

4. Liver: Because liver biopsy specimens are usually small, the same criteria used for the bone marrow are used to determine hepatic involvement by HD. In the absence of splenic involvement, the liver is involved only exceptionally by HD.

5. Miscellaneous: In any tissues sampled during the staging of HD, non-necrotizing (sarcoidal) granulomas may be encountered (*see* Fig. 2–22). In the absence of RSCs or variants, these findings are not indicative of involvement by HD; when compared with patients without granulomas, patients with granulomas have better relapse-free survival and overall survival rates.

Differential Diagnosis

1. Reactive lymphoid hyperplasia in the spleen: Finding a small number of immunoblasts, usually at the junction of the red and white pulp, is common in spleens removed at staging laparotomy in patients with HD. In infectious mononucleosis and other florid inflammatory conditions, however, immunoblasts may be abundant and some may resemble RSCs. Thus, as in other sites, a diagnosis of HD in the spleen should be based on the identification of RSCs and variants in the appropriate background. In difficult cases, immunohistochemical analysis may be helpful (Fig. 5–16).

References

Carbone PP, Kaplan HS, Musshoff K, *et al*: Report of the Committee on Hodgkin's Disease Staging. Cancer Res 31:1860–1861, 1971.

Rappaport H, Berard CW, Butler JJ, *et al*: Report of the Committee on Histopathological Criteria Contributing to Staging of Hodgkin's Disease. Cancer Res 31:1864–1865, 1971.

Sacks EL, Donaldson SS, Gordon J, Dorfman RF: Epithelioid granulomas associated with Hodgkin's disease. Clinical correlations in 55 previously untreated patients. Cancer 41:562–567, 1978.

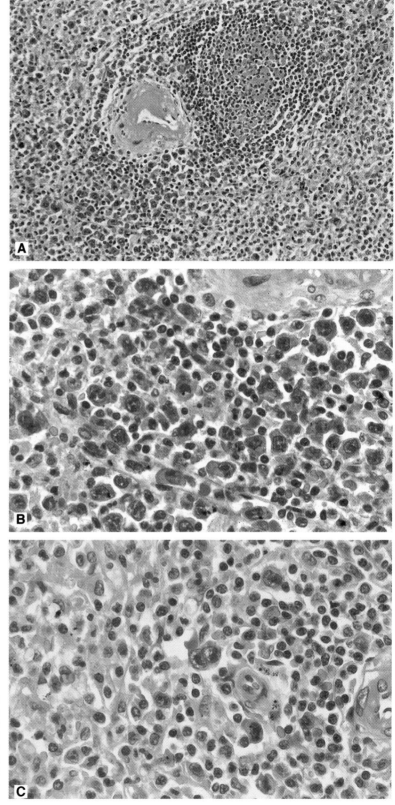

Figure 5–16. Spleen with an immunoblastic reaction in a patient with *Escherichia coli* sepsis. *A,* The spleen was enlarged only slightly, and white pulp does not appear expanded (H&E stain). *B,* High power examination shows numerous immunoblasts at the junction of the white and the red pulp (H&E stain). *C,* Occasional Reed-Sternberg-like cells are also present *(center).* The large cells in this case were CD30+ but CD15−, and many expressed B-cell antigens (H&E stain).

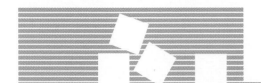

CHAPTER 6

Lymphoid Hyperplasia and Lymphoma in Abnormal Immune States

Congenital and Inherited Immunodeficiency Syndromes

COMMON VARIABLE IMMUNODEFICIENCY (CVID)

Clinical Features

Patients are usually adults at the time of diagnosis of common variable immunodeficiency (CVID). Men and women are affected equally. Serum IgG and, in some cases, IgA and IgM are decreased. Cell-mediated immunity may also be abnormal. The chief complaints relate to susceptibility to bacterial infection, especially of the respiratory tract. Some patients also become infected by mycobacteria, fungi, *Pneumocystis*, and *Giardia*. Viral infections may be severe. One in five patients develops herpes zoster. Twenty percent of patients develop various types of autoimmune diseases, most commonly Coombs+ hemolytic anemia or idiopathic thrombocytopenic purpura (ITP). Patients may also have a sprue-like malabsorption syndrome or inflammatory bowel disease. The peripheral blood in some cases reveals decreased numbers of B cells, an inverted CD4:CD8 ratio, or increased numbers of large granular lymphocytes of T lineage. The mode of genetic transmission varies and many cases are sporadic, but first-degree relatives may have IgA deficiency and an increased incidence of autoimmune disease.

Thirty percent of patients have reactive lymphoid infiltrates resulting in lymphadenopathy, splenomegaly, or nodular lymphoid hyperplasia in the gastrointestinal tract. Patients also have an increased incidence of malignancy. Of malignancies in patients with CVID, 46% are non-Hodgkin's lymphomas; 7%, Hodgkin's disease; 7%, leukemia; and the remainder, nonlymphoid tumors, among which gastric carcinoma constitutes an important subset.

The lymphomas affect patients from the first to seventh decades with a mean age in the sixth decade; most tumors are extranodal. For patients with localized disease, the prognosis may be good. Lymphomas in CVID do not appear to have the almost uniformly grim prognosis of those arising in other immunodeficiency syndromes.

Morphology

Lymphoid proliferations in patients with CVID can be divided into (1) reactive lymphoid hyperplasia; (2) atypical lymphoid hyperplasia; (3) granulomatous inflammation; and (4) malignant lymphoma; all may involve either nodal or extranodal sites. Reactive lesions are more common than lymphoma.

In reactive lymphoid hyperplasia, usually both follicles and paracortex are hyperplastic with preservation of the normal architecture. Atypical hyperplasia also usually includes both follicular and paracortical hyperplasia, but the follicles contain a predominance of blast cells with a high mitotic rate and tingible body macrophages and have attenuated or absent mantle zones; the paracortex may contain numerous immunoblasts. In lymph nodes, the architecture appears distorted at least partially, although open sinuses may be present focally. In granulomatous inflammation, various numbers of granulomas with central necrosis are surrounded by palisading histiocytes. Microorganisms may or may not be identified.

Lymphomas of various types have been reported (Fig. 6–1). Approximately half of the lymphomas have been diffuse large cell type; diffuse mixed small and large cell is the second most common type.

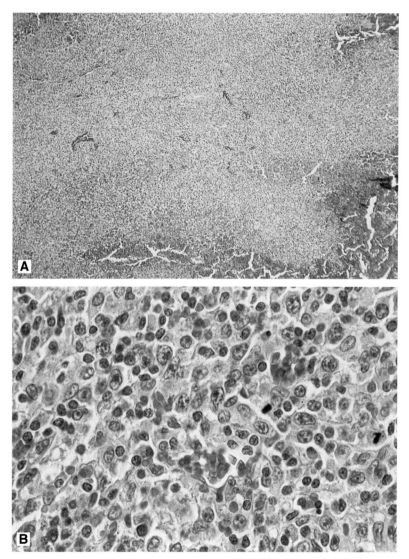

Figure 6–1. Common variable immunodeficiency; spleen with malignant lymphoma. The spleen weighed over 2000 gm. Molecular genetic analysis showed clonal rearrangement of the Ig heavy chain gene, and in situ hybridization showed the presence of EBER-1 in the neoplastic cells. *A,* White pulp is greatly expanded with coalescence of individual white pulp areas (H&E stain). *B,* In some areas, large atypical lymphoid cells predominate (H&E stain).

Illustration continued on following page.

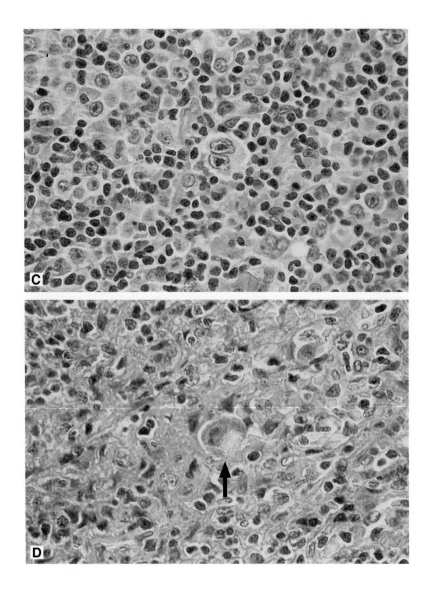

Figure 6–1. *Continued C,* In other areas, the infiltrate is polymorphous; a few cells closely resembling Reed-Sternberg cells are visible (H&E stain). *D,* Occasional cytomegalovirus-infected cells are also seen in sections from the spleen *(arrow)*; their lineage is uncertain, but they do not appear to be lymphoma cells (H&E stain).

Immunophenotype

Most lymphomas are B lineage and have expressed monotypic immunoglobulin (Ig) of IgM type. T-cell lymphomas also occur.

Genetic Features

The defect in some cases of CVID is located on chromosome 6p21.3.

In reactive hyperplasia, atypical hyperplasia, and granulomatous inflammation, T-cell-receptor (TCR) and Ig heavy chain genes are germline. B-cell lymphomas have rearranged Ig heavy chain genes. Lymphomas with Epstein-Barr virus RNA (EBV RNA) and clonal EBV genomes have been reported.

Differential Diagnosis

Atypical lymphoid hyperplasia (ALH) vs. malignant lymphoma: In cases of ALH, immunostaining delineates B- and T-cell regions, showing that nodal architecture is intact and that B cells are polytypic. In difficult cases, gene rearrangement studies should be obtained; clonal rearrangement of Ig genes is absent in ALH.

References

Buckley RH: Breakthrough in the understanding and therapy of primary immunodeficiency. Pediatr Clin North Am 41:665–690, 1994.
Cunningham-Rundles C, Lieberman P, Hellman G, Chaganti RSK: Non-Hodgkin's lymphoma in common variable immunodeficiency. Am J Hematol 37:69–74, 1991.
Filipovich AH, Mathur A, Kamat D, Shapiro RS: Primary immunodeficiencies: genetic risk factors for lymphoma. Cancer Res (Suppl) 52:5465s–5467s, 1992.
Kersey JH, Spector BD, Good RA: Primary immunodeficiencies and cancer: the immunodeficiency cancer registry. Int J Cancer 12:333–347, 1973.
Rosen FS, Cooper MD, Wedgwood RJP: The primary immunodeficiencies. (Review.) N Engl J Med 333:431–440, 1995.
Sneller MC, Strober W, Eisenstein E, et al: New insights into common variable immunodeficiency. Ann Intern Med 118:720–730, 1993.

CONGENITAL X-LINKED AGAMMAGLOBULINEMIA (BRUTON'S DISEASE)

Clinical Features

Patients have recurrent pyogenic infections, most often sinusitis and pneumonia. Autoimmune disorders are frequent. The standard treatment is prophylactic administration of immunoglobulin. The incidence of lymphoid and myeloid leukemia, and possibly of lymphoma affecting patients in the first decade seems to be increased, although only a few cases have been reported.

The disorder is caused by lack of a tyrosine kinase ("Bruton tyrosine kinase") that is important in signal transduction in B-cell differentiation.

Morphology

Circulating mature B cells are markedly decreased. Lymphoid tissues are atrophic; they lack germinal centers and plasma cells. Information on the morphology of the lymphomas is limited.

Immunophenotype

This has not been well studied, but three lymphomas in one series were T lineage.

Genetic Features

The defective tyrosine kinase gene is located on Xq22.

References

Buckley RH: Breakthrough in the understanding and therapy of primary immunodeficiency. Pediatr Clin North Am 41:665–690, 1994.
Frizzera G, Rosai J, Dehner LP, et al: Lymphoreticular disorders in primary immunodeficiencies: new findings based on an up-to-date histologic classification. Cancer 46:692–699, 1980.
Kersey JH, Spector BD, Good RA: Primary immunodeficiencies and cancer: the immunodeficiency cancer registry. Int J Cancer 12:333–347, 1973.
Rosen FS, Cooper MD, Wedgwood RJP: The primary immunodeficiencies. (Review.) N Engl J Med 333:431–440, 1995.
Sneller MC, Strober W, Eisenstein E, et al: New insights into common variable immunodeficiency. Ann Intern Med 118:720–730, 1993.

SEVERE COMBINED IMMUNODEFICIENCY DISEASE (SCID)

Clinical Features

Severe combined immunodeficiency disease (SCID) refers to a heterogeneous group of autosomal recessive or X-linked recessive disorders characterized by diminished B- and T-cell function. Causes of SCID include adenosine deaminase (ADA) deficiency, purine nucleoside phosphorylase (PRP) deficiency, or a defect in the gamma chain of the interleukin 2 receptor (IL-2R, γ chain). Boys constitute 75% of patients. They present early in life with diarrhea, oral thrush, recurrent infections, lymphopenia, and markedly reduced serum immunoglobulin.

Untreated, the immunodeficiency is usually fatal in childhood, but bone marrow transplantation may be lifesaving. Patients with ADA deficiency can be treated with injections of ADA. Patients are also at increased risk for developing malignant neoplasms, nearly all of which occur in the first decade (in accordance with the patients' short lifespans). Malignancies in the Immunodeficiency Cancer Registry include non-Hodgkin's lymphoma (74%), Hodgkin's disease (10%), and leukemia (12%).

Morphology

Lymphoid tissues, especially the thymus, show hypoplasia. The types of lymphomas have been diffuse large B-cell, immunoblastic, and unclassified. A plasmacytoma has been reported.

Immunophenotype

Most cases are B-lineage tumors.

Genetic Features

PRP deficiency is associated with a defect on chromosome 14q13.1. The gene for ADA deficiency is found at 20q13-ter, and X-linked SCID is associated with a defect at Xq13 (IL-2R, γ chain). EBV DNA has been found in some lymphomas.

References

Buckley RH: Breakthrough in the understanding and therapy of primary immunodeficiency. Pediatr Clin North Am 41:665–690, 1994.

Dictor M, Fasth A, Olling S: Abnormal B-cell proliferation associated with combined immunodeficiency, cytomegalovirus, and cultured thymus grafts. Am J Clin Pathol 82:487–490, 1984.

Frizzera G, Rosai J, Dehner LP, Spector BD, Kersey JH: Lymphoreticular disorders in primary immunodeficiencies: new findings based on an up-to-date histologic classification. Cancer 46:692–699, 1980.

Kersey JH, Shapiro RS, Filipovich AH: Relationship of immunodeficiency to lymphoid malignancy. Pediatr Infect Dis J 7:S10–S12, 1988.

Kersey JH, Spector BD, Good RA: Primary immunodeficiencies and cancer: the immunodeficiency cancer registry. Int J Cancer 12:333–347, 1973.

Rosen FS, Cooper MD, Wedgwood RJP: The primary immunodeficiencies. (Review.) N Engl J Med 333:431–440, 1995.

Seemayer TA: Molecular basis of selected primary immunodeficiency disorders. Arch Pathol Lab Med 111:1114–1117, 1987.

Watson AR, Evans DI, Marsden HB, *et al*: Purine nucleoside phosphorylase deficiency associated with a fatal lymphoproliferative disorder. Arch Dis Childhood 56:563–565, 1981.

WISKOTT-ALDRICH SYNDROME (WAS)

Clinical Features

Wiskott-Aldrich syndrome (WAS) is an X-linked recessive disorder characterized by thrombocytopenia, eczema, susceptibility to infections, lymphopenia, and increased incidence of lymphoma. Serum IgA and IgE are usually markedly elevated, whereas IgM is reduced. T-cell defects are also found. Only a few patients survive into the third decade.

In the Immunodeficiency Cancer Registry, 76% of malignancies in WAS were non-Hodgkin's lymphomas; 4%, Hodgkin's disease; 9%, leukemia; and 11%, nonlymphoid tumors. Most lymphomas occur in the first decade. They often involve extranodal sites, especially the central nervous system, and the prognosis is poor. Bone marrow transplantation may successfully treat the immunodeficiency and eliminate the excessive risk for lymphoma.

Morphology

Most malignancies are diffuse large cell lymphomas, often with a predominance of immunoblasts.

Immunophenotype

Most lymphomas are B-lineage, some with Epstein-Barr virus latent membrane protein (EBV-LMP) and Epstein-Barr nuclear antigen 2 (EBNA-2) expression. T-cell lymphoma has been reported.

Genetic Features

The defect in WAS has been mapped to Xp11.23. B-cell lymphoma with rearranged immunoglobulin heavy chain genes and monoclonally integrated EBV has been reported. In one case of B-cell lymphoma, polyclonal immunoglobulin heavy chain genes were found in most sites, with monoclonal heavy chain genes in one site. EBV genomes were clonally integrated at each site; however, the EBV termini varied in size in lesions in different areas, suggesting that the patient had a multiclonal lymphoproliferative disorder. One T-cell lymphoma was EBV-negative by Southern blot hybridization.

References

Brochstein JA, Gillio AP, Ruggiero M, *et al*: Marrow transplantation from human leukocyte antigen-identical or haploidentical donors for correction of Wiskott-Aldrich syndrome. J Pediatr 119:907–912, 1991.

Cotelingham JD, Witebsky FG, Hsu SM, *et al*: Malignant lymphoma in patients with the Wiskott-Aldrich syndrome. Cancer Invest 3:515–522, 1985.

Filipovich AH, Mathur A, Kamat D, Shapiro RS: Primary immunodeficiencies: genetic risk factors for lymphoma. Cancer Research (Suppl)52:5465s–5467s, 1992.

Frizzera G, Rosai J, Dehner LP, *et al*: Lymphoreticular disorders in primary immunodeficiencies: new findings based on an up-to-date histologic classification. Cancer 46:692–699, 1980.

Gulley ML, Chen CL, Raab-Traub N: Epstein Barr virus-related lymphomagenesis in a child with Wiskott-Aldrich syndrome. Hematol Oncol 11:139–145, 1993.

Kersey JA, Shapiro RS, Filipovich AH: Relationship of immunodeficiency to lymphoid malignancy. Pediatr Infect Dis J 7:S10–S12, 1988.

Meropol NJ, Hicks D, Brooks JJ, *et al*: Coincident Kaposi sarcoma and T-cell lymphoma in a patient with the Wiskott-Aldrich syndrome. Am J Hematol 40:126–134, 1992.

Nakanishi M, Kikuta H, Tomizawa K, et al: Distinct clonotypic Epstein-Barr virus-induced fatal lymphoproliferative disorder in a patient with Wiskott-Aldrich syndrome. Cancer 72:1376–1381, 1993.

X-LINKED LYMPHOPROLIFERATIVE DISORDER (XLP)

X-linked lymphoproliferative disorder (XLP) is an X-linked recessive disorder in which patients have a selective immunodeficiency for Epstein-Barr virus (EBV). They have an abnormal serologic reaction to EBV infection, severely impaired or absent ability to generate a cytotoxic T-cell response to EBV, abnormal peripheral blood CD4:CD8 ratio, and markedly decreased natural killer activity. At a young age, affected boys develop severe or fatal infectious mononucleosis (IM) (60%), malignant lymphoma (23%), or acquired hypo- or agammaglobulinemia (25%). To make a diagnosis of XLP on clinical grounds, a patient with one or more of the manifestations just listed must also have two affected relatives, either brothers or maternally related cousins.

XLP has been linked to a defect on the X chromosome at q24-26.

I. Infectious Mononucleosis (IM)

Clinical Features

Infectious mononucleosis (IM) in XLP affects boys from infancy to adolescence, with an approximate median age of 2.5 years. They present with fever, a maculopapular rash, generalized lymphadenopathy, hepatosplenomegaly, hepatic dysfunction, and peripheral cytopenias. IM is fatal in 85% to 90%. Causes of death include marrow failure owing to a hemophagocytic syndrome with pancytopenia, leading to overwhelming bacterial or fungal infection or hemorrhage, and fulminant EBV-induced hepatitis or meningoencephalitis. Survivors often have a profound immunodeficiency with hypogammaglobulinemia. They are at increased risk for developing non-Hodgkin's lymphoma.

Morphology

Early in the course of disease, lymph nodes show marked paracortical hyperplasia with numerous immunoblasts (some Reed-Sternberg-like) and admixed small and large lymphoid cells along with frequent infiltration of the capsule and perinodal tissue, but without architectural obliteration (sinuses remain patent). Follicles are inconspicuous or absent. Individual cell or zonal necrosis, or rarely, complete nodal necrosis, may be found. With time, immunoblasts and other lymphoid cells decrease in number. Histiocytes increase, often with sinusoidal hemophagocytosis. Necrosis may become extensive. Late in the course, lymphoid tissue is sclerotic and severely depleted; plasma cells may be relatively prominent.

Early on, the bone marrow is hyperplastic, but over time becomes infiltrated by atypical lymphoid cells followed by hemophagocytic histiocytes. The marrow becomes severely depleted and may undergo massive necrosis.

II. Malignant Lymphoma (ML)

Clinical Features

Malignant lymphoma (ML) in XLP affects boys from early childhood to adolescence (median age, 4 years).

Patients present with fever, nausea, vomiting, and abdominal pain. All have extranodal disease, usually with involvement of regional lymph nodes. The intestines are involved in 76% of cases; the ileocecal area is the single most commonly involved site. Most patients present with stage I or II disease, and therapy usually leads to complete remission. About half of patients have subsequent long term survival, but the rest die within 1 year, usually of infectious complications.

Morphology

In one series, 52.9% of the neoplasms were small noncleaved cell lymphoma (Burkitt's or Burkitt-like); 11.8%, large noncleaved; 17.6%, immunoblastic; 11.8%, small cleaved or mixed small and large cell; and 5.9%, not subclassified. Lymphomas of small noncleaved cell type were associated with a poor prognosis.

Immunophenotype and Genotype

Monotypic immunoglobulin expression and the presence of EBV genomes are reported.

Differential Diagnosis

The main problem is to distinguish infectious mononucleosis (IM) from ML. Features in favor of IM include the presence of IM-like symptoms, generalized lymphadenopathy, hepatosplenomegaly, atypical peripheral lymphocytosis, preserved architecture in lymph nodes and extranodal sites, and polymorphic lymphoid cells expressing polytypic immunoglobulin. Features supporting a diagnosis of ML in XLP include the presence of a large extranodal mass, regional lymphadenopathy, architectural effacement, and monomorphic lymphoid cells expressing monotypic immunoglobulin. In a few cases, however, patients have had IM and ML simultaneously.

References

Buckley RH: Breakthrough in the understanding and therapy of primary immunodeficiency. Pediatr Clin North Am 41:665–690, 1994.

Harrington DS, Weisenburger DD, Purtilo DT: Malignant lymphoma in the X-linked lymphoproliferative syndrome. Cancer 59:1419–1429, 1987.

Markin RS, Linder J, Zuerlein K, et al: Hepatitis in fatal infectious mononucleosis. Gastroenterology 93:1210–1217, 1987.

Mroczek EC, Weisenburger DD, Grierson HL, et al: Fatal infectious mononucleosis and virus-associated hemophagocytic syndrome. Arch Pathol Lab Med 111(6):530–535, 1987.

Tatsumi E, Purtilo DT: Epstein-Barr virus (EBV) and X-linked lymphoproliferative syndrome (XLP). AIDS Research 2(Suppl 1):S109–S113, 1986.

Acquired Immunodeficiency

HUMAN IMMUNODEFICIENCY VIRUS (HIV)-ASSOCIATED LYMPHOID LESIONS

I. Persistent Generalized Lymphadenopathy (PGL)

Clinical Features

Persistent generalized lymphadenopathy (PGL), defined as extrainguinal lymphadenopathy persisting for at least 3 months and involving at least two noncontiguous node groups, is common among HIV+ patients. PGL mainly affects adult males and is often accompanied by fever, weight loss, headaches, and malaise.

Morphology

A range of changes occurs in lymphadenopathy associated with HIV infection. Similar changes may be found in organized extranodal lymphoid tissue.

Florid follicular hyperplasia, the most common pattern, is characterized by large, irregular, germinal centers with a high mitotic rate; numerous blast cells; many tingible body macrophages; and ill-defined, attenuated, or effaced mantle zones. Follicle lysis is common. The interfollicular region contains a mixture of immunoblasts, plasma cells, lymphocytes, and histiocytes with prominent vascularity. Monocytoid B cells are often prominent. Sinus histiocytosis, epithelioid histiocytes, polykaryocytes, erythrophagocytosis, and areas with features of dermatopathic lymphadenopathy may be seen (Fig. 6–2).

Lymphoid depletion is found in late stages of PGL: lymphoid follicles are decreased in number or absent, and residual follicles are "burnt out" or regressively transformed. The interfollicular region contains scattered lymphocytes, immunoblasts, plasma cells, and many blood vessels. The presence of amorphous eosinophilic material or fibrosis make the node appear pale and depleted. The appearance may be reminiscent of Castleman's disease (Figs. 6–3 to 6–5). Lymph nodes with lymphoid depletion indicate an advanced stage of immunodeficiency; these patients frequently develop opportunistic infections, Kaposi's sarcoma, or malignant lymphoma.

In some cases, lymph nodes show changes intermediate between florid follicular hyperplasia and lymphoid depletion.

Immunophenotype

HIV-associated antigens are detected in follicular dendritic cells (FDCs) in germinal centers. Follicles contain polytypic B cells. The interfollicular region contains decreased numbers of CD4+ cells, and the CD4:CD8 ratio is usually reversed.

Genotype

HIV RNA is found in germinal centers. In most cases, Epstein-Barr virus is not detected, but when it is found, patients may be at higher risk for the development of non-Hodgkin's lymphoma.

Differential Diagnosis

1. Reactive hyperplasia in HIV− patients: No single feature or constellation of histologic features allows definitive distinction between lymph nodes from HIV+ and HIV− patients; however, polykaryocytes, epithelioid histiocytes, and mantle zone effacement may be significantly more common in HIV+ patients.
2. Non-Hodgkin's lymphoma (NHL): NHL enters the differential diagnosis in cases of florid follicular hyperplasia with follicles that have attenuated mantle zones and an interfollicular region that has numerous blasts, resulting in apparent obliteration of normal nodal architecture. Immunohistochemical stains are helpful in delineating B- and T-cell regions of the node and demonstrating polytypic follicles.
3. Castleman's disease (CD): The lymphoid depleted stage of PGL may closely resemble CD (see Castleman's Disease, Chapter 2).

II. HIV-Associated Salivary Gland Lymphoepithelial Lesion

Clinical Features

This lesion appears to represent PGL involving lymph nodes associated with salivary glands, usually the parotid. The lesions are often multiple, bilateral, and cystic. Like other HIV+ patients, patients with this disorder may develop opportunistic infections or lymphoma.

Morphology

The range of histologic changes is similar to that found in HIV-associated lymphadenopathy in other sites. The lymphoid infiltrate may extend to involve salivary gland parenchyma, with formation of epimyoepithelial islands. Ducts within lymph nodes are dilated and may show squamous metaplasia (Fig. 6–6).

Immunophenotype and Genotype

The immunophenotype and genotype are similar to findings in PGL (see preceding discussion).

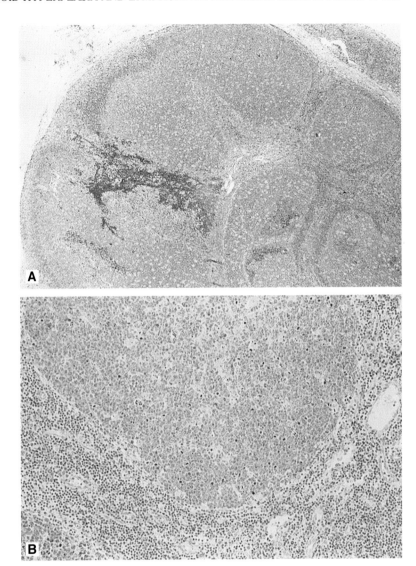

Figure 6–2. Florid follicular hyperplasia associated with HIV infection. *A,* Multiple large lymphoid follicles occupy much of the lymph node (H&E stain). *B,* This lymphoid follicle consists of a large germinal center with virtually no mantle zone (Giemsa stain).

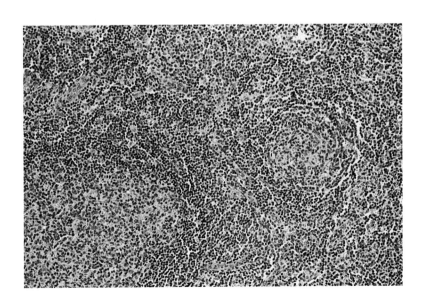

Figure 6–3. Follicular involution associated with HIV infection. The lymphoid follicles are small and have slightly sclerotic germinal centers and ill-defined mantle zones. The junction between follicles and paracortex is indistinct in some areas (H&E stain).

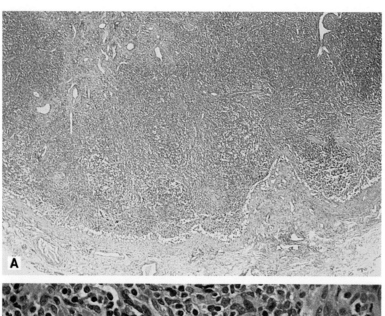

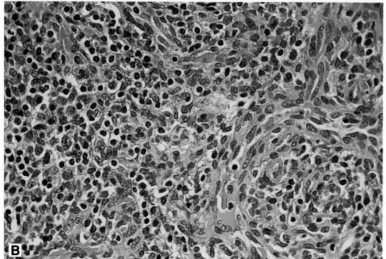

Figure 6–4. Lymph node with depletion. *A,* The capsule and the hilus are fibrotic, and intervening lymphoid tissue is more pink than usual because of loss of lymphoid elements (H&E stain). *B,* Blood vessels are prominent (H&E stain).

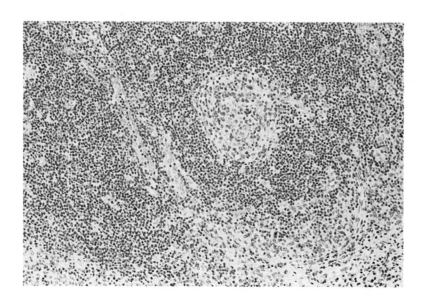

Figure 6–5. This specimen from a patient with HIV infection shows a lymphoid follicle with hyaline-vascular change. A small blood vessel pierces the germinal center *(right)* (H&E stain).

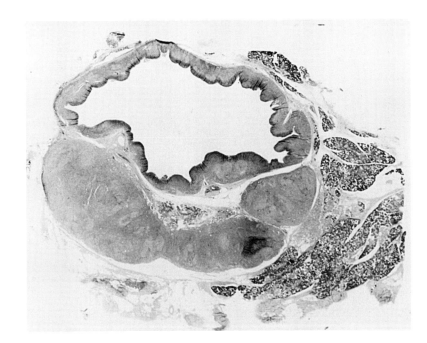

Figure 6–6. Lymphoepithelial cyst with HIV infection. A whole-mount photomicrograph shows a cyst lined by ductal epithelium and surrounded by a cuff of hyperplastic lymphoid tissue. Salivary gland parenchyma is visible at lower right (H&E stain).

III. Non-Hodgkin's Lymphoma (NHL)

Clinical features

Patients with HIV infection have an increased incidence of non-Hodgkin's lymphoma (NHL). After 6 to 8 years of HIV infection, the risk for lymphoma increases 100-fold compared to the general population. Most patients are homosexual men or intravenous drug abusers; NHL has been reported in children only infrequently. Although NHL in hemophiliacs accounts for a small proportion of HIV-associated lymphomas, lymphoma is the most common HIV-associated malignancy among hemophiliacs. Among HIV+ individuals in general, lymphoma is the second most common malignancy, after Kaposi's sarcoma. Although most patients have a diagnosis of AIDS prior to the development of NHL, the diagnosis of AIDS is rendered upon recognition of NHL in a substantial minority.

Patients with large B-cell lymphomas tend to present with a more advanced stage of immunodeficiency than those with Burkitt's and Burkitt-like lymphoma. Most patients present with stage III or IV disease, with frequent involvement of extranodal sites, including the central nervous system (Fig. 6–7), gastrointestinal tract (Figs. 6–8 and 6–9), liver, bone marrow, skin, spleen, oral cavity, and salivary glands. Rarely, lymphomas are associated with effusions from pleural, peritoneal, or pericardial cavities (primary effusion lymphoma, also known as body-cavity-based lymphoma or primary serosal large B-cell lymphoma) without formation of a discrete mass (*see* Fig. 6–12).

The prognosis is poor. Treatment is often complicated by opportunistic infections, and progressive lymphoma and opportunistic infections contribute roughly equally to mortality. Some success has been achieved using reduced dosages of combination chemotherapy, combined with growth factors such as granulocyte colony-stimulating factor (G-CSF) to promote marrow regeneration. Lymphomas of the central nervous system and primary effusion lymphomas are, however, nearly always fatal. Primary effusion lymphomas are discussed in greater detail in Chapter 3.

Morphology

The lymphomas are usually high grade tumors—diffuse large B-cell lymphoma, Burkitt's lymphoma, or high grade B-cell lymphoma, Burkitt-like. The large B-cell lymphomas, for the most part, can be divided into those with a predominance of centroblasts (large noncleaved cells) and those with a predominance of immunoblasts; plasmacytoid differentiation is frequent in the latter group (Figs. 6–7 to 6–12). Large B-cell lymphomas composed predominantly of large cleaved cells are unusual. Often the lymphomas have histologic features intermediate between immunoblastic and Burkitt's or Burkitt-like lymphoma and are difficult to subclassify. A minority of cases are anaplastic large cell lymphomas (Ki-1+ lymphomas). Some investigators have described cases with a polymorphous appearance composed of immunoblasts, plasmablasts, plasmacytoid lymphocytes, and occasional bizarre Reed-Sternberg-like cells or follicle

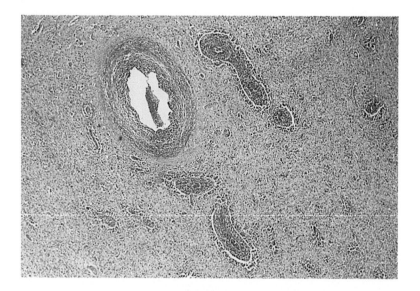

Figure 6–7. Malignant lymphoma involving the brain; the lymphoma is predominantly perivascular (H&E stain).

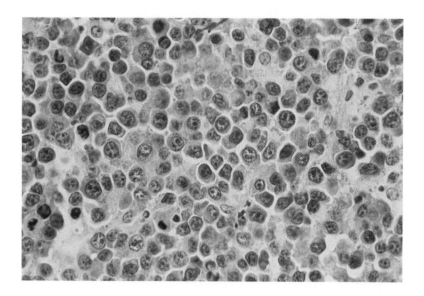

Figure 6–8. Malignant lymphoma, immunoblastic plasmacytoid type, arising in the gastrointestinal tract in a patient with AIDS (H&E stain).

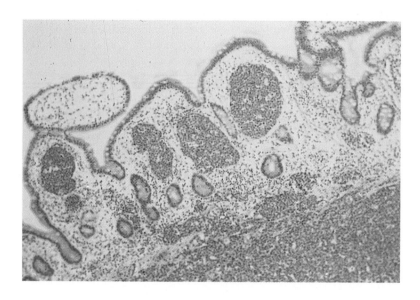

Figure 6–9. Burkitt's lymphoma of the small intestine with an unusual distribution of neoplastic cells (H&E stain).

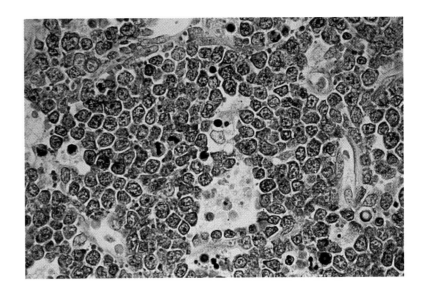

Figure 6–10. Burkitt-like lymphoma. Cells are slightly more pleomorphic than in classic Burkitt's lymphoma and have occasional distinct central nucleoli. Mitotic figures are numerous and tingible body macrophages are present (Giemsa stain).

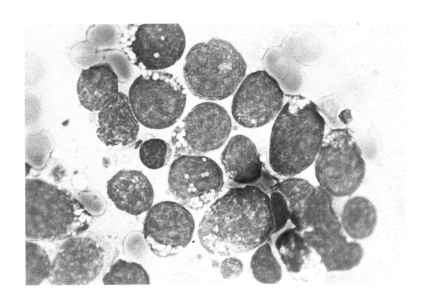

Figure 6–11. Burkitt's lymphoma involving the bone marrow in a patient with AIDS. The predominant population consists of monomorphous, intermediate-sized cells with basophilic, vacuolated cytoplasm (Wright-Giemsa stain).

center cells, reminiscent of some post-transplantation lymphomas. Low grade lymphomas have been reported in HIV+ patients, but the frequency of low grade lymphomas is not increased when compared with the normal population.

Some correlation occurs between the histologic appearance and the clinical presentation. Nearly all lymphomas in children are Burkitt's lymphoma, although large B-cell lymphoma has also been reported. Patients with lymphomas classified as small, noncleaved cell type (Burkitt's and Burkitt-like in the R.E.A.L. Classification) are much more likely to have bone marrow involvement at presentation than patients with large B-cell lymphoma. Presentation with gastrointestinal tract disease is uncommon in patients with

Burkitt's and Burkitt-like lymphoma, but is frequent in those with large B-cell lymphoma, both centroblastic and immunoblastic types. Immunoblastic lymphoma is somewhat more likely to involve the central nervous system. Patients with small noncleaved cell lymphoma are most likely to present with stage IV disease, because of the high frequency of bone marrow involvement, whereas patients with the relatively infrequent stage I disease at presentation usually have diffuse large B-cell lymphomas, most often affecting the central nervous system or the gastrointestinal tract.

After studying a large series of HIV-associated lymphomas, Knowles and coworkers concluded that small noncleaved cell lymphomas usually originate in lymph nodes,

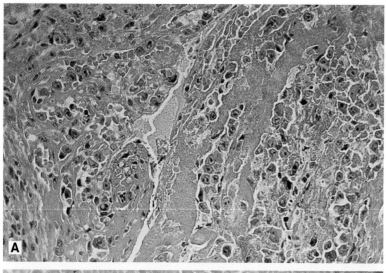

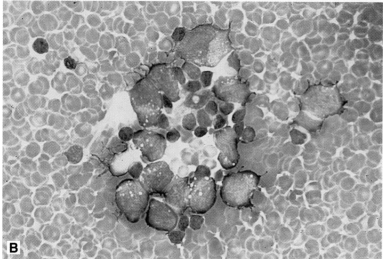

Figure 6–12. Primary effusion lymphoma in a patient with AIDS. *A,* A pleural biopsy specimen shows a thin layer of immunoblasts associated with a fibrinous exudate (H&E stain). *B,* Examination of fluid from the pleural effusion shows large, somewhat pleomorphic, atypical lymphoid cells with abundant, often vacuolated, basophilic cytoplasm (Wright stain).

and then rapidly disseminate to involve the bone marrow, other lymph nodes, and various extranodal sites. In contrast, diffuse large B-cell lymphomas (centroblastic and immunoblastic types), are more likely to arise in an extranodal site and to disseminate at a slower rate than small noncleaved cell lymphomas. The prognosis is poor for patients with any of these high grade lymphomas, but patients with immunoblastic lymphomas had the shortest survival times in this series.

Immunophenotype

Nearly all cases have been B-cell tumors, with rare cases having a T-cell or a null (non-B, non-T)-cell phenotype. The immunophenotype is similar to lymphomas of the same histologic type in immunocompetent patients. The Burkitt's lymphomas express pan-B-cell antigens, monotypic immunoglobulin (Ig) of IgM type, and CD10. The large B-cell lymphomas, especially immunoblastic lymphomas, may lack surface Ig. Monotypic cytoplasmic Ig may be detected in some surface Ig-negative cases.

Approximately a third of B-cell lymphomas of Burkitt's, Burkitt-like, and immunoblastic types are CD45RO+. CD45RO is usually thought of as a T-cell antigen, but it is normally expressed at a late stage of B-cell maturation during differentiation to plasma cells. Accordingly, CD45RO expression is especially common in immunoblastic lymphomas with plasmacytic differentiation. CD45RO expression is much more common in lymphomas in HIV-infected patients than in lymphomas in immunocompetent patients. Epithelial membrane antigen expression is also frequent in immunoblastic plasmacytoid lymphomas.

The primary effusion lymphomas usually have a null phenotype (non-B, non-T), but do express CD45 and often, CD30 and HLA-DR. Cases with the morphology of anaplastic large cell lymphoma of B and of T lineage have been described.

Most large cell lymphomas containing Epstein-Barr virus express latent membrane protein (EBV-LMP). EBV+ Burkitt's lymphomas infrequently express LMP. LMP is thought to have the capacity to induce malignant transformation of human cells. Analysis of the genetic sequence of the gene for LMP shows that, in most cases of HIV-associated, LMP-expressing lymphoma, a deletion occurs that results in a longer half-life of this oncoprotein, leading to higher cellular levels of LMP and, possibly, to a growth advantage for the infected cells.

Genetic Features

B-cell lymphomas generally show clonal Ig heavy chain gene rearrangement. In a small number of cases, the lymphomas appear to have polyclonal rearrangement of Ig heavy chain genes. Some patients have multiclonal tumors (different clones in different anatomic sites).

EBV nucleic acids are found in about half of cases; when present, the EBV is in a clonal episomal form. EBV may be clonal even when clonal Ig heavy chain gene rearrangement has not been demonstrated. EBV is found in the majority of large cell lymphomas, including nearly all primary central nervous system lymphomas. EBV is found less often in Burkitt's lymphoma (in approximately 40% of cases).

Two families of EBV (type A and type B, also known as type 1 and type 2) can be distinguished from one another on the basis of differences in the genetic sequences of EBV nuclear antigen-2 (EBNA-2). EBNA-2 is a latent gene product essential for immortalization of B cells. Type A EBV appears to immortalize B cells more efficiently in vitro and to have a greater capacity to spread beyond the oropharynx than type B EBV. The A type has a worldwide distribution. It is found in the oropharynx and in the peripheral blood lymphocytes of immunocompetent individuals. Immunocompetent patients who develop EBV-containing lymphomas have EBV type A.

The distribution of type B EBV is much more restricted, occurring mainly in the areas of Africa where endemic Burkitt's lymphoma is encountered. Endemic Burkitt's lymphoma, however, may contain EBV of either type A or type B.

In immunocompetent patients in Western countries, EBV type B can be found rarely in the oropharynx, but not in the peripheral blood. In patients who are immunosuppressed due to various causes, type B may be found not only in the oropharynx, but also in the peripheral blood. Similar to individuals with endemic Burkitt's lymphoma, roughly equal numbers of HIV+ patients with non-Hodgkin's lymphoma are infected by EBV type A or EBV type B.

C-myc rearrangement has been reported in virtually all cases of Burkitt's lymphoma; the pattern of rearrangement is typically that associated with sporadic, rather than endemic, Burkitt's lymphoma.

Alterations of bcl-6, a putative proto-oncogene that appears to be involved in the pathogenesis of large cell lymphoma in immunologically normal individuals, have been described in 20% of diffuse large B-cell lymphomas in HIV+ patients. Some cases with bcl-6 alterations contain EBV, but others do not. No c-myc mutations have been found in any case with an abnormal bcl-6 gene. Accordingly,

bcl-6 mutations have not been found in HIV-associated Burkitt's or Burkitt-like lymphoma. Mutations of p53 are frequent in Burkitt's lymphoma, but are virtually absent in large cell lymphoma. RAS mutations have been identified in a minority of both Burkitt's and large cell lymphoma.

The primary effusion lymphomas typically have Ig heavy and light chain genes rearranged, contain EBV DNA, lack c-myc rearrangement, and contain genomic sequences of Kaposi's sarcoma–associated herpes virus (also known as human herpes virus type 8 (HHV-8)). Despite their usual lack of expression of B cell–associated antigens, their genetic features indicate that they are B-lineage neoplasms.

Thus, evaluation of genetic features of HIV-associated NHL gives a clue to their pathogenesis. In different cases, c-myc rearrangement, bcl-6 mutation, p53 inactivation, RAS mutation, EBV infection, HHV-8 infection, or a combination of these factors may contribute to the development of NHL. HIV infection contributes to an increased risk for lymphoma because of the immunodeficiency it induces; it is not believed to be involved directly in lymphomagenesis.

Differential Diagnosis

Reactive lymphoid hyperplasia: See previous discussion of Persistent Generalized Lymphadenopathy.

IV. Hodgkin's Disease (HD)

Clinical Features

The incidence of Hodgkin's disease (HD) among HIV+ patients seems to be increased, although the increase is not as marked as that for non-Hodgkin's lymphoma in the United States. HD may be more frequent among patients who become infected with HIV through intravenous drug use rather than through sexual transmission. In the United States, where the major risk factor for HIV infection is homosexual contact, the ratio of HIV-associated non-Hodgkin's lymphoma to Hodgkin's disease is reported to be 11:1, whereas a study from Europe reported a ratio of 2:1 (a larger proportion of patients become infected with HIV through intravenous drug abuse in some areas of Europe). In contrast to HD in the general population, HD in HIV+ patients is usually widespread (stage III or IV) at diagnosis, with frequent bone marrow involvement. B symptoms (fever, night sweats, weight loss) are usually present. Overall, the prognosis is poor, although some patients attain durable complete remissions.

Morphology

A higher proportion of HIV+ patients have HD with mixed cellularity or lymphocyte depletion than does the general population (Figs. 6–13 and 6–14), whereas a smaller proportion have nodular sclerosis HD (NSHD). Lymphocyte predominance HD (LPHD) is unusual.

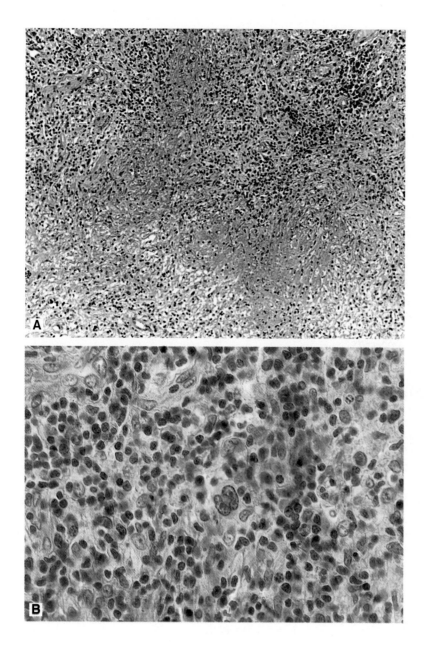

Figure 6–13. Hodgkin's disease, mixed cellularity, in a patient with AIDS, from a lymph node. *A,* A polymorphous infiltrate surrounds a large area of necrosis (H&E stain). *B,* Occasional Reed-Sternberg cells are scattered among reactive cells (H&E stain).

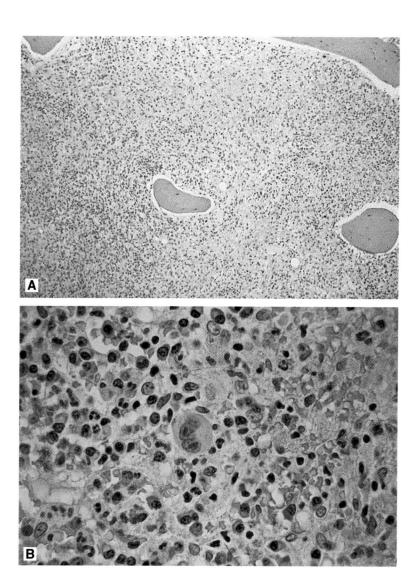

Figure 6–14. Hodgkin's disease in a patient with AIDS, from bone marrow. *A,* At low power examination, a polymorphous infiltrate appears in a sclerotic background with no residual hematopoietic elements (H&E stain). *B,* The high power view shows lymphocytes, plasma cells, granulocytes, histiocytes, and a diagnostic Reed-Sternberg cell (H&E stain).

Immunophenotype

The immunophenotype is similar to that of classic HD in immunocompetent patients (*see* Chapter 5) except that EBV latent membrane protein (EBV-LMP) is expressed by the neoplastic cells in many more cases. The background lymphocytes, which are typically predominantly CD4+ in patients without HIV infection, are frequently predominantly CD8+ in HIV+ patients.

Genetic Features

Ig heavy chain and T-cell-receptor (TCR) genes have a germline configuration. EBV genomic material is present in nearly all cases. Clonal episomal EBV has been reported.

Differential Diagnosis

Non-Hodgkin's lymphoma (NHL): Criteria for differential diagnosis are similar to those for HD and NHL in the general population (*see* Table 4–4).

V. Miscellaneous

Kaposi's Sarcoma (KS)

In the United States, KS usually affects lymph nodes in patients with relatively severe immunodeficiency and is found mainly in homosexual males. Most patients with nodal involvement also have skin disease, but occasionally, patients have a lymphadenopathic presentation. Affected nodes show a proliferation of spindle cells forming slit-like spaces with extravasated red blood cells, hemosiderin, and eosinophilic globules within the capsule, involving the subcapsular sinus, or replacing the entire lymph node. Uninvolved areas often show regressively transformed follicles, a hypervascular interfollicular region, and increased plasma cells, reminiscent of Castleman's disease (Fig. 6–15).

Kaposi's sarcoma–associated herpes virus–like sequences (KSHV, HHV-8) have been identified in more than 90% of KS cases from AIDS patients. KSHV may be involved in the pathogenesis of KS.

Differential Diagnosis

1. Vascular transformation of lymph node sinuses (VT): VT, thought to be caused by lymphatic and venous obstruction, is characterized by a proliferation of spindle cells with the formation of small vascular spaces within sinuses. Unlike KS, VT remains confined to sinuses, does not involve the capsule, is often associated with fibrosis, and typically has many well-formed vascular spaces toward the capsular aspect of the node (Fig. 6–16).

2. Bacillary angiomatosis (BA): Rarely, BA affects lymph nodes. In BA, vascular spaces are better formed than in KS, fascicular growth of spindle cells is absent, and neutrophils and large numbers of bacteria are present (*see* following discussion).

Infectious Lymphadenitis

1. Mycobacterial: Patients present most often with cervical or supraclavicular lymphadenopathy and fever, with or without pulmonary involvement. The PPD test is often negative. In most cases, *Mycobacterium tuberculosis* is the causative organism, although a substantial minority are caused by *M. avium* complex. More virulent strains of *M. tuberculosis* can infect patients with less advanced immunodeficiency and they are found more often in intravenous drug users and non-white patients, whereas atypical mycobacteria affect patients with advanced immunodeficiency. Depending on the patient's immune status, granulomas may be well or poorly formed. *M. avium-intracellulare* produces loose aggregates of histiocytes containing numerous acid-fast bacilli without formation of discrete granulomas. Because organisms are typically abundant, especially in cases of *M. avium-intracellulare* infection, the diagnosis can often be made on examination of material derived from fine needle aspiration biopsy. The microorganisms stain with a Ziehl-Neelsen stain; silver stains used for fungi may also stain *M. avium-intracellulare* (Fig. 6–17).

2. Fungal: Patients may develop fungal lymphadenitis (most often due to *Histoplasma* or *Cryptococcus* spp.), usually in the setting of disseminated disease. On routinely stained sections, the appearance is similar to that of mycobacterial infection. Special stains (silver stain, and in the case of cryptococci, mucicarmine stain) permit recognition of the fungi.

3. Bacillary angiomatosis (BA): BA is an infectious disease, usually caused by *Bartonella henselae* (the bacillus responsible for cat scratch disease) and in a minority of cases, by *Bartonella quintana* (the agent that causes trench fever). BA usually occurs in immunocompromised patients, mainly those with AIDS, and in some cases is transmitted by exposure to cats. It results in nodular, lobulated, vasoproliferative lesions containing plump, epithelioid endothelial cells, with admixed neutrophils and interstitial eosinophilic material that proves to be aggregated bacilli after Warthin-Starry staining. Patients usually present with skin lesions, but may have disseminated visceral involvement, involving the liver, spleen, and lymph nodes. Untreated, BA can be fatal, but it responds to antibiotics.

4. *Pneumocystis carinii*: Although *P. carinii* infects the lungs much more frequently than any other site, it disseminates rarely and can infect lymphoid organs (Fig. 6–18).

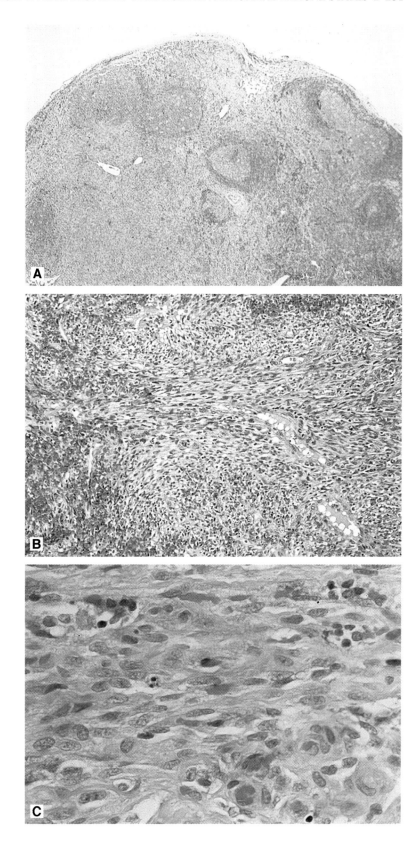

Figure 6–15. Kaposi's sarcoma (KS) involving a lymph node. *A,* KS occupies much of this lymph node, although residual hyperplastic follicles are present (H&E stain). *B,* Fascicles of spindle cells are associated with hemorrhage (H&E stain). *C,* The spindle cells form slit-like spaces but no discrete vascular channels (H&E stain).

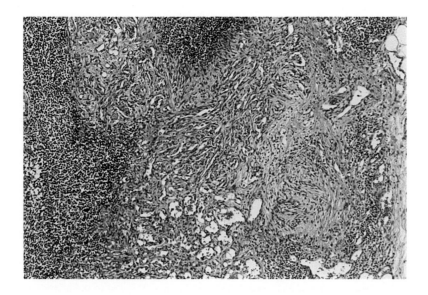

Figure 6–16. Vascular transformation of lymph node sinuses. The subcapsular sinus and a cortical sinus are occupied by blood vessels that are well-formed overall and range from slit-like to dilated (H&E stain).

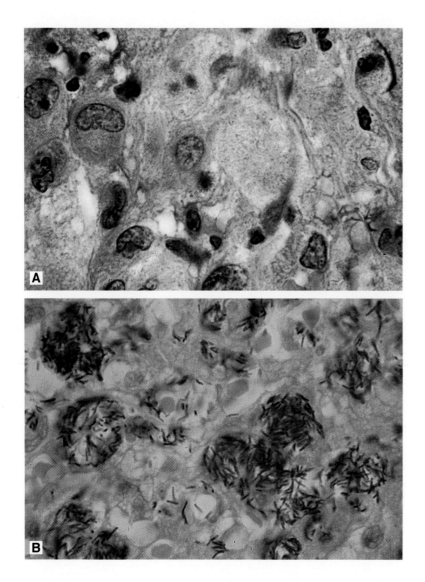

Figure 6–17. *Mycobacterium avium-intracellulare* infection in AIDS; needle aspiration biopsy of an abdominal mass. *A,* Histiocytes have abundant, finely granular cytoplasm (H&E stain). *B,* Numerous acid-fast bacilli fill the cytoplasm of the histiocytes (Ziehl-Neelsen stain).

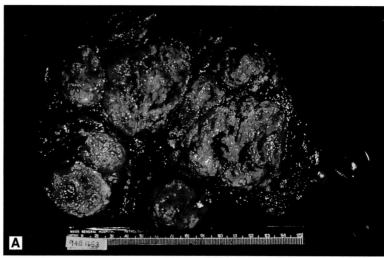

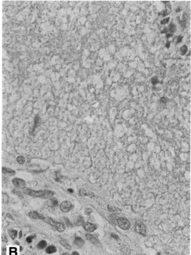
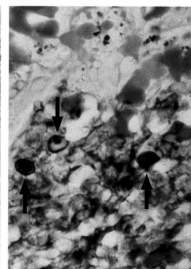

Figure 6–18. *Pneumocystis carinii* infection of spleen in a patient with AIDS. *A,* Large, soft tan-yellow nodules are visible on a cross-section of this 976-gm spleen. *B,* On microscopic examination, the nodules contain abundant finely granular to foamy material (*left,* H&E stain). Occasional microorganisms (*arrows*) are visible with a Grocott methenamine silver stain (*right*).

References

Alfonso F, Gallo L, Winkler B, Suhrland MJ: Fine needle aspiration cytology of peripheral lymph node cryptococcosis. A report of three cases. Acta Cytologica 38(3):459–462, 1994.

Ames ED, Conjalka MS, Goldberg AF, et al: Hodgkin's disease and AIDS. Twenty-three new cases and a review of the literature. Hematol Oncol Clin North Am 5:343–356, 1991.

Ansari MQ, Dawson DB, Nador R, et al: Primary body cavity-based AIDS-related lymphomas. Am J Clin Pathol 105:221–229, 1996.

Bacchi CE, Bacchi MM, Rabenhorst SH, et al: AIDS-related lymphoma in Brazil. Histopathology, immunophenotype, and association with Epstein-Barr virus. Am J Clin Pathol 105:230–237, 1996.

Boiocchi M, De Re V, Gloghini A, et al: High incidence of monoclonal EBV episomes in Hodgkin's disease and anaplastic large-cell Ki-1-positive lymphomas in HIV-1-positive patients. Int J Cancer 54:53, 1993.

Carbone A, Gloghini A, Gaidano G, et al: AIDS-related Burkitt's lymphoma. Morphologic and immunophenotypic study of biopsy specimens. Am J Clin Pathol 103:561–567, 1995.

Carbone A, Tirelli U, Vaccher E, et al: A clinicopathologic study of lymphoid neoplasia associated with human immunodeficiency virus infection in Italy. Cancer 68:842, 1991.

Cesarman E, Chang Y, Moore PS, et al: Kaposi's sarcoma-associated her-

pes virus-like DNA sequences in AIDS-related body-cavity-based lymphomas. N Engl J Med 332:1186–1191, 1995.

Chan JKC, Lewin KJ, Lombard CM, et al: Histopathology of bacillary angiomatosis of lymph node. Am J Surg Pathol 15:430–437, 1991.

Chan JKC, Warnke RA, Dorfman R: Vascular transformation of sinuses in lymph nodes. A study of its morphological spectrum and distinction from Kaposi's sarcoma. Am J Surg Pathol 15:732–743, 1991.

Chang Y, Cesarman E, Pessin MS, et al: Identification of herpes virus-like DNA sequences in AIDS-associated Kaposi's sarcoma. Science 266:1865–1869, 1994.

Cotell SL, Noskin GA: Bacillary angiomatosis. Clinical and histologic features, diagnosis and treatment. Arch Intern Med 154:524–528, 1994.

DiGiuseppe JA, Wu T-C, Corio RL: Analysis of Epstein-Barr virus-encoded small RNA 1 expression in benign lymphoepithelial salivary gland lesions. Mod Pathol 7:555–559, 1994.

Elliott JN, Oertel YC: Lymphoepithelial cysts of the salivary gland. Histologic and cytologic features. Am J Clin Pathol 93:39–43, 1990.

Gaidano G, Lo Coco F, Ye BH, et al: Rearrangements of the BCL-6 gene in acquired immunodeficiency syndrome-associated non-Hodgkin's lymphoma: association with diffuse large-cell type. Blood 84:397–402, 1994.

Gloghini A, De Paoli P, Gaidano G, Franceschi S, Carbone A: High frequency of CD45RO expression in AIDS-related B-cell non-Hodgkin's lymphomas. Am J Clin Pathol 104:680–688, 1995.

Hamilton-Dutoit S, Pallesen G, Franzmann M, *et al*: AIDS-related lymphoma. Histopathology, immunophenotype, and association with Epstein-Barr virus as demonstrated by in situ nucleic acid hybridization. Am J Pathol 138:149–163, 1991.

Hamilton-Dutoit SJ, Rea D, Raphael M, *et al*: Epstein-Barr virus-latent gene expression and tumor cell phenotype in acquired immunodeficiency syndrome-related non-Hodgkin's lymphoma. Correlation of lymphoma phenotype with three distinct patterns of viral latency. Am J Pathol 143(4):1072–1085, 1993.

Harris NL: Hypervascular follicular hyperplasia and Kaposi's sarcoma in patients at risk for AIDS. N Engl J Med 310:462–463, 1984.

Ioachim HL, Cronin W, Roy M, Maya M: Persistent lymphadenopathies in people at high risk for HIV infection. Clinicopathologic correlations and long-term follow-up in 79 cases. Am J Clin Pathol 93:208–218, 1990.

Knecht H, Raphael M, McQuain C, *et al*: Deletion variants within the NF-κB activation domain of the LMP1 oncogene prevail in acquired immunodeficiency syndrome-related large cell lymphomas and human immunodeficiency virus-negative atypical lymphoproliferations. Blood 87(3):876–881, 1996.

Knowles DM, Chamulak G, Subar M, *et al*: Clinicopathologic, immunophenotypic and molecular genetic analysis of AIDS-associated lymphoid neoplasia. Clinical and biologic implications. Pathol Ann Part 2:33–67, 1988.

Labouyrie E, Merlio JPH, Beylot-Barry M, *et al*: Human immunodeficiency virus type 1 replication within cystic lymphoepithelial lesion of the salivary gland. Am J Clin Pathol 100:41–46, 1993.

Medeiros LJ, Greiner TC: Hodgkin's disease. Cancer 75(Suppl 1):357–369, 1995.

Nadal D, Caduff R, Frey E, *et al*: Non-Hodgkin's lymphoma in four children infected with the human immunodeficiency virus. Cancer 73:224–230, 1994.

Neri A, Barriga F, Inghirami G, *et al*: Epstein-Barr virus infection precedes clonal expansion in Burkitt's and acquired immunodeficiency syndrome-associated lymphoma. Blood 77:1092, 1991.

Newcom SR, Ward M, Napoli VM, *et al*: Treatment of human immunodeficiency virus-associated Hodgkin disease. Is there a clue regarding the cause of Hodgkin's disease? Cancer 71:3138–3145, 1993.

O'Murchadha MT, Wolf BC, Neiman RS: The histologic features of hyperplastic lymphadenopathy in AIDS-related complex are nonspecific. Am J Surg Pathol 11:94–99, 1987.

Pinkus GS, Lones M, Shintaku IP, Said JW: Immunohistochemical detection of Epstein-Barr virus-encoded latent membrane protein in Reed-Sternberg cells and variants of Hodgkin's disease. Mod Pathol 7:454–461, 1994.

Raphael MM, Audouin J, Lamine M, *et al*: Immunophenotypic and genotypic analysis of acquired immunodeficiency syndrome-related non-Hodgkin's lymphomas. Correlation with histologic features in 36 cases. Am J Clin Pathol 101:773–782, 1994.

Ryan JR, Ioachim HL, Marmer J, Loubeau JM: Acquired immune deficiency syndrome-related lymphadenopathies presenting in the salivary gland lymph nodes. Arch Otolaryngol 111:554–556, 1985.

Shibata D, Weiss LM, Hernandez AM, *et al*: Epstein-Barr virus-associated non-Hodgkin's lymphoma in patients infected with the human immunodeficiency virus. Blood 81:2102–2109, 1993.

Shibata D, Weiss LM, Nathwani BN, *et al*: Epstein-Barr virus in benign lymph node biopsies from individuals infected with the human immunodeficiency virus is associated with concurrent or subsequent development of non-Hodgkin's lymphoma. Blood 77:1527–1533, 1991.

Simon HB: Infections due to mycobacteria. Infect Dis 7:1–25, 1995.

Smith FB, Rajdeo H, Panesar N, *et al*: Benign lymphoepithelial lesion of the parotid gland in intravenous drug users. Arch Pathol Lab Med 112:742–745, 1988.

Tirelli V, Errante D, Dolcetti R, *et al*: Hodgkin's disease and human immunodeficiency virus infection: clinicopathologic and virologic features of 114 patients from the Italian Cooperative Group on AIDS and Tumors. J Clin Oncol 13:1758–1767, 1995.

Tirelli V, Vaccher E, Zagonel V, *et al*: CD30 (Ki-1)-positive anaplastic large-cell lymphomas in 13 patients with and 27 patients without human immunodeficiency. J Clin Oncol 13:373–380, 1995.

Wang CY, Snow JL, Su WP: Lymphoma associated with human immunodeficiency virus infection. (Review.) Mayo Clin Proc 70:665–672, 1995.

POST-TRANSPLANTATION LYMPHOPROLIFERATIVE DISORDERS (PTLD)

Clinical Features

Allograft recipients have an increased incidence of B-lineage lymphoproliferative disorders (B-PTLD) (Figs. 6–19 to 6–23). Among solid-organ recipients immunosuppressed with azathioprine-based regimens, the mean interval to PTLD following transplant is 48 months, and the PTLDs tend to involve extranodal sites, including the allograft and the central nervous system. Patients treated with cyclosporine-based regimens develop PTLDs that occur earlier (mean interval, 15 months) and that tend to involve lymph nodes and the gastrointestinal tract (*see* Figs. 6–19, 6–22, and 6–23), but are infrequent in the central nervous system. The overall risk for PTLD is approximately 1%, but the risk is higher among nonrenal allograft recipients and patients who are heavily immunosuppressed.

Patients treated with either regimen may present with an infectious mononucleosis-like illness, constitutional symptoms, lymphadenopathy, palpable extranodal masses, organomegaly, neurologic abnormalities, pulmonary symptoms, or gastrointestinal symptoms. Infrequently, PTLD may be an incidental finding at autopsy. Epstein-Barr virus (EBV) appears to play a critical role in the development of PTLDs of B lineage. Nearly all patients have serologic evidence of primary or reactivated EBV infection at the time of diagnosis of the PTLD, and in nearly all cases, immunophenotypic or genetic studies reveal evidence of EBV infection of the PTLD itself.

The prognosis of PTLD is highly variable and difficult to predict in individual cases. In general, a better outcome has been associated with disease confined to lymph nodes or to a single organ, resectable gastrointestinal tract disease, polymorphous histology, polyclonality, and donor-origin tumors, whereas a worse outcome is associated with presentation with organ dysfunction, central nervous system disease, disseminated disease, monomorphous or monoclonal tumors, host-origin tumors, and concurrent opportunistic infections. Some PTLDs, usually polymorphous polyclonal lesions, resolve with decreased immunosuppression alone. Others, particularly monomorphous, monoclonal tumors, require treatment similar to that used for high grade lymphoma in the general population. Even allograft recipients who have illnesses that in an immunologically normal patient would usually be self-limited, such as infectious mononucleosis, may experience progression to an overwhelming, fatal lymphoproliferative disorder; therefore, even the most innocuous appearing lymphoid infiltrate warrants careful pathologic examination and close clinical follow-up. A review of the literature shows that the mortality of B-PTLD is approximately 54% overall.

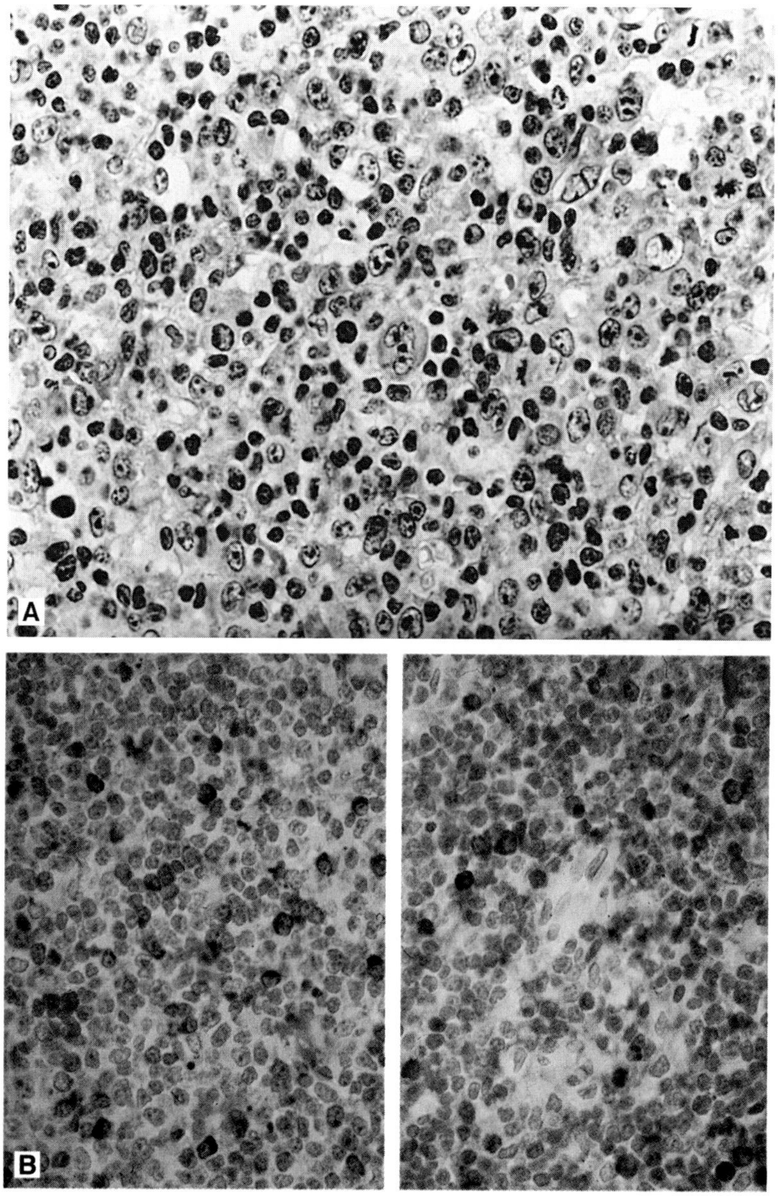

Figure 6–19. Post-transplantation lymphoproliferative disorder (PTLD), polymorphous, polyclonal (polymorphous B-cell hyperplasia), involving a lymph node in a patient with a cardiac transplant. The lesion regressed with decreased immunosuppression. *A,* The PTLD is composed of lymphocytes, plasma cells, plasmablasts, and a few immunoblasts, some of which are atypical *(center)* (H&E stain). (From Ferry JA, Harris NL: Lymphoproliferative disorders following organ transplantation. Adv Pathol Lab Med 7:359–387, 1994.) *B,* A mixture of κ+ *(left)* and λ+ *(right)* cells is present (immunoperoxidase technique on paraffin sections).

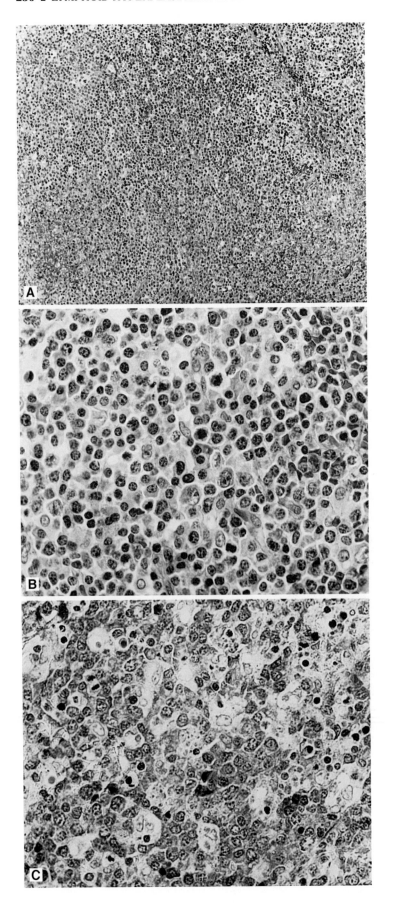

Figure 6–20. Post-transplantation lymphoproliferative disorder (PTLD), polymorphous, with polytypic Ig expression but clonal Ig gene rearrangement (polymorphous B-cell lymphoma), in a patient with a cardiac transplant treated with cyclosporine. *A,* Low power examination shows an infiltrate of lymphoid cells of various sizes and scattered histiocytes (H&E stain). *B,* In some areas, the infiltrate consists of a mixture of lymphocytes, plasmacytoid lymphocytes, numerous plasma cells, and a few immunoblasts (H&E stain). *C,* in other areas, plasmacytic differentiation is less striking, and the lymphoid population appears more monomorphous, with large numbers of tingible body macrophages (H&E stain).

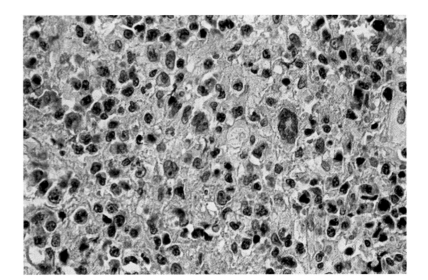

Figure 6–21. Post-transplantation lymphoproliferative disorder (PTLD), polymorphous (polymorphous B-cell lymphoma) involving the tonsils and adenoids of a child with a renal transplant. The specimen shows an infiltrate of small lymphocytes and atypical intermediate- and large-sized cells (H&E stain).

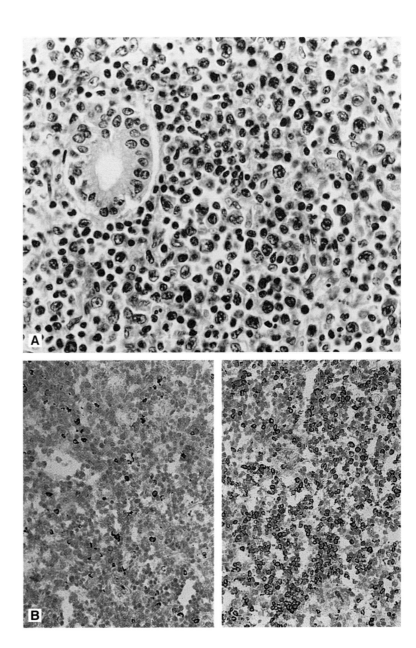

Figure 6–22. Post-transplantation lymphoproliferative disorder (PTLD), polymorphous, monoclonal, in a renal transplant recipient. *A,* A specimen from the stomach shows a dense, diffuse infiltrate of small-, intermediate-, and large-sized atypical lymphoid cells, with a suggestion of plasmacytic differentiation (H&E stain). *B,* The lymphoma expressed monotypic λ light chain (κ, *left*; λ, *right*; immunoperoxidase technique on frozen sections).

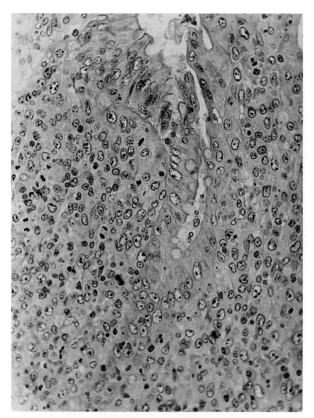

Figure 6–23. Post-transplantation lymphoproliferative disorder (PTLD), monomorphous, with monoclonal immunoglobulin expression, involving the colon of a renal allograft recipient treated with cyclosporine. A dense, diffuse infiltrate of centroblasts with a high mitotic rate is visible (H&E stain).

In allogeneic marrow recipients, the risk for PTLD is approximately 1%, although the risk is much higher when patients receive T-cell-depleted, mismatched marrow or anti-CD3 monoclonal antibody for treatment of graft-versus-host disease. Patients typically present with widespread disease and have a poor prognosis. A higher proportion of bone marrow transplant patients with PTLD die of their disease than do solid-organ allograft recipients.

A small proportion of PTLDs in both solid-organ and marrow recipients have a T lineage. The interval to the development of T-PTLD is longer, on average, than the interval to B-PTLD. Most patients have presented with disease in extranodal sites, including skin, heart, mediastinum, liver, vulva, and central nervous system; a few have presented with lymphadenopathy. The prognosis appears to be slightly worse than that for B-lineage PTLD. Two cases of T-PTLD seen at Massachusetts General Hospital were associated with hemophagocytic syndrome and a rapidly fatal course (Fig. 6–24).

Morphology

The histologic features of B-PLTD often differ from those of lymphoma in the general population. PTLDs show a range of changes, from hyperplastic processes resembling infectious mononucleosis to monomorphous infiltrates with the appearance of high grade lymphoma (see Figs. 6–19 to 6–23). Between these two extremes are the problematic cases: atypical lymphoid infiltrates that are more polymorphous than the usual lymphoma, but show a greater degree of architectural effacement and more cytologic atypia than expected in reactive lymphoid hyperplasia. Subclassification is controversial, and several different groups have proposed classification systems (Tables 6–1 and 6–2). The classification proposed at the University of Pittsburgh has three categories: polymorphous, minimally polymorphous, and monomorphous (see Table 6–1). The polymorphous category is characterized by an infiltrate of lymphoid cells representing a broad spectrum of B-cell maturation, including small lymphocytes, centrocytes (cleaved cells), centroblasts (large noncleaved cells), immunoblasts, and plasma cells. In the minimally polymorphous category, the infiltrate consists of plasma cells and lymphoid cells with plasmacytic features. Most monomorphous cases consist of a diffuse infiltrate of centroblasts, immunoblasts, or small noncleaved cells. The appearance may be indistinguishable from diffuse large B-cell lymphoma or Burkitt's lymphoma in the general population.

Five categories appear in the classification devised by Frizzera and Knowles and their co-workers (see Table 6–2). The first, plasmacytic hyperplasia, occurs mainly in the oropharynx and lymph nodes. The architecture of the lymph node or extranodal tissue is preserved. The infiltrate consists of plasma cells, plasmacytoid lymphocytes, and a few immunoblasts. The remaining four categories all differ from plasmacytic hyperplasia by displaying architectural effacement by the lymphoid infiltrate and by consistently demonstrating clonal immunoglobulin gene rearrangement and clonal EBV. The second category, polymorphic B-cell hyperplasia (PBCH), is composed of plasma cells, plasmacytoid lymphocytes, and immunoblasts; it affects lymph nodes or extranodal sites. The third category, polymorphic B-cell lymphoma (PBCL), differs from PBCH mainly by the presence of atypical immunoblasts and prominent necrosis. The fourth category, immunoblastic lymphoma (IBL), is characterized by a population of large atypical lymphoid cells. In some cases, these atypical cells have the appearance of a relatively monomorphous population of immunoblasts, sometimes with plasmacytic differentiation; in other cases, they have the appearance of bizarre, pleomorphic, anaplastic large lymphoid cells. The fifth category, multiple myeloma, is characterized by a population of atypical plasma cells. Both IBL and multiple myeloma tend to produce disseminated disease.

Because of the overlap in clinical and pathologic features between PBCH and PBCL and between IBL and multiple

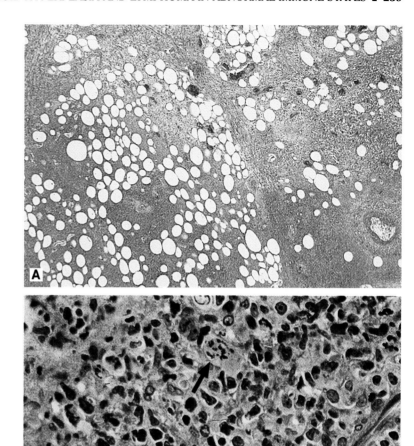

Figure 6–24. Post-transplantation lymphoproliferative disorder (PTLD) of T-cell lineage involving the vulva of a renal transplant recipient, possibly an example of subcutaneous panniculitic T-cell lymphoma. *A,* The subcutaneous tissue is extensively involved by lymphoma (H&E stain). *B,* The lymphoma consists of large, pleomorphic lymphoid cells. An atypical mitotic figure is present (*arrow,* H&E stain).

Illustration continued on following page.

myeloma, the categories have been combined, so that the Frizzera-Knowles Classification has three main diagnostic groups: (1) plasmacytic hyperplasia; (2) PBCH/PBCL; and (3) IBL/multiple myeloma. The PBCH/PBCL category, and perhaps some cases of plasmacytic hyperplasia, correspond to the University of Pittsburgh polymorphous category; IBL corresponds to the monomorphous category. It is not clear that cases in the multiple myeloma category have an equivalent in the University of Pittsburgh Classification. In studies using both classifications, the same patient could have PTLD of one type in one anatomic site or at one time, and PTLD with a different appearance in another anatomic site or at a different time.

For reasons that are not certain, the histologic types of B-PTLD vary substantially from one medical center to another, with some reporting a high proportion of polymorphic lesions and others, a predominance of monomorphic lesions.

Table 6–1
CLASSIFICATION OF PTLD, UNIVERSITY OF PITTSBURGH

Category	Lymphoid Population	Monotypic Ig	IgH-R*
Polymorphous	Small lymphocytes, plasma cells, cleaved & non-cleaved cells, immunoblasts	Some cases	Some cases
Minimally polymorphous	Plasma cells, lymphoid cells with plasmacytic features	Majority	Majority
Monomorphous	Usually large non-cleaved cells or small noncleaved cells	Nearly all†	All

*Clonal Ig heavy chain gene rearrangement.
†Some monomorphous PTLDs are Ig-negative.

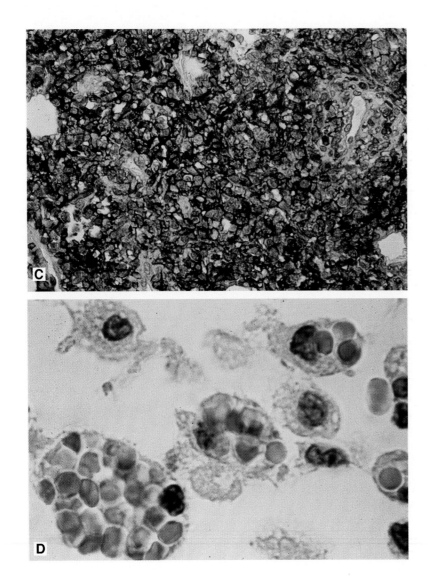

Figure 6–24. *Continued C,* The neoplastic cells are strongly positive for CD45RO, consistent with T-lineage (immunoperoxidase technique on paraffin sections). *D,* The lymphoma was rapidly fatal, and at autopsy, the individual was found to have extensive hemophagocytosis, shown here in the sinuses of a lymph node (H&E stain).

Table 6–2
CLASSIFICATION OF POST-TRANSPLANTATION LYMPHOPROLIFERATIVE DISORDER (PTLD), FRIZZERA AND KNOWLES

Category*	Involved Sites	Architecture	Cellular Composition	Clonality (Ig)	Clonality (EBV)	N-ras or p53 Mutations	c-myc Rearrangement
Plasmacytic hyperplasia	Oropharynx, lymph nodes	Preserved	Plasma cells, plasma-cytoid lymphocytes, few immunoblasts	Almost always polyclonal	Polyclonal with/without small monoclonal population	Absent	Absent
Polymorphic B-cell hyperplasia (PBCH)	Lymph nodes, extranodal sites	Effaced	Plasma cells, plasma-cytoid lymphocytes, immunoblasts; at most, small foci of necrosis	Monoclonal	Almost always monoclonal	Absent	Absent
Polymorphic B-cell lymphoma (PBCL)	Lymph nodes, extranodal sites	Effaced	Mixture of atypical lymphoid cells without striking plasmacytic differentiation and with atypical immunoblasts; extensive necrosis	Monoclonal	Monoclonal	Absent	Absent
Immuno-blastic lymphoma (IBL)	Disseminated	Effaced	Monomorphous population of large atypical lymphoid cells with/without bizarre, pleomorphic nuclei or plasmacytic features	Monoclonal	Monoclonal	Sometimes	Sometimes
Multiple myeloma (MM)	Disseminated	Effaced	Monomorphous population of atypical plasma cells	Monoclonal	Monoclonal	Sometimes	Minority

*Because of features shared by PBCH and PBCL, and by IBL and MM, these categories can be combined to obtain three main diagnostic groups: (1) plasmacytic hyperplasia; (2) PBCH/PBCL; and (3) IBL/MM.

The classifications just described include almost all cases of B-PTLD. A few cases, however, have been described as having the appearance of T-cell-rich B-cell lymphoma, isolated plasmacytoma, and lymphomatoid granulomatosis.

At our institution, we make a diagnosis of reactive lymphoid hyperplasia in cases without enough cytologic or architectural atypia to raise the question of lymphoma. For cases that fulfill the standard criteria for a diagnosis of lymphoma, we make a diagnosis of malignant lymphoma, subclassified according to the R.E.A.L. Classification, consistent with PTLD, monomorphous (occasionally polymorphous), and report the results of immunophenotyping or genetic studies, which virtually always confirm monoclonality. For atypical cases that do not fulfill standard criteria for a diagnosis of lymphoma, we make a diagnosis of atypical lymphoid infiltrate, consistent with PTLD, polymorphous, and report results of immunophenotyping and genetic studies (polyclonal or monoclonal).

Unlike B-PTLDs, T-PTLDs usually have histologic features similar to those seen in T-cell lymphomas in immunocompetent patients. Several T-lineage PTLDs have been lymphoblastic lymphomas. The remainder have been peripheral T-cell lymphomas and have included anaplastic large cell lymphoma, intestinal T-cell lymphoma (associated with celiac disease), mycosis fungoides, adult T-cell lymphoma/leukemia, and peripheral T-cell lymphoma, unspeci-

fied. One of the cases seen at Massachusetts General Hospital most likely represents a subcutaneous panniculitic T-cell lymphoma, although it had greater cytologic atypia and appeared to be a higher grade lymphoma than most previously described cases in this category (see Fig. 6–24). It is possible that some cases of T-PTLD may be T-cell lymphomas occurring sporadically, rather than being directly related to prior transplantation.

Immunophenotype

Monomorphous B-PTLDs (including immunoblastic lymphoma and multiple myeloma in the Frizzera-Knowles Classification) either express monotypic immunoglobulin (Ig) or are immunoglobulin negative (see Fig. 6–23). Certain polymorphous B-PTLDs express monotypic Ig (see Fig. 6–22), whereas other polymorphous B-PTLDs express polytypic Ig (see Fig. 6–19). Examination of immunostained frozen sections is optimal for detection of surface immunoglobulin, but paraffin section immunohistochemistry is better for detection of cytoplasmic immunoglobulin. Because many B-PTLDs show plasmacytic differentiation, we frequently obtain both frozen and paraffin section immunohistochemical studies to assess immunoglobulin expression more precisely. EBV-LMP and EBNA expression is often found in both monomorphous and polymorphous lesions.

The immunophenotype of T-PTLD is similar to that of the corresponding type of T-cell lymphoma in the general population (see Fig. 6–24C).

Genetic Features

Virtually all monomorphous PTLDs and the majority of polymorphous PTLDs (including many cases that appear to express polytypic immunoglobulin) show Ig gene rearrangement. In the Frizzera-Knowles plasmacytic hyperplasia category, clonal Ig gene rearrangement is usually absent. Southern blot hybridization is a much more sensitive method than immunophenotyping (detecting clonal populations of cells of 5% or less); therefore, a monoclonal population will be found in a higher proportion of polymorphous cases by using this technique than by using immunophenotyping (see Fig. 6–20).

EBV DNA is found in nearly all cases. In one study that used a probe to the fused termini of episomal EBV, the EBV DNA was in a monoclonal episomal form in 79% of cases, which is consistent with a clonal population latently infected by EBV. In 15% of cases, oligoclonal EBV was present; in 4%, only linear, replicating virus was found; and in 2%, no EBV genetic material was identified. Clonal EBV is found in virtually all monomorphous (including immunoblastic lymphoma and multiple myeloma) and polymorphous B-PTLDs. In the plasmacytic hyperplasia category, polyclonal EBV is usually evident; if a monoclonal population is present, it is small.

Assessment of EBV clonality is an even more sensitive way of identifying a clonal population in PTLDs than evaluation of immunoglobulin genes. Some cases that appear to be polyclonal by immunoglobulin gene rearrangement contain a population of cells infected by monoclonal EBV. Possible explanations for these observations are the following: (1) Assessment of EBV clonality is more sensitive than evaluating immunoglobulin genes—this could be the case if multiple copies of EBV were present in each cell of a small clonal population; (2) EBV infection occurred at an early stage in B-cell development, prior to completion of immunoglobulin gene rearrangement.

In a few cases, tissue from PTLDs from different sites (or from different times) from the same patient have been available for evaluation. In some of these cases, different immunoglobulin gene rearrangements were found in tissue from the different sites, suggesting these patients had multiple, independent PTLDs. When EBV clonality of the different lesions was determined, however, at least in some cases, the same clonal EBV was found in the different sites, indicating that the PTLDs were clonally related. In other cases, different clonal populations of EBV have been found in different sites, consistent with clonally unrelated PTLDs.

A highly sensitive and relatively rapid and easy method of demonstrating the presence of latent EBV infection is using in situ hybridization to detect EBV-encoded small RNA (EBER). The EBV found in PTLD has been A type, rather than B type; this result is similar to that seen in EBV+ lymphomas in the general population. EBV type B tends to be encountered in lymphomas only when patients are immunosuppressed. In endemic Burkitt's lymphoma and in HIV-associated lymphomas, for example, EBV of either type A or B can be found. It is thus somewhat surprising that EBV type B is not found in PTLD, which is associated so strongly with immunosuppression.

A few cases of monomorphous PTLD (or, in the Frizzera-Knowles Classification, immunoblastic lymphoma and multiple myeloma) have had abnormalities of p53 and N-ras, or have had c-myc rearrangement of the type associated with sporadic Burkitt's lymphoma. These genetic alterations have not been described in any polymorphous B-PTLDs or in plasmacytic hyperplasia.

Only rare T-PTLDs contain EBV; thus EBV is not considered to be important in the pathogenesis of most T-PTLDs.

In a minority of cases of PTLD, the origin of the tumor (donor versus recipient) has been determined. Among solid-organ allograft recipients, the majority of PTLDs (approximately 75%) have been of recipient origin. Although follow-up has been available in only a small number of cases, the minority of patients with donor-origin tumors appear to have a better outcome, possibly because decreasing their immunosuppressive therapy allows their immune system to better recognize the PTLD as "foreign" and thereby "reject" the tumor.

In contrast, among bone marrow recipients, most PTLDs have been of donor origin. PTLDs in this group are usually fatal, and no subset has an apparent survival advantage.

Differential Diagnosis

1. Reactive lymphoid hyperplasia, including rejection: PTLDs with a polymorphous composition can be considered in the differential diagnosis of reactive hyperplasia. Features in favor of a diagnosis of PTLD include obliteration of normal architecture, high proportion of large lymphoid cells, or atypical cells, high proportion of B cells, zonal necrosis, presence of EBV in many cells, and evidence of a monoclonal population of lymphoid cells by immunophenotyping or genetic studies.

   Some hyperplastic lesions can be followed by aggressive PTLD, and therapy for rejection may increase the chance for developing PTLD, so that patients with seemingly innocuous reactive lesions should undergo additional biopsies if they subsequently develop lesions clinically suggestive of PTLD.

2. Hodgkin's disease (HD): Polymorphous PTLDs contain a variety of cell types, including lymphocytes, plasma cells, and occasionally, atypical immunoblasts with an appearance reminiscent of Reed-Sternberg cells, and can mimic Hodgkin's disease. In addition, rare cases of B-PTLDs have the appearance of T-cell-rich B-cell lymphomas, and the differential diagnosis can be especially

problematic. A diagnosis of HD should be made only with caution in an allograft recipient. Confirmation of the immunophenotype is suggested to avoid misdiagnosis.

References

Cesarman E, Chadburn A, Frizzera G, et al: Molecular genetic analysis of post-transplantation lymphoproliferative disorders (PT-LPDs). Mod Pathol 7:104A, 1994.

Chen JM, Barr ML, Chadburn A, et al: Management of lymphoproliferative disorders after cardiac transplantation. Ann Thorac Surg 56: 527–538, 1993.

Cleary ML, Nalesnik MA, Shearer WT, et al: Clonal analysis of transplant-associated lymphoproliferations based on the structure of the genomic termini of the Epstein-Barr virus. Blood 72:349–352, 1988.

D'Amore ESG, Manivel JC, Gajl-Peczalska KJ, et al: B-cell lymphoproliferative disorders after bone marrow transplant: an analysis of ten cases with emphasis on Epstein-Barr virus detection by in situ hybridization. Cancer 68:1285–1295, 1991.

Ferry JA, Harris NL: Pathology of posttransplant lymphoproliferative disorders. In: Solez K, Racusen LC, Billingham ME, eds. Solid organ transplant rejection. Mechanisms, pathology and diagnosis. New York: Marcel Dekker, 1996;277–301.

Ferry JA, Jacobson JO, Conti D, et al: Lymphoproliferative disorders and hematologic malignancies following organ transplantation. Mod Pathol 2:583–592, 1989.

Frank D, Cesarman E, Liu YF, et al: Post-transplantation lymphoproliferative disorders frequently contain type A and not type B Epstein-Barr virus. Blood 85:1396–1403, 1995.

Frizzera G, Hanto DW, Gajl-Peczalska KJ, et al: Polymorphic diffuse B cell hyperplasias and lymphomas in renal transplant recipients. Cancer Res 41:4262–4279, 1981.

Hanto DW, Gajl-Peczalska KJ, Frizzera G, et al: Epstein-Barr virus (EBV) induced polyclonal and monoclonal B-cell lymphoproliferative diseases occurring after renal transplantation. Ann Surg 198:356–368, 1983.

Kaplan MA, Ferry JA, Harris NL, et al: Clonal analysis of post-transplant lymphoproliferative disorders, using both episomal EBV and immunoglobulin genes as markers. Am J Clin Pathol 101:590–596, 1994.

Kaplan MA, Jacobson JO, Ferry JA, et al: T-cell lymphoma of the vulva in a renal allograft recipient with associated hemophagocytosis. Am J Surg Pathol 17:842–849, 1993.

Katz BZ, Raab-Traub N, Miller G: Latent and replicating forms of Epstein-Barr virus DNA in lymphomas and lymphoproliferative diseases. J Infect Dis 160:589–598, 1989.

Knowles DM, Cesarman E, Chadburn A, et al: Correlative morphologic and molecular genetic analysis demonstrates three distinct categories of posttransplantation lymphoproliferative disorders. Blood 85:552–565, 1995.

Kowal-Vern A, Swinnen L, Pyle J, et al: Characterization of postcardiac transplant lymphomas. Histology, immunophenotyping, immunohistochemistry, and gene rearrangement. Arch Pathol Lab Med 120:41–48, 1996.

Kumar S, Kumar D, Kingma DW, et al: Epstein-Barr virus-associated T-cell lymphoma in a renal transplant patient. Am J Surg Pathol 17:1046–1053, 1993.

Locker J, Nalesnik M: Molecular genetic analysis of lymphoid tumors arising after organ transplantation. Am J Pathol 135:977–987, 1993.

Nalesnik M, Jaffe R, Starzl TE, et al: The pathology of posttransplant lymphoproliferative disorders occurring in the setting of cyclosporine A-prednisone immunosuppression. Am J Pathol 133:173–192, 1988.

Opelz G, Henderson R: Incidence of non-Hodgkin's lymphoma in kidney and heart transplant recipients. Lancet 342:1514–1516, 1993.

Penn I: The changing pattern of posttransplant malignancies. Transplant Proc 23:1101–1103, 1991.

Randhawa PS, Magnone M, Jordan M, et al: Renal allograft involvement by Epstein-Barr virus associated post-transplant lymphoproliferative disease. Am J Surg Pathol 20(5):563–571, 1996.

Rosendale B, Yousem SA: Discrimination of Epstein-Barr virus-related posttransplantation lymphoproliferations from acute rejection in lung allograft recipients. Arch Pathol Lab Med 119:418–423, 1995.

Swinnen LJ, Costanzo-Nordin MR, Fisher S, et al: Increased incidence of lymphoproliferative disorder after immunosuppression with the monoclonal antibody OKT3 in cardiac transplant recipients. N Engl J Med 323:1723–1728, 1990.

Weissmann DJ, Ferry JA, Harris NL, et al: Posttransplantation lymphoproliferative disorders in solid organ recipients are predominantly aggressive tumors of host origin. Am J Clin Pathol 103:748–755, 1995.

Lymphoma in Chromosome Breakage Syndromes

Chromosome breakage syndromes (CBS) are associated with an increased incidence of malignancy, often accompanied by immunodeficiency. The malignancies seem to be primarily caused by the tendency for chromosomal damage, rather than the immunodeficiency. Ataxia-telangiectasia, Bloom's syndrome, and Nijmegen breakage syndrome are discussed in this section. Fanconi's anemia and xeroderma pigmentosum are CBS characterized by increased risk for leukemia and cutaneous malignancies, respectively, but not for lymphoma; therefore they are not included.

ATAXIA-TELANGIECTASIA (AT)

Clinical Features

Ataxia-telangiectasia (AT) is an autosomal recessive disorder characterized by progressive cerebellar ataxia, ocular and cutaneous telangiectasia, chronic sinopulmonary infections, poor intellectual development, and variable immunodeficiency often affecting both B and T cells. B-cell defects are usually manifested as deficiency of IgG, IgA, or

IgE. Most patients also have a deficiency of cell-mediated immunity.

These patients have a striking increase in the incidence of lymphoma and lymphoid leukemia, as well as a smaller increase in certain carcinomas, nearly all of which present during the first two decades of life, in accordance with patients' shortened lifespans. In one large series, 46% of malignancies in AT patients were non-Hodgkin's lymphomas; 21%, leukemias; and 11%, Hodgkin's disease. The remainder were nonlymphoid neoplasms.

Among cases of non-Hodgkin's lymphoma, males are affected nearly twice as often as females, the median age at diagnosis is 8.5 years, and nodal or extranodal sites are affected. Patients are overly sensitive to radiation and chemotherapy, thus malignancies are especially difficult to treat and are often fatal. Although some patients reach adulthood, the lifespan is shortened significantly. Approximately 1% of the population are AT heterozygotes; these individuals also have an increased incidence of malignancy, although the risk is much less than that of AT homozygotes. Heterozygotes have an increased risk for leukemia and lymphoma, as well as for carcinomas commonly found in adults, including ovarian, gastric, breast, and other carcinomas. As many as 8% of all breast carcinomas may occur in AT heterozygotes. AT heterozygotes may represent more than 5% of all persons dying of carcinoma before age 45.

Morphology

The lymphomas are of a variety of types, both high and low grade non-Hodgkin's lymphomas. Lymphoid leukemias are of both acute lymphoblastic and chronic lymphocytic types. The majority of lymphomas are diffuse large B-cell type (Fig. 6–25), but there is greater diversity in the types of lymphoma in AT than in other immunodeficiency syndromes.

Lymphoid tissues have a depleted appearance and lack germinal centers. The thymus is atrophic and lacks Hassall's corpuscles. Bizarre, multinucleated, aneuploid cells may be found in many organs, and are thought to be due to defective ability to repair DNA. The cerebellum is small.

Immunophenotype

Lymphomas and leukemias of B- and T-cell types are described. Epstein-Barr virus nuclear antigen (EBNA) expression has been reported.

Genetic Features

The AT gene has been mapped to chromosome 11q22-23; the defective gene codes for a protein with similarities to phosphatidylinositol-3 kinases, which are important in sig-

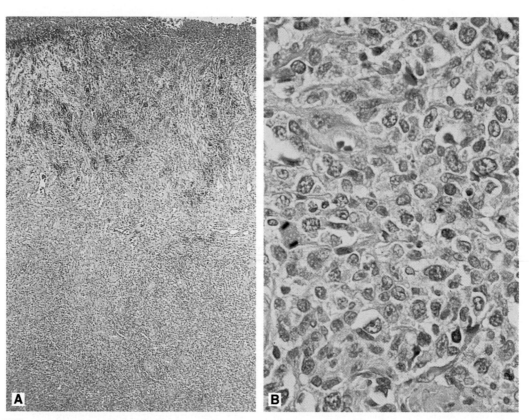

Figure 6–25. Diffuse large B-cell lymphoma involving the tonsil in ataxia-telangiectasia. *A,* The tonsil is ulcerated; the lymphoma lies beneath a thick layer of granulation tissue (H&E stain). *B,* The lymphoma is composed predominantly of centroblasts (H&E stain).

nal transduction for cellular growth control, and to a group of proteins that block cellular division until damaged DNA is repaired.

EBV DNA has been found in AT-associated non-Hodgkin's lymphoma. Non-neoplastic cells show a high frequency of chromosomal breaks on chromosomes 7 and 14 in the region of T-cell-receptor (TCR) and Ig genes.

Differential Diagnosis

The differential diagnosis is the same as that for lymphoma in the general population.

References

Case Records of the Massachusetts General Hospital, Case 2-1987. N Engl J Med 316:91–100, 1987.
Filipovich AH, Mathur A, Kamat D, Shapiro RS: Primary immunodeficiencies: genetic risk factors for lymphoma. Cancer Research (Suppl)52:5465s–5467s, 1992.
Frizzera G, Rosai J, Dehner LP, et al: Lymphoreticular disorders in primary immunodeficiencies: new findings based on an up-to-date histologic classification. Cancer 46:692–699, 1980.
Hecht F, Hecht BK: Cancer in ataxia-telangiectasia patients. Cancer Genet Cytogenet 46:9–19, 1990.
Kersey JH, Spector BD, Good RA: Primary immunodeficiencies and cancer: the immunodeficiency cancer registry. Int J Cancer 12:333–347, 1973.
Nowak R: Discovery of AT gene sparks biomedical research bonanza. (Editorial.) Science 268:1700–1701, 1995.
Okano M, Osato T, Koizumi S, et al: Epstein-Barr virus infection and oncogenesis in primary immunodeficiency. Aids Research 2(Suppl 1):S115–S119, 1986.
Savitsky K, Bar-Shira A, Gilad S, et al: A single ataxia-telangiectasia gene with a product similar to PI-3 kinase. Science 268:1749–1753, 1995.
Swift M, Sholman L, Perry M, Chase C: Malignant neoplasms in the families of patients with ataxia-telangiectasia. Cancer Res 36:209–215, 1976.

BLOOM'S SYNDROME

Clinical Features

Bloom's syndrome is an unusual autosomal recessive disorder with an increased incidence among Ashkenazy Jews. Patients have low birth weight, growth retardation, narrow faces, sun sensitivity with malar telangiectasia, café au lait spots, immunodeficiency, and an increased incidence of malignancy. Approximately one-fourth develop malignancy before age 20. In one series of 27 tumors, 7 were non-Hodgkin's lymphoma; 1, Hodgkin's disease; 10, acute leukemias (5 lymphocytic, 5 nonlymphocytic); 8, carcinomas of types commonly seen in adults; and 1, Wilms' tumor. Life span is shortened.

Morphology and Immunophenotype

Limited information on lymphoma in Bloom's syndrome is available. Burkitt's and Burkitt-like lymphoma, however, and diffuse large cell lymphoma have been reported. Immunophenotyping has shown B lineage in some cases.

Genetic Features

Patients have a high frequency of spontaneous chromosomal breakage believed to be caused by defective DNA ligase I activity; translocations tend to occur between homologous chromosomes. Immunoglobulin heavy chain rearrangement has been reported, and EBV DNA is sometimes found in the lymphomas.

References

German J, Bloom D, Passarge E: Bloom's syndrome. VII. Progress report for 1978. Clinical Genetics 15:361–367, 1979.
Gretzula JC, Hevia O, Weber PJ: Bloom's syndrome. J Am Acad Dermatol 17:479–488, 1987.
Ota S, Miyamoto S, Kudoh F, et al: Treatment for B-cell-type lymphoma in a girl associated with Bloom's syndrome. Clin Genet 41:46–50, 1992.
Vandenberghe E, Van Hove J, Brock P: Non-endemic Burkitt's lymphoma in a patient with Bloom's syndrome. Leuk Lymphoma 10:377–382, 1993.
Wright DH, Isaacson P: Follicular center cell lymphoma of childhood: a report of three cases and a discussion of its relationship to Burkitt's lymphoma. Cancer 47:915–925, 1981.

NIJMEGEN BREAKAGE SYNDROME (NBS)

Clinical Features

Patients have microcephaly, mental retardation, short stature, bird-like facial features, immunodeficiency, and café au lait spots. Six of 19 known patients have developed non-Hodgkin's lymphoma. Lymphoma and pneumonia are the most common causes of death in NBS. Sensitivity to ionizing radiation is increased. The etiology of this rare disorder seems to be a defect in DNA processing similar to that found in ataxia-telangiectasia.

Morphology and Immunophenotype

The lymphomas have been diffuse high grade B-cell lymphomas.

Genetic Features

The incidence of spontaneous chromosomal breakage is high, often involving chromosomes 7 and 14. Genetic features of the lymphomas have been studied in only a few cases, but clonal immunoglobulin heavy chain gene rearrangement has been reported, and lymphomas have been EBV-negative.

References

Taylor AMR, McConville CM, Byrd PJ: Cancer and DNA processing disorders. Br Med Bull 50:708–717, 1994.
Van de Kaa CA, Weemaes CMR, Wesseling P, et al: Postmortem findings in the Nijmegen breakage syndrome. Pediatric Pathol 14:787–796, 1994.
Weemaes CMR, Hustinx TWJ, Scheres JMJC, et al: A new chromosomal instability disorder: the Nijmegen breakage syndrome. Acta Paediatr Scand 70:557–564, 1981.

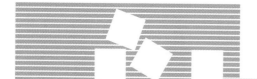

CHAPTER 7

Hematologic Disorders
That Mimic Lymphoma

Nonlymphoid disorders are often considered in the differential diagnosis of lymphoma. Three unusual disorders—granulocytic sarcoma, mast cell disease, and plasmacytoid monocyte proliferation—present special problems in this context, and for this reason, they are discussed here.

GRANULOCYTIC SARCOMA

Clinical Features

Granulocytic sarcoma (chloroma) occurs in one of three settings: (1) in patients known to have acute myeloid leukemia; (2) in patients with chronic myeloproliferative disorders or myelodysplastic syndromes; and (3) in patients with no prior hematologic disease. In patients with a myeloproliferative disorder, the development of granulocytic sarcoma coincides with a high risk of blast crisis. In patients with myelodysplasia, the presence of a granulocytic sarcoma frequently heralds development of acute myeloid leukemia. Most patients with granulocytic sarcoma and no prior evidence of hematologic disease will also develop acute myeloid leukemia unless they are treated aggressively.

Granulocytic sarcomas may involve a wide variety of sites, including bone, soft tissue, lymph nodes, skin, male and female genital tracts, nasal cavity, and others.

Morphology

Granulocytic sarcomas are tumors of immature myeloid cells. The neoplastic cells may show evidence of myeloid differentiation, including nuclear indentation or segmentation, or an admixture of cells recognizable as eosinophil precursors, but more often, they are almost exclusively blasts with round to oval nuclei; fine, evenly dispersed chromatin; small nucleoli; and scant, agranular cytoplasm. The tumor cells infiltrate tissue diffusely, with some tendency to spare the underlying architecture. Some cases are associated with

sclerosis, which is usually mild, but occasionally may be marked. The mitotic rate is usually high (Figs. 7–1 to 7–5).

Enzyme Histochemistry and Immunophenotype

With a chloroacetate esterase (CAE) stain, the neoplastic cells show pink to red granular staining (Fig. 7–3B). Only a few cells stain in some cases, however, and careful examination may be required to make the diagnosis.

Using immunohistochemical stains on paraffin sections, the neoplastic cells are usually at least focally myeloperoxidase+, lysozyme+, or CD43+, and may express CD45 or CD68 (Fig. 7–5B). On frozen sections, tumor cells are CD45+, CD13+, CD33+, and CD15+/−. They are usually negative for B-cell markers and for T-associated antigens (other than CD43).

Differential Diagnosis

1. Malignant lymphoma: The most common misdiagnosis in cases of granulocytic sarcoma is lymphoma, usually diffuse large cell type. Immature myeloid cells have more finely dispersed chromatin, cytoplasm that may have an eosinophilic blush, and in some cases, evidence of myeloid differentiation such as eosinophilic myelocytes. Immunohistochemical stains or a CAE stain can establish the diagnosis in difficult cases.
2. Plasmacytoma: Uncommonly, granulocytic sarcomas may contain a prominent component of myelocytes, with somewhat eccentrically placed nuclei and relatively abundant cytoplasm. The appearance may mimic an infiltrate of immature plasma cells. Finding cytoplasm that is pink to red and granular supports a diagnosis of granulocytic sarcoma; cytoplasm that is homogeneous and amphophilic, or deep blue on a Giemsa stain, with a prominent hof supports plasmacytoma. Enzyme or immunohistochemical stains can establish a diagnosis in difficult cases. Clinical features may also be helpful in differential diagnosis (*see* Fig. 7–5).

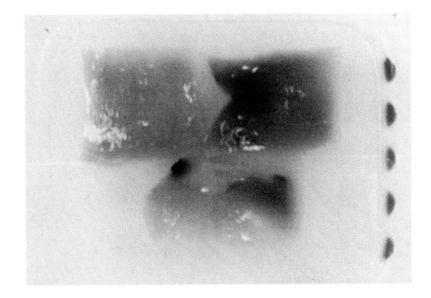

Figure 7–1. Granulocytic sarcoma. When initially sectioned, the paraffin-embedded tissue was bright green, so the designation of chloroma is warranted. The green color faded with time. (Courtesy of Dr. Jaime Prat, Hospital de la Santa Creu i Sant Pau, Barcelona, Spain.)

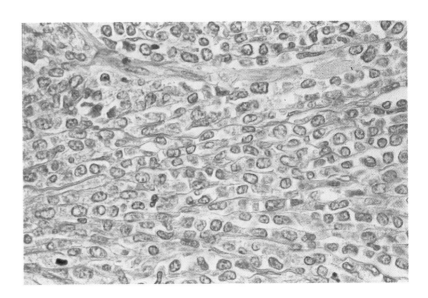

Figure 7–2. Granulocytic sarcoma. A monomorphous population of primitive cells has fine chromatin, small nucleoli, and scant cytoplasm associated with delicate sclerosis (H&E stain).

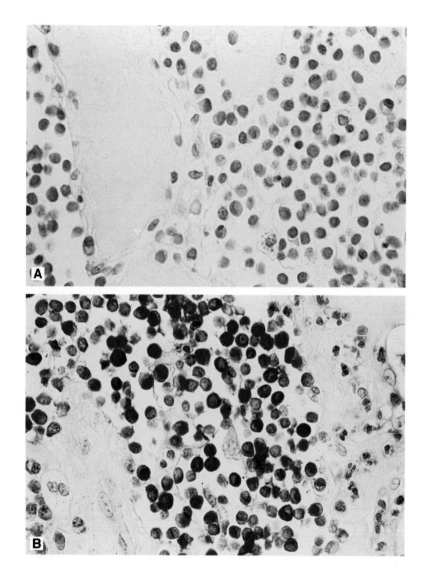

Figure 7–3. Granulocytic sarcoma of the vagina. *A*, Neoplastic cells show incomplete but definite myeloid differentiation, with indentation of nuclei and the acquisition of pink cytoplasm (H&E stain). *B*, Staining for chloroacetate esterase (CAE) is unusually intense in this case.

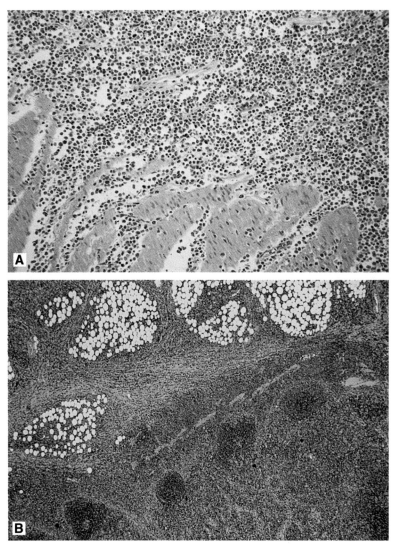

Figure 7–4. Granulocytic sarcoma (GS) of the ileum in a patient with acute myeloid leukemia. *A,* The patient presented with a tumor that deeply infiltrated the ileum; this specimen shows invasion of the muscularis propria (H&E stain). *B,* The GS also involved mesenteric lymph nodes. In this photomicrograph, GS surrounds a lymph node *(lower right)* and extensively infiltrates perinodal soft tissue *(upper left)* (H&E stain).

Illustration continued on following page.

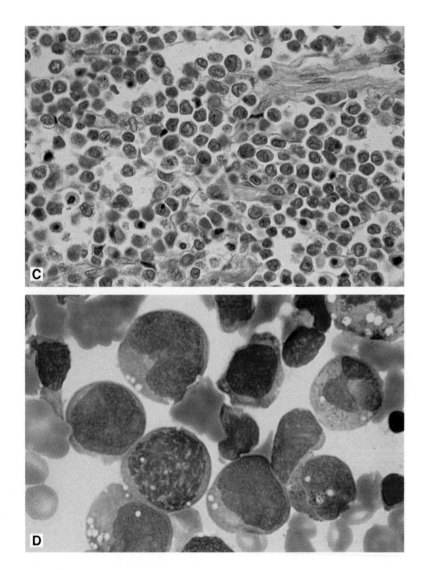

Figure 7–4. *Continued C,* High power examination shows medium to large discohesive cells with finely dispersed chromatin and small nucleoli (H&E stain). *D,* A bone marrow aspirate smear shows a predominance of myeloblasts, which have a high nuclear:cytoplasmic ratio; large, round, or folded nuclei; and pale blue cytoplasm with occasional small, azurophilic granules (Wright-Giemsa stain).

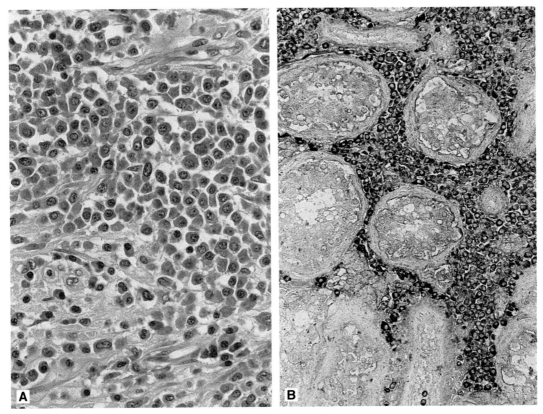

Figure 7–5. Granulocytic sarcoma of the testis, mimicking plasmacytoma. *A,* In this case, myelocytes with eccentrically placed cytoplasm predominate. A few mature plasma cells, with smaller, more heterochromatic nuclei, appear at the bottom of the field for comparison (H&E stain). *B,* Neoplastic cells infiltrating between seminiferous tubules are strongly positive for myeloperoxidase (immunoperoxidase technique on paraffin sections).

3. Carcinoma: In cases in which granulocytic sarcoma is associated with sclerosis, neoplastic cells may appear to grow in cords, mimicking the Indian-file pattern of breast carcinoma. A CAE stain, a stain for mucin, or immunohistochemical stains are useful in establishing the diagnosis.

References

Imrie KR, Kovass MJ, Selby D, *et al*: Isolated chloroma: the effect of early antileukemic therapy. Ann Intern Med 123(5):351–353, 1995.

Neiman RS, Barcos M, Berard C, *et al*: Granulocytic sarcoma: a clinicopathologic study of 61 biopsied cases. Cancer 48:1426–1437, 1981.

Quintanilla-Martinez L, Zukerberg LR, Ferry JA, Harris NL: Extramedullary tumors of lymphoid or myeloid blasts. The role of immunohistology in diagnosis and classification. Am J Clin Pathol 104:431–443, 1995.

Roth MJ, Medeiros LJ, Elenitoba-Johnson K, *et al*: Extramedullary myeloid cell tumors. An immunohistochemical study of 29 cases using routinely fixed and processed paraffin-embedded tissue sections. Arch Pathol Lab Med 119:790–798, 1995.

Segal G, Stoler M, Tubbs R: The "CD43 only" phenotype. An aberrant, nonspecific immunophenotype requiring comprehensive analysis for lineage resolution. Am J Clin Pathol 97:861–865, 1992.

MAST CELL DISEASE

Clinical Features

Mast cell disease (MCD) occurs in two major forms: cutaneous MCD, an indolent disorder confined to skin; and systemic MCD, a disease with an indolent or an aggressive course involving two or more different tissues. Patients with systemic MCD, who are usually adults, may have skin lesions, flushing, weight loss, fatigue, skeletal involvement (bone pain, demineralization, osteosclerosis, fractures), gastrointestinal symptoms, hepatosplenomegaly, lymphadenopathy, cardiovascular abnormalities (hypertension, angina, tachycardia), neuropsychiatric changes, peripheral cytopenias, eosinophilia, or a combination of these. Patients appear to have an increased incidence of hematolymphoid disorders, including myelodysplasia, chronic myeloproliferative disorders, acute myeloid leukemia, and lymphoma.

A higher mortality rate has been associated with older age at presentation, absence of skin lesions, cytopenias, hepatosplenomegaly, and associated leukemia or preleukemic disorders. A rare form of MCD, called lymphadenopathic mastocytosis with eosinophilia, is an aggressive disorder characterized by hepatosplenomegaly, anemia, marrow involvement, lymphadenopathy, and eosinophilia. Rarely, patients develop mast cell leukemia, which is typically rapidly fatal. In many fatal cases of MCD, the cause of death is the associated leukemic or preleukemic disorder, rather than MCD itself.

Morphology

Lymph nodes: Lymph nodes are often partially involved. Mast cells in tight clusters or sheets may occupy the paracortex, surround or infiltrate follicles, infiltrate medullary cords, fill sinuses, or surround blood vessels. The nodes may also show eosinophilia, plasmacytosis, fibrosis, follicular hyperplasia, and increased numbers of small blood vessels. The mast cells are round, oval, or fusiform; have oval, reniform, or infrequently, lobated nuclei; and have finely dispersed chromatin, inconspicuous nucleoli, and occasional distinct chromocenters. Cytoplasm is clear or lightly eosinophilic, and cell borders are usually sharp. Mitoses are rare or absent in nearly all cases (Fig. 7–6).

Spleen: The spleen usually shows thickened, fibrotic trabeculae infiltrated by mast cells. In addition, there may be peritrabecular aggregates, or diffuse red pulp, white pulp, or perifollicular involvement. The capsule is usually fibrotic, and eosinophils are typically present. The cytologic features are the same as those described for lymph node involvement. Extramedullary hematopoiesis may be prominent.

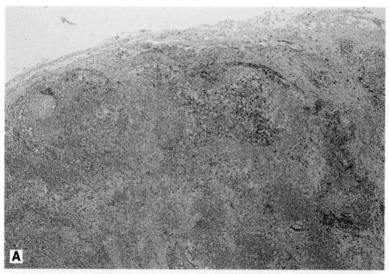

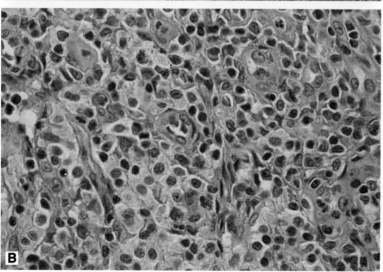

Figure 7–6. Mast cell disease, lymph node. In addition to lymphadenopathy, this patient had hepatosplenomegaly and skin lesions, which are consistent with systemic mastocytosis. *A,* The nodal architecture is preserved overall, but multiple pale aggregates of neoplastic mast cells appear in the paracortex, adjacent to sinuses, in the capsule, and around blood vessels (H&E stain). *B,* The mast cells have round nuclei, fine chromatin, and abundant pale cytoplasm. Eosinophils are present and the number of small blood vessels is increased (H&E stain).

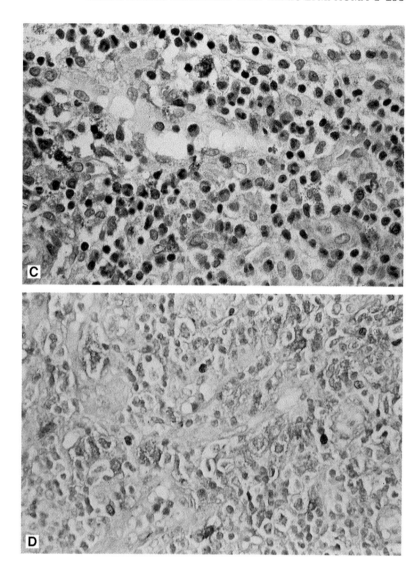

Figure 7–6. *C,* Mast cells have small, purple cytoplasmic granules; eosinophils are readily visible with a Giemsa stain. *D,* With a chloroacetate esterase stain, some mast cells show fine red-violet granularity.

Bone marrow: In the marrow, MCD forms paratrabecular, perivascular, or interstitial aggregates; less often, diffuse infiltrates of mast cells are surrounded by, or intermixed with, eosinophils and lymphocytes. Spindle-shaped mast cells are more common than oval mast cells in the marrow. Bony trabeculae may be thin or sclerotic. The marrow also shows myeloid hyperplasia in most cases (Fig. 7–7).

Histochemical Features, Immunophenotype, and Ultrastructural Features

Neoplastic mast cells have cytoplasmic granules on Giemsa, toluidine blue, and chloroacetate esterase (CAE) stained sections (Fig. 7–6 *C* and *D*, and 7–7*C*); one or more of these stains should be performed to confirm the diagnosis. Granules, however, are often fewer and smaller than in normal mast cells. Careful study may be required to identify positive staining.

Immunohistochemical staining is difficult because of problems with nonspecific staining; it is not considered helpful.

Ultrastructural examination reveals granules with distinctive scroll-like, lamellar, and rope-like inclusions.

Differential Diagnosis

The differential diagnosis of MCD is broad. In categories 2 through 9 in the following list, Giemsa, toluidine blue, and CAE stains are useful for confirming or excluding the mast cell nature of the infiltrate.

1. Reactive mastocytosis: An increase in mast cells occurs in a wide variety of conditions. In general, normal mast cells are present as scattered single cells; neoplastic mast cells form clusters. Normal mast cells are typically heavily granulated on Giemsa-stained sections; neoplastic mast cells may contain only sparse granules.

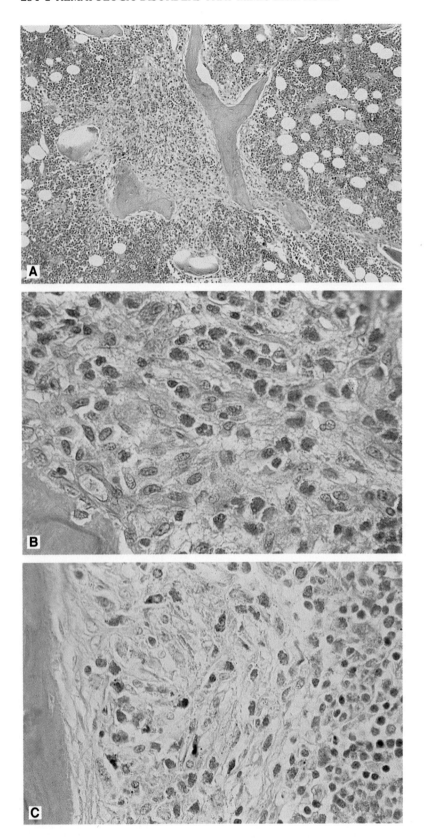

Figure 7–7. Mast cell disease of bone marrow. *A,* A paratrabecular infiltrate of cells is pale in comparison to the surrounding hematopoietic marrow (H&E stain). *B,* The neoplastic cells have oval to slightly elongate nuclei and relatively abundant pale cytoplasm. Eosinophils are prominent (H&E stain). *C,* With a Giemsa stain, very fine cytoplasmic granularity is visible in the spindle-shaped mast cells.

2. Hairy cell leukemia (HCL): In cases of MCD with diffuse splenic red pulp involvement, HCL enters the differential diagnosis. Although cytologic features overlap somewhat, HCL is not associated with thickened fibrous trabeculae or eosinophilia. HCL is Ig+ and B-associated antigen+.

3. Monocytoid B-cell lymphoma (MBCL) and hyperplasia of monocytoid B cells: Small aggregates of neoplastic mast cells in lymph nodes may mimic hyperplastic monocytoid B cells, and diffuse infiltrates may mimic MBCL. Eosinophilia and fibrosis favor MCD. B-antigen expression rules out MCD.

4. Follicle center lymphoma (FCL): When mast cells infiltrate and replace follicles in lymph nodes, the appearance can mimic FCL, especially at low power examination. Follicle center cells have less cytoplasm and irregular, heterochromatic (cleaved) or vesicular (noncleaved) nuclei in contrast to mast cells. Eosinophilia is unusual in FCL; B-antigen expression supports FCL.

5. Angioimmunoblastic T-cell lymphoma (AIL-TCL): The "clear cells" of AIL-TCL are intermediate-sized cells with relatively abundant pale cytoplasm. High endothelial venules are increased, and eosinophils may be numerous, creating a picture that overlaps the morphology of MCD. In contrast to MCD, however, neoplastic T cells are not typically uniform, may be quite pleomorphic, and usually show mitotic activity. T-antigen expression supports T-cell lymphoma.

6. Fibrosis: When mast cells have a spindle shape, especially when they form paratrabecular aggregates in the marrow, they may be mistaken for fibroblasts. The presence of eosinophils and lymphocytes should raise the question of MCD. Also, mast cells tend to have nuclei that are more rounded than those of fibroblasts.

7. Myelofibrosis: When mast cells have a spindle shape and diffusely infiltrate the marrow, the appearance can mimic idiopathic myelofibrosis. The features just described for fibrosis (no. 6) may be helpful in diagnosis.

8. Other chronic myeloproliferative disorders (MPD): Because bone marrow specimens with MCD usually show hyperplasia of the hematopoietic elements, the changes may suggest MPD, and the possibility of MCD may be overlooked. A diagnosis of MPD should be made using strict criteria, clinical findings, peripheral blood findings, and results of cytogenetic analysis. Conversely, because MCD is associated with an increased incidence of MPD, this possibility should be considered when evaluating marrow specimens with MCD.

9. Histiocytic lesions (sinus histiocytosis, Langerhans' cell histiocytosis, and granulomas): Infiltrates of mast cells confined to nodal sinuses may be interpreted as sinus histiocytosis or as Langerhans' cell histiocytosis. Cytologic features and the presence of eosinophilia may be helpful in excluding sinus histiocytosis. Langerhans' cells have much more complex nuclear clefts and folds

than mast cells. Aggregates of mast cells may resemble granulomas, but their appearance is less epithelioid and they lack necrosis and multinucleated cells.

10. Granulocytic sarcoma (GS): The cells of GS have a higher nuclear:cytoplasmic ratio and a higher mitotic rate than MCD. MCD typically contains mature eosinophils. Some GS contain cells of the eosinophil lineage, but they are usually immature. GS and MCD both may show granular staining using Giemsa and CAE stains. Myeloid cell granules are pink to red on both special stains, whereas mast cell granules are purple on Giemsa stain and red-violet on CAE stain. GS are usually myeloperoxidase+, lysozyme+, and CD43+.

References

Brunning RD, McKenna RW, Rosai J, et al: Systemic mastocytosis. Extracutaneous manifestations. Am J Surg Pathol 7:425–438, 1983.
Friedman B, Darling G, Norton J, et al: Splenectomy in the management of systemic mast cell disease. Surgery 107:94–100, 1990.
Horny H-P, Kaiserling E, Parwaresch MR, Lennert K: Lymph node findings in generalized mastocytosis. Histopathology 21:439–446, 1992.
Lawrence JB, Friedman BS, Travis WD, et al: Hematologic manifestations of systemic mast cell disease: a prospective study of laboratory and morphologic features and their relation to prognosis. Am J Med 91:612–624, 1991.
Lennert K, Parwaresch MR: Mast cells and mast cell neoplasia: a review. Histopathology 3:349–365, 1979.
Longley J, Duffy TP, Kohn S: The mast cell and mast cell disease. J Am Acad Dermatol 32(4):545–561, 1995.
Webb TA, Li C-Y, Yam LT: Systemic mast cell disease: a clinical and hematopathologic study of 26 cases. Cancer 49:927–938, 1982.

PLASMACYTOID MONOCYTE PROLIFERATION

Synonyms and Related Terms: Plasmacytoid T-cell lymphoma; plasmacytoid T-zone cell proliferation; plasmacytoid monocyte proliferation associated with myeloproliferative disorder.

Plasmacytoid monocytes are a distinctive type of cell that are found in lymph nodes and in certain extranodal sites in a variety of reactive conditions, including Kikuchi's disease, Castleman's disease, granulomatous lymphadenitis, and nonspecific lymphoid hyperplasia. Plasmacytoid monocytes have the distinction of having had a larger number of names, corresponding to a variety of postulated lineages and stages of differentiation, than perhaps any other lymph node-based cell. Plasmacytoid monocytes were first recognized in 1958 by Lennert and Remmele, who called them "lymphoblasts in clusters." Subsequently, ultrastructural studies revealed that plasmacytoid monocytes have abundant rough endoplasmic reticulum and a well-developed Golgi apparatus, reminiscent of a plasma cell. This, in combination with the usual location of plasmacytoid monocytes in the lymph node paracortex, led to their being designated "T-associated plasma cells." Immunohistochemical studies then revealed that plasmacytoid monocytes did not express immunoglobulin, acquired the name "plasmacytoid T cells." Because plasmacytoid monocytes expressed only a limited number of T-cell-associated, but not T-cell-specific, antigens, and had markers associated with other cell types, particularly monocytes and macrophages, the term "plasmacytoid T-zone cell," which did not indicate a definite lineage, was suggested. Emphasis was then placed on the expression of monocyte and macrophage-associated antigens, and the term "plasmacytoid monocyte" has become most popular.

Rarely, proliferations of plasmacytoid monocytes that appear to be neoplastic have been reported. These cases have distinctive clinical and pathologic features.

Clinical Features

Fewer than ten cases of tumor-like plasmacytoid monocyte proliferation have been described. Almost all patients are elderly, with a male preponderance. In all reported cases, at some point in their clinical course, patients have some form of myeloid neoplasia: a myelodysplastic syndrome (chronic myelomonocytic leukemia in two cases); a myeloproliferative disorder (idiopathic myelofibrosis in two cases); or acute myeloid leukemia, which may be myelomonocytic or monocytic. The bone marrow disorder usually predates the plasmacytoid monocyte proliferation, but it may appear concurrently or be discovered after the plasmacytoid monocyte proliferation.

At the time of presentation with plasmacytoid monocyte proliferation, patients have constitutional symptoms, generalized lymphadenopathy, and often hepatosplenomegaly. The clinical picture is highly suggestive of lymphoma. In some cases, plasmacytoid monocyte proliferation has coincided with the development of an accelerated phase or blast crisis in a previously stable myeloproliferative disorder or myelodysplastic syndrome. Treatment has varied, but overall the prognosis is poor, with most patients succumbing to their illness. In general, the myeloid neoplasia is the principal cause of death, whereas the plasmacytoid monocyte proliferation does not appear to contribute substantially to mortality. In the case reported by Harris and Demirjian, the patient received busulfan and prednisone with resolution of lymphadenopathy, but later died of chronic myelomonocytic leukemia that progressed to acute leukemia.

Morphology

The normal architecture of the lymph nodes is distorted by a diffuse, occasionally vaguely nodular infiltrate of plasmacytoid monocytes involving the paracortex and the medulla (Fig. 7–8). Lymphoid follicles may remain at the periphery of the node, and a few sinuses may be patent. Plasmacytoid monocytes in these proliferations usually resemble normal plasmacytoid monocytes. They are uniform, medium-sized cells with round, oval, or slightly irregular nuclei, evenly dispersed to finely granular chromatin, and one to three small, inconspicuous nucleoli. The nuclei

are centrally or slightly eccentrically placed; the cytoplasm is pale eosinophilic (light gray-blue on a Giemsa stain) and relatively abundant. Rarely, there is an admixture of slightly enlarged, pleomorphic plasmacytoid monocytes. A few pyknotic cells and tingible body macrophages are often admixed with the plasmacytoid monocytes. The number of high endothelial venules may be increased; mitotic figures are rare to absent. Extramedullary hematopoiesis or sparse infiltrates of abnormal myeloid cells may be found, but the plasmacytoid monocyte proliferation predominates in lymph nodes.

In the spleen, plasmactoid monocytes may be found in aggregates around the periphery of the white pulp (Fig. 7–8B). Plasmacytoid monocytes may also be found in the bone marrow biopsy specimen or on the aspirate smear. In one case, plasmacytoid monocytes formed a small paratrabecular aggregate. In another, they surrounded a lymphoid aggregate. In general, in both the spleen and the bone marrow, the involvement by the associated myeloid disorder is more prominent than that of the plasmacytoid monocyte proliferation. In one case in which an autopsy was performed, leukemic infiltration was found throughout the body, and small numbers of plasmacytoid monocytes were found in association with the leukemic infiltrate in all sites.

Immunophenotype and Enzyme Histochemistry

Normal and neoplastic plasmacytoid monocytes are consistently CD4+, CD43+, CD45+, CD68+ and HLA-DR+ (Fig. 7–8D). Typically, they are negative for B-cell antigens, other T-cell antigens, lysozyme, chloroacetate esterase, myeloperoxidase, and nonspecific esterase. Finely granular staining for acid phosphatase has been described. In some proliferations, plasmacytoid monocytes express CD2, CD5, CD10, or CD14. In one study, the plasmacytoid monocyte proliferation strongly expressed L-selectin, which is responsible for the binding of lymphocytes to high endothelial venules, and the authors suggested that L-selectin expression was responsible for the preferential localization in lymph nodes of the plasmacytoid monocytes.

Genetic Features

Immunoglobulin heavy chain and T-cell-receptor genes are in the germline configuration.

Summary

The nature of the plasmacytoid monocyte proliferation in these unusual cases is uncertain. The associated bone marrow disorders can be thought of as stem cell disorders; thus, the plasmacytoid monocyte proliferation can be considered differentiation of the neoplastic clone in a somewhat unusual direction. With this hypothesis, one can suggest that neoplastic plasmacytoid monocytes migrate to lymph nodes like normal plasmacytoid monocytes, thereby producing

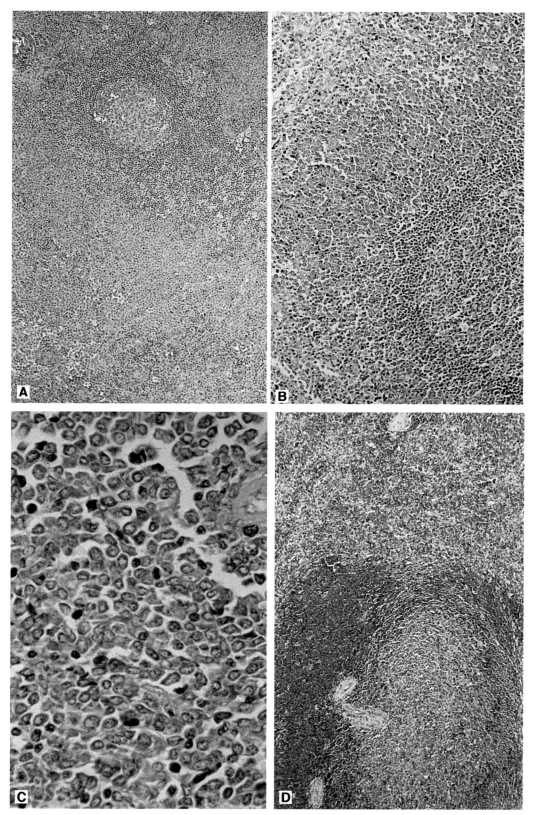

Figure 7–8. Plasmacytoid monocyte (PM) proliferation. The patient also had chronic myelomonocytic leukemia. *A,* In a lymph node, sheets of PMs expand the paracortex and surround a reactive lymphoid follicle *(top)* (H&E stain). *B,* In the spleen, numerous PMs are found at the periphery of white pulp containing a reactive follicle *(lower right)* (Giemsa stain). *C,* Higher power view shows PMs with uniform, round to oval, pale nuclei and a moderate amount of pale cytoplasm. A few admixed pyknotic cells are seen (Giemsa stain). *D,* PMs surrounding a follicle are strongly CD43+ (immunoperoxidase technique on paraffin sections).

like normal plasmacytoid monocytes, thereby producing lymphadenopathy. Alternatively, because the plasmacytoid monocyte proliferation shows little or no cytologic atypia or mitotic activity and contributes little to mortality, the possibility that it represents an unusual reactive process cannot be wholly excluded.

Differential Diagnosis

1. Lymphoblastic lymphoma (LBL): Plasmacytoid monocytes are slightly larger than small lymphocytes and have finely dispersed chromatin, an appearance that may suggest lymphoblasts. In contrast to plasmacytoid monocytes, LBL has a high mitotic rate, scant cytoplasm, and an immunophenotype incompatible with a diagnosis of plasmacytoid monocyte proliferation. With rare exceptions, patients with LBL do not have myeloid neoplasia.
2. Plasmacytoma, plasma cell myeloma: Neoplastic plasma cells usually have larger nuclei and more abundant, more deeply staining cytoplasm than plasmacytoid monocytes. The plasma cell nuclei are either coarsely heterochromatic or vesicular and have prominent nucleoli. Plasma cells express cytoplasmic immunoglobulin. Unlike plasmacytoid monocyte proliferation, plasma cell neoplasia is not associated with myeloid neoplasia. The distribution of disease seen in plasmacytoid monocyte proliferation, with its generalized lymphadenopathy, would be exceedingly unusual in plasmacytoma or plasma cell myeloma.
3. Mast cell disease (MCD): Lymphadenopathic mastocytosis may enter the differential diagnosis of plasmacytoid monocyte proliferation. Eosinophils, plasma cells, and fibrosis are not usually found in plasmacytoid monocyte proliferations, in contrast to mast cell disease. Bone marrow involvement is common, and has a distinctive appearance in MCD, but it is inconspicuous in plasmacytoid monocyte proliferation. In contrast to plasmacytoid monocytes, mast cells have cytoplasmic granularity with Giemsa and chloroacetate esterase stains. Plasmacytoid monocytes have a distinct immunophenotypic profile not encountered in mast cells.

References

Baddoura FK, Hanson C, Chan WC: Plasmacytoid monocyte proliferation associated with myeloproliferative disorders. Cancer 69(6):1457–1467, 1992.

Facchetti F, De Wolf-Peeters C, Kennes C, et al: Leukemia-associated lymph node infiltrates of plasmacytoid monocytes (so-called plasmacytoid T cells). Evidence for two distinct histological and immunophenotypical patterns. Am J Surg Pathol 14:101–112, 1990.

Harris NL, Demirjian Z: Plasmacytoid T-zone cell proliferation in a patient with chronic myelomonocytic leukemia. Histologic and immunohistologic characterization. Am J Surg Pathol 15:87–95, 1991.

Horny HP, Kaiserling E, Handgretinger R, et al: Evidence for a lymphotropic nature of circulating plasmacytoid monocytes: findings from a case of CD56+ chronic myelomonocytic leukemia. Eur J Haematol 54:209–216, 1995.

Lennert K, Remmele W: Karyometrische Untersuchungen an Lymphknotenzellen des Menschen: I. Mitt. Germinoblasten, Lymphoblasten und Lymphozyten. Acta Haematol (Basel) 19:99–113, 1958.

Müller-Hermelink HK, Stein H, Steinmann G, Lennert K: Malignant lymphoma of plasmacytoid T-cells. Morphologic and immunologic studies characterizing a special type of T-cell. Am J Surg Pathol 7:849–862, 1983.

Thomas JO, Beiske K, Hann I, et al: Immunohistological diagnosis of "plasmacytoid T cell lymphoma" in paraffin wax sections. Am J Clin Pathol 93(6):822–827, 1990.

APPENDIX

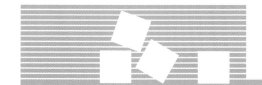

Processing of Lymph Nodes and Other Tissues with Possible Involvement by Lymphoma

At the Massachusetts General Hospital, when a biopsy specimen is submitted in which lymphoma is considered in the differential diagnosis, we perform the following "lymphoma work-up":

1. Fresh tissue kept moist with a small amount of saline is submitted promptly to the frozen section laboratory. If a delay in delivery of the tissue is unavoidable, it must be refrigerated.

2. The specimen is sectioned. A lymph node greater than 1 cm in diameter should be sectioned crosswise, yielding multiple sections each showing cortex, paracortex, medulla, and hilus. If a lymph node is bisected longitudinally and the cut is made slightly off-center, all the nodal compartments, particularly the hilus, may not be apparent, causing an impression of abnormal architecture. If the lymph node is small (<1 cm), it may be bisected on the longitudinal axis.

3. One section is frozen, and a frozen section is cut and stained to give a preliminary impression of the adequacy of the specimen and to guide further processing. This block is kept frozen in OCT mounting medium at a temperature of −70°C for possible immunohistochemical and genetic studies.

4. A section is also taken for flow cytometric analysis in selected cases.

5. In selected cases, touch preparations are made. Air dried touch preparations can be stained with a Wright-Giemsa stain or be saved for possible enzyme histochemical stains. Fixed touch preparations can be stained with hematoxylin and eosin. Immediate fixation helps avoid air-drying artifacts.

6. If the frozen section suggests the presence of lymphoma, the remainder of the tissue is divided; one or more slices are fixed in B-5 fixative and the rest in formalin. B-5-fixed sections must be cut very thin be-cause B-5 penetrates tissue poorly. A thickness of 2 mm is optimal, and 4 mm is the maximum. If it is difficult to cut such thin slices, thicker slices may be fixed briefly (5 to 10 minutes), resectioned, and returned to B-5 fixative. Total B-5 fixation time is 2 hours, after which the tissue is transferred to formalin until further processing is undertaken. A longer period of exposure to B-5 will yield tissue too brittle to section and may affect antigen expression.

Tissue fixed in formalin alone is fixed overnight to obtain optimal morphology.

If the tissue is insufficient for both B-5 and formalin fixation, B-5 fixation alone is usually preferred in cases in which the clinical situation does not permit a delay for overnight fixation with formalin. In other situations, the preference of the pathologist and the capabilities of the histology laboratory usually determine whether the tissue should be fixed in formalin or B-5. Formalin-fixed tissue should be available in cases of suspected cat scratch disease (*see* no. 8 following).

7. If examination of the frozen section shows a poorly differentiated malignant tumor, in addition to the steps already described, tissue specimens may be prepared for electron microscopy.

8. If examination of the frozen section suggests an inflammatory or infectious process, a tissue specimen obtained by the surgeon from the operating room is sent for cultures if possible; alternatively, the pathologist may submit tissue for culture if sufficient tissue is available for this purpose. If examination of the frozen section reveals granulomas and cat scratch disease is considered in the differential diagnosis, adequate tissue is fixed in formalin, because silver stains for cat scratch disease do not work on tissue fixed in B-5.

9. If the frozen section examination indicates that the tissue submitted may be inadequate for diagnosis (for

example, too small or extensively necrotic), more tissue is requested from the surgeon.

10. In cases in which there is not sufficient tissue to prepare both a frozen block and fixed tissue, such as small biopsy specimens of the brain or orbit, the entire specimen is frozen and either of the following steps are taken: (1) 15 to 20 frozen sections are cut on Histostix for immunostaining, and the frozen block is thawed and fixed for permanent sections; or (2) the entire specimen is frozen and saved in the frozen state until all necessary special studies are obtained. If the morphology of the frozen section and the results of immunophenotyping are not adequate to make a diagnosis, the frozen block can be thawed and processed for a permanent section.

11. In cases in which a prior biopsy examination showed changes suggesting lymphoma, but in which no frozen tissue was saved, another biopsy may be performed specifically to obtain tissue for immunohistochemical studies. In such cases, assuming the morphology of the first specimen was adequate for study, we often freeze the entire new specimen and save it for immunohistochemical studies. When only multiple tissue fragments are available for examination, we sequentially freeze the fragments and examine a frozen section of each until we are certain that there is adequate tissue for marker studies.

12. A modified lymphoma work-up is also performed on cytologic specimens when lymphoma is considered in the differential diagnosis.

    a. Fluid derived from effusions, cerebrospinal fluid, and other fluids in excess of that required for routine studies can be submitted for flow cytometric analysis.

    b. Fine needle aspiration specimens may yield both fluid and small fragments of tissue for study. The fluid specimen is processed as just described. Any fragments of tissue too large for routine cytologic preparation are submitted to the frozen section laboratory, where they are handled like other small biopsy specimens (*see* no. 10). If there are multiple tissue fragments, some can be fixed for permanent sections after examining a frozen section and ensuring that the frozen tissue is adequate for immunohistochemical studies.

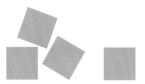

INDEX

Note: Page numbers in *italics* refer to illustrations; page numbers followed by t refer to tables.

A

Abbreviations, 65t
Abdominal lymph node(s), splenic marginal zone lymphoma involving, 103, *105*
Abscess, suppurative lymphadenitis with, vs. cat scratch disease, 17, *20*
Acquired immunodeficiency, 220–243
Acquired immunodeficiency syndrome (AIDS). See *Human immunodeficiency virus (HIV) infection.*
Acute myelogenous leukemia, vs. plasmacytoma/plasma cell myeloma, 112
Acute myeloid leukemia, vs. B-lymphoblastic lymphoma, 70
Adult T-cell lymphoma/leukemia (ATLL), 177, *178–179*
  vs. large granular lymphocyte leukemia, 147
  vs. mycosis fungoides/Sézary syndrome, 149
  vs. T-cell chronic lymphocytic leukemia, 145
Agammaglobulinemia, congenital X-linked (Bruton's disease), 217
AIDS (acquired immunodeficiency syndrome). See *Human immunodeficiency virus (HIV) infection.*
AIL-TCL. See *Angioimmunoblastic T-cell lymphoma (AIL-TCL).*
ALCL. See *Anaplastic large cell lymphoma (ALCL).*
Anaplastic large cell lymphoma (ALCL), 180–188
  clinical features of, 180
  cutaneous, *185*
  differential diagnosis of, 183–184, 184t
  genetics of, 182–183
  histiocyte-rich variant of, 180, *187*
  Hodgkin's-related, 204, *206–209*
  immunophenotype of, 182
  morphology of, 180, *181–183*, *185–188*
  neutrophil-rich, *188*
  small-cell variant of, 180, *186*
  synonyms for, 180
  vs. nodular sclerosis Hodgkin's disease, 198
Angiocentric (nasal-type) lymphoma, 164–167
  clinical features of, 164
  differential diagnosis of, 167, *168*
  genetics of, 167, *167*
  immunophenotype of, 167
  morphology of, 164, *165–166*
  synonyms for, 164
  vs. intestinal T-cell lymphoma, 176
  vs. intravascular large B-cell lymphoma, 126

Angiocentric (*Continued*)
  vs. lymphomatoid granulomatosis, 171
  vs. subcutaneous panniculitic T-cell lymphoma, 155
Angioimmunoblastic T-cell lymphoma (AIL-TCL), 156–163
  clinical features of, 156–157
  differential diagnosis of, 157
  genetic features of, 157
  immunophenotype of, 157
  morphology of, 157, *158–163*
  synonyms for, 156
  vs. hyaline-vascular variant of Castleman's disease, 55–56
  vs. mast cell disease, 255
Angiolymphoid hyperplasia, with eosinophilia, vs. Kimura's disease, 58–59, *60*
Angiomatosis, bacillary, in AIDS patients, 230
  vs. Kaposi's sarcoma, 230, *232*
Ann Arbor staging, of Hodgkin's disease, 209, 209t, *210–211*, 212
Appendicitis, immunoblastic lymph node reaction due to, 12, *13*
Arthritis, rheumatoid, 36, *37*
  vs. plasma cell variant of Castleman's disease, 56
AT gene, in ataxia-telangiectasia, 244–245
Ataxia-telangiectasia, clinical features of, 243–244
  immunophenotype and genotype of, 244–245
  morphology of, 244, *244*
ATLL. See *Adult T-cell lymphoma/leukemia (ATLL).*
Autoimmune disease(s), rheumatoid arthritis as, 36, *37*
  systemic lupus erythematosus as, 33, *34–35*. See also *Systemic lupus erythematosus.*
Axillary lymph node(s), cat scratch disease affecting, *18*
  T-cell chronic lymphocytic leukemia affecting, *145*
Azzopardi phenomenon, 41

B

B cells, 1
  activation of, in paracortex, 4
  differentiation of, postulated pathway of, *2*
    with postulated neoplastic counterparts, *68*
  in Castleman's disease, *51*, 52
  in dermatopathic lymphadenopathy, 61

Reactive lymphoid hyperplasia, 9–62
  etiology of, autoimmune, 33, *34–35*,
      36, *37*
    bacterial, 17–27. See also specific infec-
      tion, e.g., *Cat scratch disease.*
    fungal, 27, *28–29*
    histiocytic lesions in, 38–48. See also spe-
      cific disorder, e.g., *Sarcoidosis.*
    miscellaneous, 48–62. See also specific
      disorder, e.g., *Castleman's disease.*
    predominant pattern by, 9t
    protozoal, 30, *31–32*
    viral, 9–16. See also specific viral infec-
      tion, e.g., *Infectious mononucleosis.*
  in HIV infection, 220
  of spleen, 212, *213*
  vs. anaplastic large cell lymphoma, 184
  vs. follicle center lymphoma, 89–90
  vs. lymphocyte predominance Hodgkin's dis-
    ease, 194
  vs. peripheral T-cell lymphoma, 151
  vs. post-transplantation lymphoproliferative
    disorder, 242
Reactive mastocytosis, vs. mast cell disease,
  253
Reactive paracortical hyperplasia, vs. T-cell-
  rich large B-cell lymphoma, 126
Reactive plasmacytosis, vs.
  plasmacytoma/plasma cell myeloma, 112
R.E.A.L. (Revised European-American Lymphoma) classification, of B-cell neoplasms, 63t
  of T-cell neoplasms, 139t
Reed-Sternberg cells, in B-cell chronic lymphocytic leukemia, 75, *76*
  in Hodgkin's disease, 209
  in infectious mononucleosis, 9, *11*
  in nodular sclerosis Hodgkin's disease, *197*,
    198
  in T-cell-rich large B-cell lymphoma, 123
Renal transplant, lymphoproliferative disorder
  following, *237–238*
Revised European-American Lymphoma
  (R.E.A.L.) classification, of B-cell neoplasms, 63t
  of T-cell neoplasms, 139t
Rheumatoid arthritis, 36, *37*
  follicle lysis in, *6*
  vs. plasma cell variant of Castleman's dis-
    ease, 56
Richter's syndrome, 72, *74–75*
  analysis of, 77
  trisomy 12 associated with, 75
Rosai-Dorfman disease. See *Sinus histiocytosis,
  with massive lymphadenopathy.*
Russell bodies, in plasma cell variant of Castleman's disease, 52, *53*

S

Salivary gland(s), lymphoepithelial lesions of,
  HIV-associated, 220, *223*
Sarcoidosis, clinical features of, 38
  differential diagnosis of, 38, *40*
  immunophenotype of, 38
  morphology of, 38, *39*

Sarcoidosis (*Continued*)
  vs. mycobacterial infection, 21
  vs. Whipple's disease, 27
Sarcoma, granulocytic, 246–251
  clinical features of, 246
  differential diagnosis of, 246, 251
  enzyme histochemistry and immunophe-
    notype of, 246, *248*
  morphology of, 246, *247–251*
  vs. diffuse large B-cell lymphoma, 118
  vs. mast cell disease, 255
  Kaposi's, *131*, 230, *231*
  spindle cell, vs. diffuse large B-cell lym-
    phoma, 118–119, *119*
SCID (severe combined immunodeficiency disease), 217–218
Secondary lymphomatous effusions, vs. primary effusion lymphoma, 130
Seminoma, vs. diffuse large B-cell lymphoma,
  118
Severe combined immunodeficiency disease
  (SCID), 217–218
Sinus(es), lymph node, 8
  vascular transformation of, vs. Kaposi's
    sarcoma, 230
Sinus histiocytosis, vs. mast cell disease, 255
  with lipogranulomas, 46, *47*
  with massive lymphadenopathy, clinical fea-
    tures of, 44
    differential diagnosis of, 46
    immunophenotype of, 46
    morphology of, 44–45, *45*
Skin, anaplastic large cell lymphoma of, *185*
  mycosis fungoides of, *148*
Small intestine, Burkitt's lymphoma of, *224*
  immunoproliferative disease of, 99–100, *100*
Small lymphocytic lymphoma (B-SLL), 72
  vs. lymphocyte predominance Hodgkin's dis-
    ease, 194
Soft tissue, intravascular large B-cell lymphoma of, *127–128*
Spindle cell sarcoma, vs. diffuse large B-cell
  lymphoma, 118–119, *119*
Spleen, diffuse large B-cell lymphoma of, *118*
  hairy cell leukemia of, 107, *109*
  Hodgkin's disease of, staging of, 209, *210*
  large granular lymphocyte leukemia of, *147*
  mantle cell lymphoma of, 83, *85*
  marginal zone B-cell lymphoma of, 103,
    104–106
  mast cell disease of, 252
  Pneumocystis carinii infection of, *233*
  reactive lymphoid hyperplasia of, 212, *213*
Squamous cell carcinoma, vs. nasal-type T/NK-
  cell lymphoma, 167, *168*
Staging, Ann Arbor, of Hodgkin's disease, 209,
  209t, *210–211*, 212
Stomach, mucosa-associated lymphoid tissue
  (MALT) lymphoma of, *93–95*
Subcutaneous panniculitic T-cell lymphoma,
  155, *156*
Syphilis, vs. plasma cell variant of Castleman's
  disease, 56
  vs. rheumatoid arthritis, 36
Systemic lupus erythematosus, 33, *34–35*
  vs. herpes simplex lymphadenitis, 14
  vs. Kikuchi's disease, 41

ATLASES IN DIAGNOSTIC SURGICAL PATHOLOGY

- **Atlas of Orthopedic Pathology** *(Wold, McLeod, Sim & Unni)*
  Order #W2911-3

- **Atlas of Pulmonary Surgical Pathology** *(Colby, Lombard, Yousem & Kitaichi)*
  Order #W2893-1

- **Atlas of Liver Pathology** *(Kanel & Korula)*
  Order #W2657-2

- **Atlas of Gastrointestinal Pathology** *(Owen & Kelly)*
  Order #W6730-9

- **Atlas of Head and Neck Pathology** *(Wenig)*
  Order #W4032-X

- **Atlas of Cardiovascular Pathology** *(Virmani, Burke & Farb)*
  Order #W4476-7

- **Atlas of Surgical Pathology of the Male Reproductive Tract** *(Ro, Grignon, Amin & Ayala)*
  Order #W5284-0

- **Atlas of Endocrine Pathology** *(Wenig, Heffess & Adair)*
  Order #W5917-9

- **Atlas of Lymphoid Hyperplasia and Lymphoma** *(Ferry & Harris)*
  Order #W5907-1

ENROLL TODAY!
SEE REVERSE SIDE FOR DETAILS.

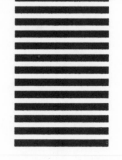